Postmortal Society

Throughout history mankind has struggled to reconcile itself with the inescapability of its own mortality. This book explores the themes of immortality and survivalism in contemporary culture, shedding light on the varied and ingenious ways in which humans and human societies aspire to confront and deal with death, or even seek to outlive it, as it were.

Bringing together theoretical and empirical work from internationally acclaimed scholars across a range of disciplines, *Postmortal Society* offers studies of the strategies adopted and means available in modern society for trying to 'cheat' death or prolong life, the status of the dead in the modern Western world, the effects of beliefs that address the terror of death in other areas of life, the 'immortalisation' of celebrities, the veneration of the dead in virtual worlds, symbolic immortality through work, the implications of understanding 'immortality' in chemical-neuronal terms, and the apparent paradox of our greater reverence for the dead in increasingly secular, capitalist societies.

A fascinating collection of studies that explore humanity's attempts to deal with its own mortality in the modern age, this book will appeal to sociologists, anthropologists, philosophers and scholars of cultural studies with interests in death and dying.

Michael Hviid Jacobsen is Professor of Sociology at Aalborg University, Denmark. He is the editor of *The Poetics of Crime* and *Beyond Bauman: Creative Excursions and Critical Engagements*, and co-editor of *The Sociology of Zygmunt Bauman*; *The Transformation of Modernity*; *Utopia: Social Theory and the Future*; and *Imaginative Methodologies: Creativity, Poetics and Rhetoric in Social Research* (all available from Routledge).

Studies in Death, Materiality and the Origin of Time

Series editors:
Dorthe Refslund Christensen, *Aarhus University, Denmark*
Rane Willerslev, *Aarhus University, Denmark*

Eventually we all die – and we experience death head-on when someone close to us dies. This series, Studies in Death, Materiality and the Origin of Time, identifies this fact as constitutive of the origin of human conceptions of time. Time permeates everything, but except for time itself all things are perishable – yet, it is only through the perishable world of things and bodies that we sense time. Bringing together scholarly work across a range of disciplines, the series explores the fact that human experiences and conceptions of time inherently hinge on the material world, and that time as a socially experienced phenomenon cannot be understood as separate from material form or expression. As such, it departs from a persistent current within Western thinking. Philosophy, biology and physics, among other disciplines, have studied time as an essential, ethereal and abstract concept. In the same way, death has often been conceived of in abstract and sometimes transcendental terms as occupying one extreme margin of human life. As an alternative, this series examines the ways in which bodily death and material decay are central points of reference in social life, which offer key insights into human perceptions of time.

Postmortal Society
Towards a Sociology of Immortality

Edited by Michael Hviid Jacobsen

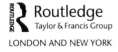

LONDON AND NEW YORK

First published 2017
by Routledge
2 Park Square, Milton Park, Abingdon, Oxon OX14 4RN

and by Routledge
711 Third Avenue, New York, NY 10017

Routledge is an imprint of the Taylor & Francis Group, an informa business

British Library Cataloguing in Publication Data
A catalogue record for this book is available from the British Library

Library of Congress Cataloguing in Publication Data
A catalogue record for this book is available from the Library of Congress

ISBN: 978-1-4724-8558-8 (hbk)
ISBN: 978-1-3156-0170-0 (ebk)

Typeset in Times New Roman
by Out of House Publishing

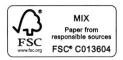

MIX
Paper from
responsible sources
FSC
www.fsc.org   FSC® C013604

Printed and bound by CPI Group (UK) Ltd, Croydon, CR0 4YY

Dedicated to the undying memory of Michael C. Kearl (1949–2015)

Contents

Illustrations

Figures

Tables

Contributors

William Sims Bainbridge is a programme director at the National Science Foundation, Arlington, Virginia, United States. His research combines social and information sciences as reported in: *The Virtual Future* (2011), *eGods: Faith Versus Fantasy in Computer Gaming* (2013), *An Information Technology Surrogate for Religion: The Veneration of Deceased Family in Online Games* (2014), *Personality Capture and Emulation* (2014), *The Meaning and Value of Spaceflight* (2015), *Virtual Sociocultural Convergence* (2016) and *Star Worlds: Freedom Versus Control in Online Gameworlds* (2017).

Nunzia Bonifati is a scientific journalist and Adjunct Professor of Philosophy at the University of Rome Tor Vergata, Italy. Her scientific interests are mainly devoted to the moral implications and consequences of human–robot interaction, human enhancement and new technologies. On such topics she has published several papers and books including: *Et voilà i robot* (2010) and – with Giuseppe O. Longo – *Homo Immortalis* (2012).

Guy Brown is a Professor of Cellular Biochemistry at the University of Cambridge, United Kingdom. His research interests include: cell death, mitochondria, microglia, neuroinflammation and the diseases of ageing. From a social perspective, he is interested in end-of-life and the future of death. He has written numerous papers and five books, including: *The Living End: The Future of Death, Aging and Immortality* (2007) and *Living Too Long* (2015).

Allison Gibson is an Assistant Professor of Social Work at Winthrop University in Rock Hill, South Carolina, United States. Her research interests include: technology and social work practice, digital immortality, persons with Alzheimer's disease and community-based programmes for older adults. She has worked previously for the Alzheimer's Association, in hospice and palliative care and in behavioural health crisis services.

David Giles is a Reader in Media Psychology at the University of Winchester, United Kingdom. His published books include: *Illusions of Immortality*

(2000), *Media Psychology* (2003) and *Psychology of the Media* (2010). His current research is largely focused on the relationship between audiences and celebrities and the changes to this brought about by social media. He has published more broadly on the microanalysis of online data, particularly discussion forums.

Jeff Greenberg is a Professor of Psychology at the University of Arizona, United States. He co-developed terror management theory, which explains how awareness of mortality influences many aspects of human behaviour. His research focuses on prejudice, self-esteem, political preferences, aggression, ageing, religion, attitudes towards animals and existential isolation. His recent co-authored books include: *Death in Classic and Contemporary Film: Fade to Black* (2013), *The Worm at the Core* (2015) and *Social Psychology: The Science of Everyday Life* (2015).

Peter J. Helm is a doctoral student at the University of Arizona, United States, under the mentorship of Jeff Greenberg. His research focuses on existential isolation, self-esteem, aggression, self-presentation, meaning and political preferences.

Michael Hviid Jacobsen is a Professor of Sociology at Aalborg University, Denmark. His research interests include: death and dying, palliative care, ethics, sexuality, deviance, crime, social theory, poetic sociology, emotions and research methodology. Recent authored, co-authored and edited books include: *Deconstructing Death* (2013), *Erving Goffman* (2014), *Poetics of Crime* (2015), *Framing Law and Crime* (2016), *Liquid Criminology* (2016), *Beyond Bauman* (2016), *The Interactionist Imagination* (2017) and *Emotions and Everyday Life* (2017).

Michael C. Kearl was Professor of Sociology at Trinity University, San Antonio, Texas, United States. His seminal contribution to the field of the sociology of death and dying consisted in *Endings: A Sociology of Death and Dying* (1989), and his work also counted several important journal articles dealing with immortality and the proliferation of postselves and skulls in contemporary popular and civic culture. Michael C. Kearl passed away in March 2015.

Uri Lifshin is a doctoral student at the University of Arizona, United States, working under the mentorship of Jeff Greenberg. His research interests include: terror management theory, motivation, self-esteem, aggression, religion, prejudice and the human–animal relationship.

Gianfranco Pecchinenda is Professor of Sociology of Knowledge at Naples University Federico II, Italy. His research interests include: identity, memory, neurosciences, narrative, time and death. He is also a novelist. Recent books include: *Videogames and Simulation Culture* (2010), *Homunculus: A Sociology of Identity* (2012) and *The Mimetic System* (2014).

Danielle R. Silberman is a recent graduate from the Master of Social Work Program at Winthrop University in Rock Hill, South Carolina, United States. She currently works as a social worker for the Hospice and Palliative Care Charlotte Region in Charlotte, North Carolina. Her research interests include: digital immortality and older adults who have experienced early life trauma. She has previous experience working with survivors of domestic violence and children with behavioural and emotional disorders.

Carla J. Sofka is a Professor of Social Work at Siena College in Loudonville, New York, United States. Her research interests include the role of digital/ social media in coping with illness, death and grief, thanatology in pop culture, digital survivor advocacy, digital immortality and museums as healing spaces. She co-edited and contributed to the book *Dying, Death and Grief in an Online Universe: For Counselors and Educators* (2012).

Adriana Teodorescu is a PhD, Vice-President of the Romanian Death Studies Association and a member of the Association for the Study of Death and Society (ASDS). Her interests include: death studies, comparative literature, gender studies, ageing and old age. Recent books include: *Dying and Death in 18th–21st Century Europe* (2011), *Dying and Death in 18th–21st Century Europe, Volume 2* (2014) and *Death Representations in Literature: Forms and Theories* (2015).

Tony Walter is Honorary Professor of Death Studies, University of Bath, United Kingdom. His research interests include: comparative sociology, the place of the dead in society, funerals and communications media. Books include: *Funerals* (1990), *Pilgrimage in Popular Culture* (1993), *The Revival of Death* (1994), *The Eclipse of Eternity* (1996), *On Bereavement* (1999) and *Social Death* (2016). He is currently working on three new books on different aspects of death in the modern world.

Preface and acknowledgements

We will all die; the evidence supporting this prospect is as overwhelming as it is unpleasant and discouraging. Quite possibly, our deaths mark an ending, perhaps even a definitive ending to what we call 'our lives'. Of the billions of people who have lived and died before us throughout human history, the endless ranks of other mortal beings, no one ever seems to have returned again. To be human, it seems, is to be mortal. Nevertheless, *before* we die we are allowed to entertain ideas about life immortal – a life in which death is defeated – and even to entertain the most futile, unlikely and absurd ideas. This book is about some of these ideas and how they have developed in and changed throughout our culture. The book was supposed to be a joint venture between me and my dear colleague and friend, Michael C. Kearl. Unfortunately, his unexpected and untimely death cut that collaboration short, but the project survived and is now published. This book is dedicated to Michael C. Kearl and his vision of a sociology taking death, dying and immortality seriously – and also a vision of a sociology that despite its morbid topic was supposed to be fun, inspirational and lively. I am grateful in the production process to my two editors at Routledge, Neil Jordan and Shannon Kneis, for an unusually professional and carefree collaboration.

Michael Hviid Jacobsen
Aalborg University, Denmark

Introduction: Towards a postmortal society

Paving the pathway for a sociology of immortality

Michael Hviid Jacobsen

Introduction

When I started writing these lines, my eyes strangely scanned the many pictures, clippings of memorable philosophical and poetic quotations, birthday cards, invitations and other items collected throughout the years and now attached to my pin-up board in my office at the university. Many immortal words by great thinkers mixed with the pictures of friends and family, most fortunately still alive and kicking, others now passed away. One of these pictures is of my good friend and colleague, Michael C. Kearl, prominent sociologist of death and dying, who died unexpectedly a few years ago, and whose kind eyes gaze down upon my desk daily. Doing this book was our joint idea – an idea he never saw materialise. Writing these lines also made me contemplate my own mortality and it made me think about how this is matched by the mortality of everybody else – the billions of people who have gone before me as well as the mortality of everybody I know who is now alive, and the billions of people who will live and die in the future after my own death.

Crudely speaking, this world of ours can be divided into two relatively large and distinct groups of people. The 'Mortalists' – who think that we need to reconcile ourselves with the inescapable reality of death (including our very own death) and that to be human is to be mortal – and the 'Immortalists' – who are determined to conceive of even the most imaginative and improbable ways to cheat death. I belong to the former group as I believe that we are all mortal – whether we like it or not. Death, in my view, is not only the Great Equaliser, it is also the Great Humaniser, because it makes us realise that we are indeed all mortal and that there is no escape from death. It is human to be mortal. Moreover, there is still no convincing empirical evidence to support claims to immortality or to suggest that somebody some time has lived forever. And immortality in fact, as Shelly Kagan suggested in her book *Death*, 'means not just living a very long time or even an extraordinarily long time, but literally living *forever*' (Kagan 2012:239, original emphasis). And yet, despite overwhelming and incontrovertible evidence to the contrary – the fact that we must all die and nobody seems to live forever – people still cannot stop believing or hoping that we might be able to defeat or cheat death in the end. One of the quotation clippings on the pin-up board in my office is from Albert Camus's opening page of *The Myth of Sisyphus* quoting the ancient Greek poet Pindar's words from *Pythian*: 'O my soul, do not aspire to immortal life, but exhaust the limits of the possible'. In hindsight it seems as if Pindar's words fell on deaf ears. Throughout human history numerous ways to counter or postpone death have been conceived and, always in vain, tried and tested. The search for immortality has been part of human society and human striving for thousands of years. Even in the ancient world – a world not yet seduced by medical marvels and technological wonders intended to end the so-called 'natural causes' of death and extend human life – religious rituals and practices were used to create a sense of order and continuity in a world being continuously and helplessly deprived of life (see, e.g., Renfrew *et al.* 2015). Today, life-prolonging technologies, gene therapies, stem cell research, cloning, cryonics and digitalised immortality on the Internet now seem to honour some of our hopes to live forever.

Deep down, this hope for immortality is a very human thing – something hardly found among any other species. Humanity's dream of immortality undoubtedly dates back to and is interwoven with its unique awareness of inevitable death. Humans not only know that they must die – they also know that they know (Bauman 1992:12). This knowledge is as terrifying as it is unpleasant – and it is one of the main reasons for our continued and desperate search for a remedy for death. Cross-culturally, eternal existence has primarily been an attribute of the gods and those currying their favour. Moving into the second decade of the twenty-first century, humanity's prospects for super-longevity (if not immortality) have never been more promising than today, and longevitists such as Aubrey de Grey believe that the prospect of people living for hundreds of years is seemingly just around the corner (see, e.g., Appleyard 2007). The last few years have witnessed how biologists, by eliminating two genes promoting ageing and limiting diet, created a baker's yeast capable of living to 800 years (in yeast time) without any negative side effects. We have also seen how Russian billionaire Dmitry Itskov was funding research on inserting human minds into the everlasting artificial bodies of cyborgs. In 2011, a *Time* magazine cover story boldly proclaimed: '2045: The Year Man Becomes Immortal'. But detractors outnumber proponents of the death of death. Philosophers argue, for instance, how mortality and awareness of it is exactly what defines our species and motivates its civilisation-building quests. Social scientists observe how death is the wellspring of socio-cultural change just as biologists see it as the required mechanism for evolutionary development. Whether belonging to the camp of the detractors or the proponents of immortality, the very topic seems to spawn an intense and undying interest among different groups of scientists – an interest undoubtedly matched by the thoughts and hopes of most ordinary mortal people.

In the chapters that follow in this book, we delve into and contemplate questions of how and what if such death-transcending practices and technologies were to be developed. What do our ideas of immortality look like? How do we practise immortality? How differently would lives be lived and how different would the societies wherein they are lived be if immortality was indeed possible? For instance, given the genetic diversity of the population, compounded by unique experiences and exposures, there will never be some standardised, over-the-counter vitamin-like pill producing immortality. Observing the economics associated with the rise of customised pharmaceuticals, the price tag for quality superannuated existences (e.g. *sans* arthritis, dementia, diminished sex drive, diminished sexual desirability) will be extremely high. The affluent and those on the higher rungs of status hierarchies have always been the longer-lived. Super-longevity and immortality will first be their province. Contrariwise, those at the bottom of the social ladder may often find their paths to personalised immortality blocked or limited. Apparently, there seems to be an element of social stratification in our hopes to attain immortality. Questions and discussions of this nature – as well as many more – will be explored in more detail in what follows later in this book. But before we move into these matters, let us first look briefly into the topics of life, death, immortality and the coming of a 'postmortal society'.

Thoughts on life, death and immortality

On my desk at work I have a skull – obviously not a real skull, but a rather realistic plastic replica bought cheaply in a small tourist shop in Mexico. It is morbid and macabre, according to many of my students and colleagues, however still somewhat fascinating, thus showing our mixed and conflicting human feelings about death. My own preoccupation with death and immortality started early – it dates back to my master's dissertation in sociology, in which I explored the so-called 'deathwork' performed by orderlies working in a hospital mortuary in which they tried to create a sense of meaning in their professional work life informed, as it was, by daily experiences of and exposures to death and dying (Jacobsen 1997). Even though the encounter with death and dying is not an everyday experience to most people nowadays, the awareness of death is not reserved only for such specialised groups. Everybody thinks about, is touched by and will eventually experience death, dying and loss. There is no life without death. In this way, life is tragedy waiting to happen. In the wonderful words of French philosopher Jacques Derrida (1992), when someone dies, an entire and irreplaceable world disappears. It is this loss of worlds that makes death so terrible and unbearable. Although we, compared to earlier historical times, have been able quite effectively to minimise our first-hand contact with death and dying in modern society, death is still and remains something that we cannot escape. Death is an integral – indeed an invaluable – part of any human society and any human life. Death makes the world go around because it ensures that nothing lasts forever, that nothing stands in the way of development and progress too long or that nothing outlives its potential or natural life course. In fact, we would be unable to get by or get anything meaningful done without death lurking somewhere in the horizon of each and every human life.

Throughout history, many famous words of wisdom and aphorisms have been coined in order to capture the intimate connection between life, death and immortality. 'Life is the beginning of death', as German idealist poet and philosopher Novalis once suggested. 'Death is the beginning of immortality', French revolutionary Maximilien Robespierre proclaimed, and Polish poet Stanisław Jerzy Lec poignantly proposed that 'the first condition of immortality is death'. Moreover, Mexican poet Octavio Paz once claimed that death is the mirror reflecting the vain gesticulations of the living. In the same way, immortality, one might say, is the mirror reflecting the glorious illusions and hopeful wishes of those who will eventually die. Life, death and immortality are indeed inextricably linked, each giving meaning to and deriving its own meaning from the other two. According to German-English sociologist Norbert Elias, death is the problem of the living as dead people obviously have no problems. We humans are the only species that knows it is going to die and who will have to live with this knowledge. The knowledge of our own mortality creates an existential need for suspending this awareness – and this, in Elias's view, is the main reason why entertaining ideas and fantasies of immortality continues to be so important to us (Elias 1985/2001:35–40; see also Partridge 2015). Perhaps it is indeed our fundamental human sense of 'thanatophobia' – the deep-seated psychological fear of death stemming from the utter unimaginability of existence without us – that spirals us into nourishing illusions and imageries of immortality (Hall 1915). As already observed by Polish philosopher Wincency Lutoslawski in his intriguing discussion of the 'ethical consequences of the doctrine of immortality', 'many of our most important practical decisions are made with a view to preventing our death and the death of those dear to us' (Lutoslawski 1895:309). This knowledge of death, and the fear of death, thus spur and shape many of our motives. Naturally, the awareness of death is not a constant in human life. To most children, for example, the awareness of death is not well-developed and they often lack the experience of knowing people who die. This is why American poet and playwright Edna St. Vincent Millay once called childhood the 'kingdom where nobody dies'. Later in life, however, this awareness gradually matures or is suddenly awakened when somebody we know actually dies or when we ourselves become seriously ill, grow old or become 'terminal'. Sociologists Peter L. Berger and Thomas Luckmann thus once suggested how the awareness that we are constantly changed by 'objective time' (getting older by the minute and always one step closer to death) meant that our appreciation of 'subjective time' also changed accordingly, and that death therefore gradually became a still more important part of our life-plans and projects (Berger & Luckmann 1966). Things, events and actions suddenly take on a new meaning in the shadow of death. Following this lead, American philosopher Martha Nussbaum once memorably observed:

The intensity and dedication with which very many human activities are pursued cannot be explained without reference to the awareness that our opportunities are finite, that we cannot choose these activities indefinitely many times. In raising a child, in cherishing a lover, in performing a demanding task of work or thought or artistic creation, we are aware, at some level, of the thought that each of these efforts is structured and constrained by finite time.

(Nussbaum 1994:229)

Interestingly though, Canadian sociologist Erving Goffman has mused how we are normally able to go about our everyday business without being too overtly disturbed or distracted by this knowledge of awaiting death and the fact that the minutes and seconds of our lives are incessantly ticking away (Goffman 1967:261). This kind of 'everyday immortality' ensures that we are not paralysed by the awareness of death and are capable of creating and living meaningful lives despite the fact that the Grim Reaper is constantly looking over our shoulders. As Austrian psychoanalyst Sigmund Freud stated on our ability to suspend our knowledge of death and on our need for believing in immortality: 'Our unconscious does not believe in its own death; it behaves as if immortal ... We have shown an unmistakable tendency to put death aside, to eliminate it from life' (Freud 1918/1963:107–109). In a similar vein, French historian of so-called 'death mentalities', Philippe Ariès once observed how this was not only an individual achievement but in fact a more comprehensive cultural phenomenon perhaps particularly characteristic of contemporary society:

Everything ... goes on as if neither I nor those who are dear to me are any longer mortal. Technically, we admit that we might die; we take out insurance on our lives to protect our families from poverty. But really, at heart we feel we are non-mortals.

(Ariès 1974:106)

Because human life is lived in the shadow not only of death but also in the shadow of our awareness of death, humans will go to great lengths in order to avoid or postpone the dreamless sleep of death. But as most of us are well aware, the bidding for actual immortality (to become, in the words of Ariès, 'non-mortals'), either for the individual person or for mankind as a whole, is hardly realistic. We can, however, still glimpse it in the rise of the new science of immortality, in the anti-ageing industry's search for eternal youth and in promises of eternal life delivered throughout history by alchemists, preachers and prophets, plastic surgeons, cryogeneticists, cloning proponents, gerontologists and genetics researchers (see, e.g., Appleyard 2007; Brown 2008; Gruman 1966; Hentsch 2004; Immortality Institute 2004; Krüger 2010; Reanney 1991; Shostak 2003; Young 1988; Weiner 2010). Since we – or at least many of us – find it difficult or perhaps even dangerous to buy into such fanciful promises, various types of so-called 'symbolic immortality' are often sought out to compensate for the inability to achieve real or actual immortality. We might say that the hope for an eternal life is replaced by the idea of experiencing a sense of immortality in this life (Kellenberger 2015). For instance, these types of symbolic or vicarious immortality include the biological reproduction of the human race through procreation, religious beliefs in an afterlife and the hopes of resurrection, investments in fame and memorialisation as well as in experimental and ecstatic out-of-body experiences through hedonistic pleasure, sexual acts, narcotics and mysticism (see, e.g., Lifton 1968, 1973; Toynbee 1980). Although claims to or strategies of 'symbolic immortality' are indeed difficult to capture or validate in research, because they are often unacknowledged as such or remain relatively unarticulated, attempts to operationalise the concept have made it amenable to empirical testing (see, e.g., Mathews & Mister 1988).

On the one hand, these never-ending quests for immortality, whether actual or symbolic, are, as mentioned earlier, a very human thing – perhaps that which definitively separates us from our animal ancestry. Apart from biological procreation, humans are the only creatures, presumably, that are concerned with immortalising themselves by projecting their lives, identities and ideas into the future through the production of lasting pieces of work, fame and fortune or through carefully preparing and nurturing their self-images for memorialisation after their deaths. They are also the only ones who momentarily seek to experience immortality through death-defying acts of transcendence. On the other hand, however, immortality is also a very inhuman thing – it is normally something attributed only to deities, saints or to those few and amazingly artistic souls who have left a lasting imprint on humanity. For example, German writer Hermann Hesse's so-called 'Immortals' from his famous book *Steppenwolf* (1927/1969) included the incomparable likes of Mozart and Goethe – both gifted with an almost inhuman talent that is rarely found. But whether regarded as a human or an inhuman thing, the quest for immortality has captured the human imagination for millennia.

The topic of immortality from fiction to sociology

Immortality has always been a powerful impulse in human civilisation, whether in the shape of magic, religion or science (Cave 2012; Gollner 2013). Perhaps unsurprisingly then, immortality has always attracted the attention of and been a motivational force in different forms of creative expression and artistic imagination. For thousands of years, in fact at least as far back as the Gilgamesh Epic, written some 4,000 years ago, the topic has appeared in poetry and literature. Among ancient Egyptian, Indian, Roman and Greek scribes, the human quest to become immortal – a status most often allotted exclusively to the gods – was a frequently occurring theme. The same goes for the detailed and poetic treatment of immortality in more modern times in the classic works of such great writers as Dante, John Milton, William Shakespeare and Ralph Waldo Emerson. Particularly novelists from the great Romantic period toyed with how humans may possibly try to achieve the tantalising yet intangible and unattainable status of immortal and experience undying love. Especially within the horror story and science fiction genres has the topic of immortality been a powerful and recurrent feature (Clark 1995). From Dr Frankenstein's attempt to revive dead human matter in Mary Shelley's classic novel *Frankenstein* from 1818 (in which, in Kenneth Branagh's filmic adaptation of the novel, Victor Frankenstein confidently states that 'No one need ever die') to the equally eccentric scientist Joe Messenger in Peter James's book *Host* (1993), who downloads the contents of human brains into a supercomputer that can store, preserve and possibly also revive dead people's intelligence, we see vivid and mindboggling descriptions of how humans, aided and abetted by experimental science and technology, continue to entertain impossible dreams of immortality.

This human quest for immortality, and not least its often tragic and inhuman consequences, has also been described in a lot of literature. For example, in British author Aldous Huxley's satirical novel *After Many a Summer* (1939), we follow the death-fearing Hollywood millionaire Jo Stoyte who, presumably in vain, goes to great lengths to secure his own immortality, assisted by an obscure scientist who had studied the secrets to long life in various animal species. Although a work of fiction, Huxley's book also reads as an incisive critique of American celebrity culture and its quest to immortalise its heroes. An equally critical account of immortality is found in Argentinian writer Jorge Luis Borges's (1970) wonderful short story, 'The Immortal', which shows how, if people were ever to become truly immortal, as the main protagonist in the story who in the City of Immortals encounters the long-dead Homer, everything would merely turn out to be echoes and repetitions of past events and ennui and inertia would eventually set in. More recently, in American journalist and novelist Drew Magary's wonderful futuristic debut novel *The Postmortal* (2011), he shows how living a postmortal life – as is the case of the main character in the book, John Farrell – is not without its own serious costs. Farrell has received the cure that will ensure that he will not age or die of natural causes. In a world where nobody ages or dies, nobody ever retires and everybody has to work constantly, women will continue to have periods and, since a 'natural death' is no longer possible, only death through accidents, starvation, disease or murder await people at some point in their inhumanly extended lifetime. A related topic is described in Portuguese Nobel Prize-winner José Saramago's novel *Death with Interruptions* (2008). In the book he imaginatively toys with the idea of the ending of death and how this affects society. Saramago shows how the initial celebration of the ending of death is quickly replaced by a deep-seated despair, because the dying of death is accompanied by serious demographic, social and economic problems that illustrate how death is in fact a necessity. Eventually, under the threat of world collapse, an underground group named the 'maphia' undertakes killing people in order to avoid the problems of overpopulation.

Film-makers and movie script-writers have always been enticed by the theme of immortality, perhaps particularly within the adventure, fantasy and science fiction genres. The hugely popular *Star Trek*, *Harry Potter* and *Lord of the Rings* film series each in their own way deals with the possibility of immortality. There is indeed no shortage of films dealing with death-transcendence and immortality. For example, the classic *Cocoon* (1985) depicted the rejuvenation of a group of elderly people in a retirement home who, through the intervention of aliens from another planet, experienced immortal bliss, whereas in *The Green Mile* (1999) we saw how immortal life – outliving everybody you know and love – does not necessarily guarantee happiness. More recently, in *The Age of Adaline* (2015), a similar thought-provoking story unfolds about how immortality realised leads to a tormented and lonely life.

But whereas immortality has constituted a recurrent and potent theme in many parts of classic and contemporary popular culture, sociology instead seems to have neglected or avoided the topic. Searching for a 'sociology of immortality' on the Internet, one will be disappointed and surprised to discover that very little indeed – in fact almost nothing – seems to be published under this specific heading. Apart from within the specialised sub-disciplines of the 'sociology of religion' and the 'sociology of death and dying', studies of immortality – and human conceptions of ways to cheat, counter or circumvent death – have never held a prominent position in sociology as such. In truth, studying death was not a great concern for the classical sociologists. However, they did in fact all touch – albeit in a roundabout way – upon the theme of immortality. Karl Marx deemed religion, and with it the promise of heavenly redemption, 'the opiate of the masses', which detracted from the daily toil as well as the urgency of the class struggle. Max Weber studied how the Calvinists sought signs of salvation by way of hard work and asceticism, and his work also contained in-depth studies of the otherworldly ideas of various world religions. To Émile Durkheim, society itself – consisting of so-called material and immaterial 'social facts' – was immortal, and even that which seemed to challenge or threaten the cohesion and continuation of society, such as anomie, was ultimately regarded as something that showed the ultimate survival strength of the social. Georg Simmel, in some detail in his more metaphysical essays, discussed the limited yet transcendence-seeking nature of human life (elegantly expressed in the notion of 'more-than-life'), and he also pointed out how immortality from the very outset was built into human existence (Simmel 2010). So although not entirely absent, the topic of immortality was never really the main trademark of sociological analysis. Anthropologists, historians and archaeologists have always taken a keen interest in studying the cultural importance and historical dimensions of death and immortality beliefs. In sociology, such studies have been few and far between. Every now and then a sociological study pops up scrutinising the topic of immortality. Two important and valuable exceptions to this general neglect is Tony Walter's *The Eclipse of Eternity* (1996), which provides an in-depth introduction to changing conceptions of the afterlife, and Zygmunt Bauman's *Mortality, Immortality and Other Life Strategies* (1992), which analyses the different ways modern and postmodern society construct and deconstruct death and immortality, thereby showing that death and immortality – or at least our understanding of these phenomena – do not stand still (see also Jacobsen 2013, 2016). Obviously, the topic is also touched upon in various other books, book chapters and journal articles, but there is still no comprehensive body of sociological knowledge about immortality – no actual 'sociology of immortality'. Hence we could and should take a much more genuine and systematic interest in immortality, because it seems to be such an important notion in the lives of individuals as well as in the way societies, cultures, religions and collective value-systems work. Just as sociology back in the 1990s finally began to take the study of death and dying seriously, sociology should also begin to embrace immortality as a topic deserving of attention and systematised research. The often simplistic diagnosis and description of a process of 'secularisation' in the Western world, which results in the gradual undermining of ideas and beliefs about immortality with the advent of modern society and the advances of the modern scientific mentality, will hardly suffice. I rather suggest that studying the idea of the coming of a so-called 'postmortal society' might be one – but surely not the only – place to start.

Towards a postmortal society

We now live in a world of 'posts'. Apparently, there is always something new awaiting us after something else – something now deemed outdated, useless or yesterday's news – has stopped, disappeared or passed away. Hence the popularity of 'post' terms in many descriptions of recent social changes such as postmodernism, postindustrialism, postemotionalism, postcolonialism, posthumanism and now also 'postmortalism'. The last of these notions obviously suggests that there *is* something *after* mortality, something that succeeds death and that death is therefore no longer the last sentence. As mentioned above, humanity has always entertained such futile ideas, but the apparently new thing is that we are perhaps closer than ever before in not only speculating about some heavenly afterlife but in expanding human life almost indefinitely and also in reviving those already dead. Scientific breakthroughs such as gene testing, immune therapy, regenerative technology, cures for a wide range of previously incurable and deadly diseases and the discovery of the role of the hormone melatonin in delaying or even preventing the ageing process is apparently on the verge of revolutionising our understanding of and approach to diseases, average lifespans and natural causes of death, which, as a consequence, also challenges our conventional conceptions of the boundaries between life, death and immortality (see, e.g., Reanney 1991; Weiner 2010).

Admittedly, the notion of 'postmortalism' as used in the title of this book is not yet so well-defined or well-described. A few texts have already dealt with postmortality and postmortalism (see, e.g., Cetron & Davies 1998; Lafontaine 2009). They have shown how particularly scientific advances within medicine and technology will, at some time in the future, drastically prolong human life. They have also discussed how the coming of a postmortal society will have a profound impact on many different dimensions of our world. For example, in their incisive book, *Cheating Death*, social forecasters Marvin Cetron and Owen Davies (1998) stated that the postmortal society would mark a revolution in the way we organise society. It would liberate us from the shackles of death, and, 'like all great liberations, the postmortal revolution will uproot much of what has gone before' (Cetron & Davies 1998:12). Because postmortalism confronts many of the conceptions about life, death and immortality that we have taken for granted for a long time, the postmortal society also inaugurates a veritable challenge to our values, ethics, economics, beliefs and our social organisation. According to Cetron and Davies, the coming of the postmortal society will therefore bring about some radical changes within most spheres of society. In their book they described some of the preconditions for the postmortal society (such as advances in medical technology, extended life expectancies and living healthier and more secure lives), they envisioned some of the major trends that would accompany the arrival of the postmortal society (such as changes in family structures, the impact on the labour force and work lives, the pressures on welfare provisions and the creation of new social inequalities in living long lives), and they outlined a number of the challenges accompanying this development (such as how to provide decent living conditions and adequate care for an increasingly ageing population, the environmental impact of a population that lives (and consumes) longer and longer and the creation of personal meaning in a world in which everybody lives much longer than ever before). In short, a postmortal society would in most respects be a society that differs radically from the world of today. Perhaps postmortalism is on its way, even though Cetron and Davies admitted that 'the world in ten or twenty years from now may not be literally postmortal. Yet our deaths are not likely to arrive on schedule. They might not arrive at all' (Cetron & Davies 1998:11). So even though they admitted that we might not actually and literally become immortal (perhaps this is destined to remain one of humanity's most persistent pipe dreams), the postmortal society may – at least symbolically – come to inform ever larger parts of our lives and in many different respects.

We now want – even expect and almost demand – to live longer, and we want to put ever more life experience and life content into this extended life. Whereas the so-called 'resurrectionists' in the seventeenth and eighteenth centuries – who at times even stole dead bodies from graveyards – wanted to revive the dead, bringing them back to life (Haycock 2008), in our self-centred postmortal society we are more concerned with keeping the living alive longer and ensuring that we continue to live healthy and active lives until the very end – if it comes. The ideas of the postmortal society are also evident in the 'carpe-diem culture' that, contrary to the so-called 'extensionalists' and 'suspended animationists' – who want to extend life for as long as humanly possible (preferably indefinitely) and to revive dead matter some time in the future when diseases can be cured and dead bodies reanimated – insist that we need to regard every moment in mortal life as a potential glimpse of immortality and that we should actively seek out such life-transcending and near-death moments through extreme sports, acid trips, sexual escapades or other types of 'eternal nows'. More than a century ago, Swedish-American philosopher John E. Boodin suggested that the emerging type of immortality should now be labelled 'social immortality'. He insisted that 'the kingdom of heaven has now become a kingdom to be progressively realized in this world' (Boodin 1915:196). Whereas immortality in premodern tribal and traditional societies was primarily promised in the shape of an otherworldly and ethereal afterlife (particularly stressing the 'after' prefix), in the modern world immortality is increasingly linked to one's current life, thus removing it from its firm anchoring in the great unknown and instead relocating it in the here-and-now. No more procrastination, postponed satisfaction, delayed gratification or pies in the sky. We want 'instant immortality' in the same way as we crave instant coffee, instant community and instant love. The principles of a postmortal society also thrive on the Internet, where there has been an increasing interest in recent years in so-called 'digitalized immortality' or 'electronic immortality' where not only can we continue to commemorate and keep the memory of the dead alive and kicking on numerous memorial pages, but where we may also, despite being killed thousands of times in virtual reality, always restart the game again, or where we, through attempts at transferring and storing the neural energy and the memory from deceased people, may hope to keep them artificially alive even after their actual death (see, e.g., Moreman & Lewis 2014; Ntelia 2015; Rothblatt 2014; von Eckartsberg & von Eckartsberg 2011). Contemporary survival concerns also materialise concretely in the shape of so-called 'survival retreats', where people fearing nuclear annihilation, terrorism, ecological meltdown, extinction, pandemics or hordes of malicious strangers hope to be able to survive in fenced-off communities when the rest of the world has succumbed (see, e.g., Black 2011; Mitchell 2001). And it is indeed not difficult to discover or decipher many other examples and indications of postmortal thoughts and practices in contemporary society. So although the postmortal society is not yet here – and perhaps, and quite possibly, it will never materialise fully fledged as a place in which nobody ever dies – we are nevertheless capable of seeing signs and interpreting tendencies that point to the fact that postmortalism as an idea, as a movement and as a potential is very much becoming part of contemporary society.

About this book

This book is about death, dying, survivalism, immortality and postmortalism – all delicately interwoven and intricately intertwined in the lives of individuals and societies alike. Therefore, the book is in fact as much about life, as it is lived, as it is about death and immortality. The chapters included in the volume point to different types, dimensions, forms and experiences of immortality in contemporary society and with their own perspectives dissect and critically discuss the viability and desirability of our continued search for remedies, strategies, techniques or prophylaxes to prevent us from ever dying. The chapters are all written by sociologists or scholars working within neighbouring disciplines, each in their way adding valuable insights to the still youthful and underdeveloped sub-discipline of 'sociology of immortality' and to its potential for charting and understanding the, perhaps, postmortal society.

The first chapter, by Tony Walter, is concerned with outlining how the dead, despite being dead, still survive in society and how the living may engage with their dead – particularly the 'family dead' and the 'sacred dead'. In the chapter, the author sketches and discusses three different frames by means of which this is achieved – three frameworks that are related but also in potential tension with each other. First, he shows how the dead become ancestors – how we create ancestry and engage in exchanges with our ancestors. Second, it is presented how the dead become immortal as offered by world religions. Third, the author describes how the dead survive in the secular memories of the living. Moreover, Walter also distinguishes between two types of culture – 'care cultures' in which the living and the dead look after each other in some kind of dynamic exchange, and 'memory cultures' concerned with remembrance.

Chapter 2, by Guy Brown, follows up on this cultural dimension by outlining different pathways to surviving and obtaining some sort of immortality. Starting out with the ancient Gilgamesh Epic that dealt with death and immortality, Brown proposes four central ways through which humans have always attempted to achieve immortality. First, by staying alive as long as possible, which has been the realm of medicine and magic. Second, by surviving the death of the body in some accentuated spiritual form, which is traditionally the concern of many religions. Third, by surviving through one's children and one's children's children, which is the realm of genetics and family. Fourth, by our earthly work and deeds embedded in society and memory, which is the realm of memetics and culture. Each in their own way, these four forms continue to promise its users some hope for obtaining immortality.

In Chapter 3, by Michael Hviid Jacobsen, we are introduced to the inspirational ideas of death and immortality in the sociology of Zygmunt Bauman. In the chapter, the author outlines the contours of Bauman's original thinking about immortality as a rather overlooked yet important contribution to the theorising on 'symbolic immortality'. According to Bauman, the author shows, immortality is an integral part of human culture and society, and through the study of the quest for immortality or so-called 'life strategies' we may come to understand more encompassing and important aspects of society. The chapter presents and discusses Bauman's ideas about immortality and shows how his critical diagnosis of liquid-modern individualisation also informs his understanding of contemporary attempts at achieving immortality through fitness, health and 'self-care'.

Chapter 4 is written by Uri Lifshin, Peter J. Helm and Jeff Greenberg. Building on a long tradition of thought, the so-called 'terror management theory' proposes that maintaining faith in a symbolic, meaning-imbuing conception of reality provided by one's culture and sustaining the sense that one is a significant participant in that meaningful reality helps people feel transcendent of their own physical deaths and thereby allows them to cope with the awareness of their own mortality. Various hypotheses have been derived from this theory and have by now been supported by substantial amounts of experimental research. In this chapter, the authors provide an overview of terror management theory, highlight some of the empirical evidence supporting its basic ideas and show some of the implications for contemporary society.

Chapter 5, by David Giles, looks into how fame is one of the major motors for claims to immortality. Fame, stardom and celebrity status have always been important carriers for obtaining some sort of immortalisation, memorialisation and remembrance in posterity. In this chapter, the author presents and discusses some of the techniques and technologies that have evolved throughout history for bestowing immortality on individuals, and examines these in the light of the ever more crowded world of contemporary celebrity. Some of the techniques discussed are 'visual representation', 'impersonation' and 'naming practices'. The author also outlines a number of the reasons for these immortalisation attempts, such as 'ideological and nationalistic purposes', 'economic purposes' and 'sentimental reasons'.

In Chapter 6, Adriana Teodorescu shows how work represents a fundamental human experience, whose understanding and socio-cultural practice is performed more and more from the point of view of its ability to provide personal meaning to people. Her chapter points out how one of the fundamental vectors that construct the contemporary Western imaginary of work is the pursuit of symbolic immortality, and shows that this is achieved by overusing three essential features of postmodernity – narcissism, the imperative of breaking the limits and the (new) infantilisation of the employee – which are promoted by contemporary corporate discourse. As Teodorescu suggests, in the construction of this type of discourse, one can easily detect different techniques that seek to underline the relationship between work and meaning (that work gives meaning to life) and which seek to place this relationship within the symbolic immortality imaginary.

In Chapter 7, by Gianfranco Pecchinenda, we are introduced to an interesting typology of different 'cultures of immortality' that each in their own way has informed the way humans have thought about and tried to obtain immortality throughout history. According to the author, every society passes on to its members a certain image of man, an idea of himself and his identity, together with a vision of the sense of the existence and a culture of immortality. In the chapter, Pecchinenda outlines these different cultures under the headings of the 'Natural Aristotelian Man', the 'Cartesian Man', the 'Structural Man', the 'Communicating Man', the 'Genoma Man' and the 'Neuronal Man', which are all figures or images of man that represent some important ideas about how humans are related to death in different socio-historical configurations. At the end of the chapter, some considerations on the social impact of these changes in immortality are presented.

The topic of the impact of science and technology on ideas of immortality is also pursued in Chapter 8 by Nunzia Bonifati, who discusses the impact of the fast-paced development of science and technology (biomedicine, bioengineering, bioinformatics, nanotechnology, satellite technology, robotics, genomics, synthetic biology and so on), which allows humankind to hope for a potential overcoming of its own biological limits – such as death. In the chapter, the author specifically focuses on this movement towards the 'post-human' through the development of a number of 'human enhancement technologies' – wearable technologies, organs and tissues, drugs and hormones, implantable devices, genetically modified babies and so on – which all, each in their own way, extend the human potential to live longer and perform better. Bonifati also outlines some of the philosophical ideas underpinning this 'post-human' development within science and technology intended to promote human immortality. Moreover, the author ends her chapter by pointing to some of the paradoxical and indeed undesirable consequences of this development.

Chapter 9 is written by Carla J. Sofka, Allison Gibson and Danielle R. Silberman and investigates different dimensions of the brave new world of digitalised immortality now on offer and available on the Internet. Digital and social media perform increasingly important roles in our daily lives. This chapter describes various elements of one's 'digital afterlife' and the potential impact of a person's ongoing online presence on the bereaved. In the chapter, current policies of online service providers regarding deceased user accounts will also be summarised and implications of these policies for the deceased's next of kin are discussed. Moreover, the authors present some of the strategies available to encourage the proactive creation of 'digital advance directives' among digital and social media users.

The topic of the Internet is also pursued in Chapter 10 by William Sims Bainbridge, who considers the possibility that modern Internet-based technologies may allow at least a slight improvement in the possibility for ordinary people to have increased fame: for example, through massively multiplayer online games in which they can be living players or electronic avatars of persons who have in fact already died. The chapter thus explores the veneration of the dead in online gameworlds. The chapter's original approach to the topic of immortality is exemplified through three case examples in which specific deceased persons are symbolically resurrected as avatars inside virtual worlds. In each case the person was an extremely ambitious religious leader who sought power during life, as a form of 'immortality', and who possessed powerful visions that promised transcendence of the limits of material reality.

The final chapter of the book, Chapter 11, was written by Michael C. Kearl, who passed away quite recently. In the chapter, Kearl describes the new cult of 'postselves' in American civic and popular cultures that has been accentuated towards the end of the twentieth and the beginning of the twenty-first centuries. Kearl shows how – contrary to the thesis claiming the increased denial and invisibility of death in contemporary society – everyday life is in fact buzzing with the presence of the dead. According to Kearl, important driving forces behind this renewed interest in death, afterlife and transcendence are extreme individualism, capitalism and technological innovations making the construction of new types of 'postselves' possible and available to ever more people. Moreover, the tragic events of the terrorist attacks on 9/11 further fuelled the development towards the proliferation of 'postselves' and a more publicly visible memorialisation of the dead.

This book is, in fact, dedicated to the last contributor, to my good friend and colleague Michael C. Kearl, who sadly passed away unexpectedly in early 2015. Although not the first, he was one of the few of his own generation of sociologists who took the sociology of death and dying seriously as a field of research in its own right. He was a dedicated teacher who inspired students to take an interest in the topics of death, dying and immortality, who collected heaps of educative and esoteric material that he generously shared on the Internet (in the treasure trove of the still accessible homepage entitled *Kearl's Guide to the Sociology of Death and Dying*) and who wrote many insightful pieces on death, dying and immortality, particularly the pioneering book *Endings: A Sociology of Death and Dying* (1989) and his wonderful piece on 'postselves' from 2010, which is republished in this volume. As a man and as a sociologist, Mike was a giant – a giant with a big heart and unfortunately, it turned out, also a heart that failed him one morning on his way to work. He is, however, not forgotten. As has been shown recently in an article dedicated to his work, Michael C. Kearl had an important, yet surprisingly unacknowledged, impact on the development of the sociology of death and dying (Graham & Montoya 2015). This book would never have materialised without his inspirational ideas. Mike, rest peacefully, we are now passing on the baton – perhaps a small step towards immortality? And remember, as once beautifully written by Norwegian painter Edvard Munch: 'From my rotting body, flowers shall grow and I am in them and that is eternity' (Munch quoted in Thompson & Sorvig 2007:30).

References

Appleyard, Bryan (2007): *How to Live Forever or Die Trying: On the New Immortality*. New York: Simon & Schuster.

16   *M. H. Jacobsen*

Ariès, Philippe (1974): *Western Attitudes Toward Death from the Middle Ages to the Present*. Baltimore: Johns Hopkins University Press.
Bauman, Zygmunt (1992): *Mortality, Immortality and Other Life Strategies*. Cambridge: Polity Press.
Berger, Peter L. & Thomas Luckmann (1966): *The Social Construction of Reality*. London: Harmondsworth.
Black, David S. (2011): *Survival Retreats: A Practical Guide to Creating a Sustainable, Defendable Refuge*. New York: Skyhorse Publishing.
Boodin, John E. (1915): 'Social Immortality'. *International Journal of Ethics*, 25 (2):196–212.
Borges, Jorge Luis (1970): 'The Immortal', in Donald A. Yates & James E. Irby (eds): *Labyrinths: Selected Stories and Other Writings*. Harmondsworth: Penguin Books, pp. 135–149.
Brown, Guy (2008): *The Living End: The Future of Death, Aging and Immortality*. London: Palgrave/Macmillan.
Cave, Stephen (2012): *Immortality: The Quest to Live Forever and How It Drives Civilisation*. London: Biteback.
Cetron, Marvin & Owen Davies (1998): *Cheating Death: The Promise and the Future Impact of Trying to Live Forever*. New York: St. Martin's Press.
Clark, Stephen R. L. (1995): *How to Live Forever: Science Fiction and Philosophy*. London: Routledge.
Derrida, Jacques (1992): *Aporias*. Stanford, CA: Stanford University Press.
Elias, Norbert (1985/2001): *The Loneliness of the Dying*. London: Continuum.
Freud, Sigmund (1918/1963): 'Reflections on War and Death', in Philip Rieff (ed.): *Character and Culture*. New York: Collier Books, pp. 107–134.
Goffman, Erving (1967): *Interaction Ritual*. New York: Pantheon Books.
Gollner, Adam L. (2013): *The Book of Immortality: The Science, Belief and Magic Behind Living Forever*. London: Scribner.
Graham, Connor & Alfred Montoya (2015): 'Death, After-Death and the Human in the Internet Era: Remembering, Not Forgetting Professor Michael C. Kearl (1949–2015)'. *Mortality*, 20 (4):287–302.
Gruman, Gerald J. (1966): *A History of Ideas about the Prolongation of Life*. New York: Springer.
Hall, G. Stanley (1915): 'Thanatophobia and Immortality'. *American Journal of Psychology*, 26:550–613.
Haycock, David Boyd (2008): *Mortal Coil: A Short History of Living Longer*. New Haven, CT: Yale University Press.
Hentsch, Thierry (2004): *Truth or Death: The Quest for Immortality in the Western Narrative Tradition*. Vancouver, BC: Talonbooks.
Hesse, Hermann (1927/1969): *Steppenwolf*. Harmondsworth: Penguin Books.
Huxley, Aldous (1939): *After Many a Summer*. London: Chatto & Windus.
Immortality Institute (ed.) (2004): *The Scientific Conquest of Death: Essays on Infinite Lifespans*. Allen, TX: Libros En Red.
Jacobsen, Michael Hviid (1997): *The Myth of Homo Immortalis: Contours of a Thanatology of Radicalized Modernity*. Unpublished master's thesis, Aalborg University.
Jacobsen, Michael Hviid (ed.) (2013): *Deconstructing Death: Changing Cultures of Death, Dying, Bereavement and Care in the Nordic Countries*. Odense: University Press of Southern Denmark.

Jacobsen, Michael Hviid (2016): ' "Spectacular Death": Proposing a New Fifth Phase to Philippe Ariès's Admirable History of Death'. *Humanities*, 5 (19). Available online at: www.mdpi.com/2076-0787/5/2/19.

James, Peter (1993): *Host*. London: Orion.

Kagan, Shelly (2012): *Death*. New Haven, CT: Yale University Press.

Kearl, Michael C. (1989): *Endings: A Sociology of Death and Dying*. Oxford: Oxford University Press.

Kearl, Michael C. (2010): 'The Proliferation of Postselves in American Civic and Popular Cultures'. *Mortality*, 15 (1):47–63.

Kellenberger, James (2015): *The Everlasting and the Eternal*. London: Palgrave/Macmillan.

Krüger, Oliver (2010): 'The Suspension of Death: The Cryonic Utopia in the Context of the U.S. Funeral Industry'. *Marburg Journal of Religion*, 15 (1):1–19.

Lafontaine, Céline (2009): 'The Postmortal Condition: From the Biomedical Deconstruction of Death to the Extension of Longevity'. *Science as Culture*, 18 (3):297–312.

Lifton, Robert J. (1968): *Revolutionary Immortality: Mao Tse-tung and the Chinese Cultural Revolution*. London: Weidenfeld & Nicolson.

Lifton, Robert J. (1973): 'The Sense of Immortality: On Death and the Continuity of Life'. *American Journal of Psychoanalysis*, 33:3–15.

Lutoslawski, Wincenty (1895): 'The Ethical Consequences of the Doctrine of Immortality'. *International Journal of Ethics*, 5 (3):309–324.

Magary, Drew (2011): *The Postmortal*. London: Penguin Books.

Mathews, Robert C. & Rena D. Mister (1988): 'Measuring an Individual's Investment in the Future: Symbolic Immortality, Sensation Seekers and Psychic Numbness'. *Omega: Journal of Death and Dying*, 18 (3):161–173.

Mitchell Jr, Richard G. (2001): *Dancing at Armageddon: Survivalism and Chaos in Modern Times*. Chicago: University of Chicago Press.

Moreman, Christopher M. & A. David Lewis (eds) (2014): *Digital Death: Mortality and Beyond in the Online Age*. New York: Praeger.

Ntelia, Renata E. (2015): 'Death in Digital Games: A Thanatological Approach'. *Antae*, 2 (2):90–100.

Nussbaum, Martha (1994): *The Therapy of Desire*. Princeton, NJ: Princeton University Press.

Partridge, Christopher (2015): *Mortality and Music: Popular Music and the Awareness of Death*. London: Bloomsbury.

Reanney, Darryl (1991): *The Death of Forever: A New Future of Human Consciousness*. London: Souvenir Press.

Renfrew, Colin, Michael J. Boyd & Iain Morley (eds) (2015): *Death Rituals, Social Order and the Archaeology of Immortality in the Ancient World*. Cambridge: Cambridge University Press.

Rothblatt, Martine (2014): *Virtually Human: The Promise – and the Peril – of Digital Immortality*. London: St. Martin's Press.

Saramago, José (2008): *Death with Interruptions*. New York: Harcourt.

Shostak, Stanley (2003): *Becoming Immortal: Combining Cloning and Stem-Cell Therapy*. Albany, NY: State University of New York Press.

Simmel, Georg (2010): *The View of Life*. Chicago: University of Chicago Press.

Thompson, J. William & Kim Sorvig (2007): *Sustainable Landscape Construction: A Guide to Green Building Outdoors* (2nd edn). Washington, DC: Island Press.

Toynbee, Arnold (1980): 'Various Ways in Which Human Beings Have Sought to Reconcile Themselves to the Fact of Death', in Edwin S. Shneidman (ed.): *Death: Current Perspectives*. Palo Alto, CA: Mayfield, pp. 11–34.

von Eckartsberg, Rolf & Elsa von Eckartsberg (2011): 'Social and Electronic Immortality'. *Janus Head*, 12 (1):9–21.

Walter, Tony (1996): *The Eclipse of Eternity: A Sociology of the Afterlife*. London: Routledge.

Weiner, Jonathan (2010): *Long for This World: The Strange Science of Immortality*. New York: HarperCollins.

Young, Stephen (1988): 'A Glimpse of Immortality'. *New Scientist*, 15 September.

1   How the dead survive

Ancestors, immortality, memory[1]

Tony Walter

Introduction

How do the dead survive? How, if at all, may the living engage with them? The chapter sketches three of the more significant answers that have gripped human imagination and characterised particular cultures over millennia: (1) the dead become ancestors, (2) they become immortal, or (3) they survive in the memories of the living. The sketch highlights relations and tensions between the three: for example, how the immortality offered by world religions[2] has conflicted with ancestor veneration; how in the West secular memory started to replace religious care of the dead as a result of *religious* not secular innovation; the subtle relationships between remembering the dead and caring for them; and how memory of the dead in the West's more secular societies may be mutating into a new form of ancestor veneration. I argue that each imagined post-mortem state is associated with an imagined social universe for the living (family, religion, diverse groups) and a particular purpose for funeral rites (to create ancestors, immortality, memories). Each form of post-mortem survival, therefore, is connected to the everyday life of society, drawing on and legitimating particular forms of society and ritual.[3]

I do not consider all the dead. In nearly every culture there are two kinds of dead available for interaction with the living (Goss & Klass 2005): the *family* dead, and the *sacred* dead who represent bigger groups and institutions that today would include religion (e.g. Jesus, the Buddha), the nation state (e.g. the war dead), politics (e.g. Mao) and culture (e.g. Beethoven, Elvis). Though the two are related, this chapter focuses on the family dead. My aim is to develop a socio-historical typology of death, survival and immortality of the familial dead across the ages; my hope is that this will shed some light on what twenty-first-century people do with their family dead.

The chapter does not cover all kinds of afterlife belief. It barely touches on reincarnation as found in some Eastern religions, in many tribal societies or as a popular discourse in contemporary Western society. And many details and variations cannot but be skated over, which may annoy some anthropologists and historians who relish details of the particular, but I trust they will at least grant that it is legitimate to attempt to develop typologies. The critical question is whether the typology that results from this chapter's analysis is illuminating.

There is a view in social science, reflected in some of the chapters of this volume, that humans are universally anxious or fearful about their own personal survival, giving rise to the hopes of personal survival, whether literal or symbolic, to be found in most cultures. For Ernest Becker (1973) and Terror Management Theory (see Lifshin *et al.*'s chapter in this volume), such immortality strategies are not only part of culture, but a major driver of culture. This chapter's reading of a range of archaeological, anthropological, historical and sociological material, however, questions such views. It suggests, rather, that survivors' experience of the dead as temporary ancestor may be as significant as the not-yet-dead's anxiety about their own finitude, perhaps more so. Anxiety about personal finitude may prove to have characterised primarily the three-millennia-long era of the world religions (Bowker 1991), and hence has been of particular relevance to the emergence of what is often called 'civilisation' – but much less relevant to most tribal societies or to post-religious secular societies.

Family ancestors

In many agricultural societies, those whose social position in life commanded respect continue in death to be respected as ancestors. Meyer Fortes (1965) argued that in Africa what becomes an ancestor is not the person, but simply the authority that the deceased had over their descendants, and this seems also to be the case in East Asia, though authority there has long been shared between ancestors and the state. Ancestors therefore reflect and/or support authority within kinship systems rather than personal attachment, and the details of ancestral life after death are of little concern to the living (Hamilton 1998).

The universality of ancestor veneration has been a matter of some debate (Parker Pearson 1999, ch. 7). Some economic anthropologists (e.g. Lehmann & Myers 1985; Meillassoux 1972) argue that ancestors are rarely found in hunter-gatherer societies

> where the immediate returns on production provide no basis for a general sense of cultural 'indebtedness' to past generations. Agriculture is by contrast a peculiarly 'ancestral' mode of production precisely because current generations are indebted to the labour of previous generations.
>
> (Whitley 2002:121)

Lyle Steadman *et al.* (1996), however, defining ancestral spirits more widely, find evidence of ancestors in a number of immediate return hunter-gatherer groups, which raises the question of the relation of ancestors to animism. Certainly among hunter-gatherers, human spirits and nature spirits are often interconnected and reside within the physical environment. David Chidester

(2002:13) notes that for Australian aboriginal hunter-gatherers the ancestor is the totem group's mythic founder who died long ago, contrasting with African agriculturalists for whom the ancestor is 'not a cultural hero from the beginning of time but a close relative' to whom one is personally indebted. Ninian Smart (1996:32) considers it possible that ancestors comprised humans' very earliest concept of life after death. Without taking sides in this debate, we can say with confidence that ancestor veneration is very common in human history and pre-history. And it seems that ancestorhood as the post-mortem destination of those currently alive rather than the special status of a long-dead mythic hero characterises many agricultural societies. It is to these known 'family' ancestors that we now turn.

These ancestors' agency continues with them beyond the grave (Espírito Santo & Blanes 2013). In Chinese society, 'every death produces a potentially dangerous spirit. Funeral rites ... convert this volatile spirit into a tamed, domesticated ancestor' (Watson 1988:204). In many societies, the dead have power to meddle in the affairs of the living, to cause both harm and good; as well as the wise, beneficent ancestor whose guidance is valued, there is also the hungry or angry ghost out to cause trouble (Emmons 2003a; Jacobi 2003; Ochoa 2010). Trouble-making ghosts provide explanations for suffering and misfortune. Mary Douglas (2004:179) observes this was lost when monotheistic religion replaced all-too-human ancestors with a single all-loving God, thus creating the problem of theodicy: how to explain evil and suffering when the sole supernatural agent is all-powerful and all-good?

Ancestors' agency is the basis for the living to interact with the dead in ritual processes of exchange (Baudrillard 1993). Gifts and prayers to the dead ensure that the dead aid, or at least do not harm, the living (Scott 2007; Suzuki 2013:17), the logic being one of mutual care, underlain by an implicit threat: if we look after you, you will look after us. Ritual exchange is often enabled by mediums (Emmons 2003b) and shamans (Vitebsky 1992). Exchange continues not for eternity, but for a few generations until memory – of the person, or of the grave's location – fades, after which the ancestor becomes less known, less accessible, part of the ancestral collectivity or simply forgotten (Horstmann 2011; Mbiti 1970; Suzuki 2013; Watson 1988). Some ancestors, however, gain mythic status as family or clan founders, their stories told for many generations, justifying the occupation or ownership of land or enabling distant kin to be identified (Vansina 1985; Walter 2015; Watson 1988). In Canadian Pacific communities where the dead are reincarnated within the tribe, the ancestors *are* the living, giving extra force to twenty-first-century claims to ancestral land (Mills 2001).

Who becomes an ancestor, what rites create ancestors, and how long it takes for a recently dead individual ancestor to become subsumed into a more collective and impersonal body of ancestors, can vary considerably (Panagiotopoulos & Espírito Santo, forthcoming). Belinda Straight (2006:108) sketches wide variations across a range of societies: 'Some deceased persons are denied agency altogether, deliberately annihilated, or just forgotten, whereas others are remembered for a time before slowly being de-individuated as their unique personhood is overcome by a collective (yet agentive) ancestral substance'. C. J. Calhoun (1980) considers that, in some African tribes, it is ancestors' deadness, their inactivity, that detaches them from their pre-mortem unique personality and enables them to become idealised representations of authority. In several societies, it tends to be older males who, having status in life, gain post-mortem status as ancestor (Kopytoff 1971).

If veneration of family ancestors is ancient and widespread, how does it fare when subsistence agriculture encounters larger-scale social forces such as markets, cities, empires and formal religions? The answer is that ancestor veneration has been supported by some of these forces, and undermined by others. In East Asia, ancestors have continued strongly into the modern era. Confucius, unconcerned about the dead themselves, used ancestral respect to encourage respect for the living older generation (Park 2009, 2010), so that many Chinese today still demonstrate filial piety in part through ancestral rites (Bryant 2003; Watson & Rawski 1988). Likewise, Taoism and Shinto do not undermine exchanges with the family dead. Indeed, in Meiji Japan (i.e. from 1868), family became a symbolic microcosm of the nation, with family ancestor rites being used to sustain national identity. The Meiji government, instrumental in modernising the Japanese economy, 'controlled Japanese people's lives via control of death: it legitimated the household as a perpetual entity and demanded its successive performance of ancestor worship through the family grave' (Suzuki 2013:15). Animist Shinto is also a source of spirits in Japan, enabling the land of Japan (nature spirits), family (ancestral spirits) and nation (the emperor, the deified war dead) to meld together. Under post-war conditions, Japanese ancestor veneration continues to evolve (Morioka 1986; Suzuki 1998).

Other social forces, however, undermined ancestors. While Western colonists saw no conflict between modernity and Christianity, they considered spirit worship to be superstitious, backward and even evil (Endres & Lauser 2011), as did postcolonial, capitalist and Communist modernisers. Mao was concerned that family loyalty undermined loyalty to party and state, so family funerals became simple, with family no more important than workmates; only the funerals of important local or national party members (ultimately Mao himself) were on any scale. More recently, under economic liberalism, some Chinese are reverting to family ancestors but in a more egalitarian way, reflecting personal choice and personal relationships rather than pre-Mao age/gender hierarchies (Goss & Klass 2005). In several Southeast Asian countries today, ancestral and other spirits are being revitalised 'to address the risks and opportunities of economic restructuring and neo-liberal globalisation'; the modernity that is evolving is a 'spirited modernity' (Endres & Lauser 2011:3–4). A Chinese colleague described to me a medium-size business whose headquarters office block has a rooftop ancestral shrine where business decisions are checked out with the ancestors; here, Communists consult the family ancestors to ensure capitalist profits.

Religious immortality

That humans might seek not temporary ancestral status but immortality is found in the ancient Near East in the Epic of Gilgamesh and in Egyptian beliefs and mortuary practices. But it was the emergence of world religions that really challenged ancestor veneration.[4] These religions, especially as they developed over time (Bowker 1991), came to offer immortality – forever (not just for two or three generations while kin survived to perform ancestral rites) and to everyone (including the lower classes, women, children and even slaves). This has proved particularly attractive to many excluded from ancestral status, whether in Africa (Jindra & Noret 2011), Korea (Park 2010) or elsewhere in the world.

As well as offering an immortality that was new and attractive, the monotheistic Abrahamic religions actively attacked ancestor veneration. Ancestors possess agency, the power to affect social life on earth, but in monotheism only the one true God (plus his appointed angels and saints) have legitimate supernatural power. So ancestral spirits and shrines – along with animist nature spirits and shrines – posed a direct threat to monotheism (Douglas 2004). In eighteenth- and nineteenth-century Korea, as in many parts of the world, Catholic and Protestant missionaries were clear that converts could no longer worship their ancestors, so many converts were rejected by their family or even became martyrs (Park 2010). Christianity, like Mao's version of Communism, demands a total loyalty that is potentially undermined by familial love and loyalty (Mount 1982). What binds believers together across the globe is not family ancestors, but 'metaphorical common ancestors' – Abraham, Jesus, the Prophet, the Buddha (Steadman *et al.* 1996:72). The encounter between ancestral societies and Christian or Islamic missionaries has therefore often proved conflictual and sometimes bloody. Immortality in the Christian/Muslim heaven is not compatible, at least in theory, with ancestors.

Despite the resistance of some societies to having their ancestors overthrown by a foreign god, ancestors can be overthrown surprisingly easily if the conditions are right. Warfare, for example, raises the status of young warriors over old men and over the ancestors who legitimate them; when there is a permanent state of war, or endemic raiding and counter-raiding as is common among cattle-herding people, 'ancestor cults can dwindle to mere piety, or disappear' (Douglas 2004:189). Family ancestors may also appear weak in the face of colonialism or subjugation to empire. In India in the early twenty-first century, some young Sora – whose parents, via shaman mediums, dialogued with deceased relatives in order to transform them into ancestors – have become Baptists, a religion they find attractive because of its association with Western modernity. Others have embraced Hinduism, attractive for its association with Indian nationalism. Both Baptist and Hindu Sora, seeking to engage larger national and global forces, have turned their backs on local ancestors and mediums (Vitebsky 2008). World religions and their global deity can seem more powerful than family ancestors to those seeking to participate in an increasingly global world.

Christianity, Islam and Judaism, along with other world religions, therefore came to shift the social focus from family and clan to a wider and more inclusive concept of the chosen people, God's creatures or God's children. All are offered immortality.[5] That said, Islam and Christianity have often excluded unbelievers and condemned them to spiritual or even literal death. That anyone can enter heaven or gain nirvana is radical teaching for peoples who had always been told that only those with status and power could have any meaningful kind of post-mortem survival, yet too often this radical universalism has descended into bloody exclusion of unbelievers not only from heaven, but even from life on earth.

Nevertheless, there are many examples throughout the world of syncretism between immortality and family ancestors, and even incorporation of family ancestors into universalistic religions. It is understandable if people want both the eternal life/reincarnation/nirvana offered by religion, *and* to care for deceased family members and seek their advice and guidance. Many Buddhists build merit that can be transferred to deceased family members they care about. In southern Thailand, both Muslim and Buddhist villagers still believe in ancestor spirits, taking heed of both ancestral power and modern religion (Horstmann 2011). Millions of urban Japanese engage Buddhist priests to perform funeral rites whose main purpose is to turn the deceased into a family ancestor (Smith 1974). Many Shona are Christian, yet also use ancestral stories to trace the kin connections that enable them to survive in Zimbabwe's catastrophic economy (Walter 2015). In Catholicism throughout the world, not least in the Mexican Day of the Dead, saints and even the family dead can pray for the living and in turn be prayed to (Bryant 2003). In Karelia, the dead traditionally became ancestors as well as entering the Russian Orthodox heaven (Keinänen 2014). In the Church of England liturgy of the Eucharist in which believers symbolically ingest Christ through bread and wine, Douglas Davies (1993) argues that many people feel the presence of deceased relatives, finding an affinity between an absent/present Christ and an absent/present loved one. Though Christian theology speaks of the resurrected Christ dwelling within the believer, it discourages believers from contacting the spirits of the family dead; Christ is the only deceased human spirit that believers are supposed to entwine with (Hauenstein 2009). Yet, at the same time, as Davies shows, Christianity provides a liturgy symbolising Christ within the believer that readily evokes in them the family dead.

Many of these examples are found in lived, experienced or 'vernacular' religion, often not entirely approved of by priests, monks and theologians (Ladwig 2011). In South Korea, unusually, Protestant churches developed in the twentieth century a death anniversary rite that unites Christianity and ancestor veneration, though it is only after several generations of being Christian that 'those who could once only utter "my God" … could also profess "the God of my ancestors"' (Park 2010:270). Also formally addressing this issue are the Mormons, with their programme of posthumous conversion of family ancestors.

Christian views of heaven, theological as well as vernacular, have for two millennia oscillated between a heaven where souls perpetually worship God, and a heaven where souls enjoy the perpetual company of other loved family members (McDannell & Lang 2001). Nineteenth- and twentieth-century manifestations of 'family heaven' have pictured the dead residing in an ancestral hall benignly looked after by their Maker. Though Christianity is formally God-centred, its teachers know most humans to be family-centred. Christian teachers thus have had two choices: either to exclude family love from heaven for the sake of a higher love, for God, or – one way or another – to co-opt family love (Mount 1982).

Secular memory

The Catholic Church in the European Middle Ages co-opted it. Indeed, through indulgences – by which families paid priests to pray for the souls of their deceased members – the church exploited it. Attacking this abuse was at the heart of the Protestant Reformation initiated by Luther in the 1530s; in his understanding of Scripture, there is nothing that the living can do for the dead. If they are to enter heaven, it is on account of their pre-mortem faith and by the grace of God; there is nothing their grieving family can do to help.[6] His teaching radically undermined the power of the Catholic Church and offered Protestant believers direct access to God. It reduced funerals to mere acts of disposal, erasing at a stroke the medieval funeral's assistance to souls on their way to heaven (Gittings 1984). And it left a puzzle. If there is nothing we can do to care for our dead, what can we do for them? How are we to relate to them?[7]

Even if many ordinary folk in countries such as England continued after the Reformation to engage with their dead (Duffy 1992), Protestantism itself had no answer. So the answers that came to dominate were secular. We can remember the dead. We can honour them (and before long, upper-class Protestant funerals were not shy about displaying social status). We can appreciate their legacy (Cave 2012). Their genes may live on in our children (Brown 2007); their artistic, cultural or political achievements may continue to influence the living (Kearl & Rinaldi 1983); their labours create the economic infrastructure that determines future generations' standard of living (Walter, forthcoming); but Protestantism allows no exchange with the dead, exiling them as an active presence. They can do nothing for us, and we can do little or nothing for them. Thus it was no secular social movement but Luther's intensely religious reform that secularised the relationship between north-west Europe's living and their dead.

So the most that those many western Europeans and North Americans who are cultural heirs to the Reformation can do for their dead is to remember them with affection, respect or esteem. The churchyard, a place where the rural Christian community lay in anticipation of resurrection, came in time to be replaced by the cemetery, a place for remembering urban individuals. Gravestone inscriptions 'Here lies the body of ...', implying the soul had gone to heaven, gave way to 'In memory of ...' The dead were not disenchanted, but re-enchanted: 'Bodies serving a religion of memory and history would rival those gathered in communities of a transcendent God' (Laqueur 2015:238). Though devout Protestants divided people into the saved and the unsaved, they could still remember those they loved or respected, whether or not they were saved. Memory thus offered a potentially secularising and universalising discourse – erupting in recent decades in the proliferation of talk about memory (Klein 2000), reflected in the secular academy in the thriving field of memory studies.

Remembering the dead, like becoming an ancestor, requires active work by survivors, and to an extent by the pre-deceased (Unruh 1983). Yet the memory of all but a very few is far from eternal. Memory, like status as a personally known ancestor, fades as survivors themselves die. Beyond that, personal memories are transformed, for the lucky few, into remembrance, into genealogy or into history – three ways that modern people engage with those who died before anyone living was born. Even in the short run, though all humans *can* be remembered for a while, not all humans *are* remembered – and erasing memory can involve as much work as creating memory. We are all mortal, but some are more mortal, less grievable (Butler 2004; Doka 2002) than others, suffering social death soon after physical death (Jonsson 2015). Those who are ruthlessly and immediately forgotten usually belong to an out group. The very same Western modernity that now promotes human rights was built on slavery and racism, on creating the 'other' and exploiting their labour. Erasing memory of the other is central to hegemony, a powerful form of oppression, increasingly challenged today by counter-memories that reclaim erased peoples and revive their memory (Assmann 2008; Cannell 2011; Misztal 2004). Memory, it turns out, is as contested as salvation. Who is to be saved? Who is to be remembered? By whom? For how long?

Care versus memory

Above I have sketched three frames for thinking of and engaging with the dead: (1) exchange with the ancestors, (2) immortality as offered by world religions, and (3) secular memory. In all three frames, the dead may be encountered. The living may engage with the ancestral dead, they may interact with the family and saintly dead in religious practices that allow the living and the dead to care for each other, and everyone can encounter the dead in memory. At the same time, it may be helpful to distinguish two kinds of culture.

Across the world, I suggest, there are *care cultures* in which living and dead look after one another in some kind of dynamic exchange, and *memory cultures* in which all the living can do for the dead is remember them. In other words, some cultures offer the physically dead a social role and invite them back into society, while other cultures strive to separate the dead from the living (Malefijt 1968). In the former, the transformed dead can enter into exchange with the living. In the latter they cannot, for, as Epicurus argued, death is the annihilation of life, or as some religions argue, the dead have left earth entirely behind and are now reincarnated or in heaven: either way, there is no possibility of connection with the living. Some religions, and some religious practices, thus sustain a culture of memory, while others embrace a culture of reciprocal care in which the living and the dead can assist each other.

This was illustrated by Mayumi Sekizawa, a Japanese folklorist researching how Europeans and Japanese relate to their war dead. She told me: 'you Europeans remember your war dead. We Japanese care for ours.' British war remembrance (note the term 'remembrance') is saturated with the language of memory: 'We will remember them', 'Lest we forget'. By contrast, the Japanese war dead become *kami*, gods. Carved into the wall facing visitors entering Tokyo's Yūshūkan museum to the war dead is Fujita Toko's (1806–1855) *Ode to the Righteous*, describing how the spirits of the war dead live forever between heaven and earth, guiding the living 'along the path of righteousness'. In Japan, the living perform rites for the war dead; the dead guide the living. What is true of the sacred war dead is true also of the ordinary family dead. In Japan there is ritual exchange of care and guidance. In Protestant Europe, by contrast, the main language for speaking of the dead is that of memory: memorial services, *in memoriam* newspaper columns, memorial benches, memorial cairns. It is hard to talk about the dead without using the language of memory.

Of course, memory often invokes kinship and care, and vice versa: nurturing memories entails kin work (Lambek 2007) and nurturing ancestors entails memory work (Straight 2006). The popular English-language phrase 'in loving memory' leaves its meaning tantalisingly open: are the dead gone, but we can remember them with affection? Or does memory provide the means for love to continue? Despite such fuzziness between care and memory, and despite many humans both caring for and remembering their dead, most live in cultures that validate only one of these narratives. Japanese do remember their dead, and some scholars argue that nowadays Japanese 'ancestral' rites produce not ancestors but memory (Smith 2002; Suzuki 1998) – yet the language remains substantially that of ancestors. Likewise, secularised Protestant Westerners care for their dead, for example by tending the grave (Francis *et al.* 2005), yet may be embarrassed to speak of practices that imply the dead can benefit from such tending. Grieving individuals whose practices or beliefs are not given legitimacy by their culture may keep silent, question their practices, recast them in more culturally acceptable terms or use ambiguous phrases such as 'in loving memory'.

And yet in both care and memory cultures the dead may be encountered. The living may engage with the ancestral dead, they may interact with the family and saintly dead in religious practices that allow the living and the dead to care for each other, and they can encounter the dead in memory.

Continuing bonds: the return of ancestors?

The argument so far presumes that afterlife beliefs provide hope in the face not only of *my* death (what will happen to me when I die?) but also of *thy* death (what will happen to me when you die?). Philippe Ariès (1981) argued that in Western Europe the late Middle Ages were saturated with concern about *my* death – am I bound for heaven or for hell? This took a secular turn in Renaissance humanism – what will happen to me and my earthly works when I die? This fostered a heightened sense of individuality, concern with personal finitude and a desire for immortality, whether religious or secular. Ariès goes on to argue, however, that the Romantic movement of the nineteenth century added to this a concern with *thy* death. Even today, when I ask my (largely white, female British) sociology students what they most fear about death, by no means all admit to fearing their own non-existence but almost all say they fear the death of loved ones. In the English language today, there are many more popular books on living with bereavement than on confronting one's own demise. Of course, psychoanalysis might assert that anxiety about *my* death is so great that it is repressed; while not discounting this possibility, my duty as a scholar is to seek the simplest and most economical account available – which unconscious repression is not (Kellehear 2007). While we cannot say that Romantic *thy* death has entirely replaced Medieval/Renaissance *my* death, we can clearly identify clear historical, sociological and demographic reasons why – at least among many secular contemporary Westerners – *thy* death has become the more pressing concern. After the long and healthy lives many enjoy today, being dead is little to be feared – yet longevity has deepened ties with close family and friends, making their loss the greater anxiety (Lofland 1985).

Nineteenth-century Romanticism taught that the meaning of life is to be found in intimate relationships, which leaves bereavement – losing the beloved – as death's greatest threat, even greater than my own death. Romanticism also taught that love is eternal, so continues after death – the person may have died, but the relationship continues (Day 2012:62). As the inscription on a beautiful 1960 gravestone for an 11-year-old boy in an English country churchyard states: 'Life is short, but love is long'. Where are the dead? How do they survive? In our hearts. Like ancestors, like memories, the Romantic dead survive in the hearts of those who love them (Árnason 2012). This is what late-twentieth-century bereavement theorists identify as 'continuing bonds' (Klass *et al.* 1996; Moss & Moss 1984; Stroebe *et al.* 1992; Unruh 1983).

Though the deceased may live on in my heart, the experience of a continuing relationship can also foster the idea that the deceased continues to live in some other, spiritual realm. Thus, in a Romantic era, bereavement can generate afterlife beliefs and practices. This found expression in nineteenth-century America in sentimental forms of Protestantism (Kete 2000), and on both sides of the Atlantic in Spiritualism whereby mediums could contact the dead (Emmons 2003b). Spiritualism has continued to attract bereaved people through to the present day, especially when the loved one has died violently, which can raise doubts that they are 'okay' in their post-mortem existence – hence Spiritualism's popularity immediately after the First World War.

In the twentieth century, however, by far the most popular afterlife belief in Western societies was the eternal soul (McDannell & Lang 2001; Walter 1996). In this view, humans consist of body and soul; the body is mortal, but the soul – the person's essence – is immortal. Once released from the body, the soul goes to heaven where it joins, and will be joined by, other loved family members. This was the first century in which it became normal for death to occur not in childhood or childbirth but in old age, leaving a widow mourning the loss of a husband of maybe 50 or more years. With the elderly widow's own life expectancy no more than a few years, hope for reunion with her husband in heaven offered considerable comfort – assuming a good enough marriage! Romanticism plus longevity thus lent credence to soul reunion.

In many Western countries, however, the early twenty-first century has witnessed a new imagined spiritual status for the loved dead: he or she is transformed into an angel. Souls are locked up in heaven (Quartier 2011), but angels fly back and forth, guarding and guiding the living, so are particularly attractive to younger mourners with 50 or 60 years left on earth before they themselves can get to heaven to join their grandparent, parent, child or friend (Walter 2016). The angel articulates an active continuing bond in which, crucially, the dead as well as the living exert agency, mainly guiding and guarding – one of the main functions of traditional ancestors. Thus love across the grave continues for a couple of generations – for as long as there are people alive to be cared for by the dead – who then dissolve into little more than a name on the genealogist's family tree.

Angels exist in all the monotheistic religions, but these religions have all taught that angels comprise a different order of being than humans, and that angels never were human. So, although the angel concept is Christian, the idea that the dead become angels is better termed post-Christian, arising from the experience of loss and spread through social media (Walter 2016). This raises an intriguing question. As creedal belief declines, have we therefore come full circle, with the angel image allowing care discourses and ancestral practices to be revalidated in the West – a return to the family ancestors who held sway before the arrival of world religions? Several scholars have noted a dismantling of the life/death boundary in late Western modernity (Howarth 2000), a shift from separating the dead from the living towards more fluid exchanges. Does all this hint at a return of ancestors? The answer is both yes and no.

Yes: Increasing numbers of the twenty-first-century Western dead live not forever as immortal souls, but as angels looking after the living for a couple of generations until they themselves die. The dead are imagined as having agency and the capacity to guide the living – a common experience of those mourning a parent or grandparent (Marwit & Klass 1995). And the living look after the dead, for example by tending the grave or tending their memory. Recent decades in the West have also seen more talk of survivors' experiences of sensing the presence of the deceased, an often not unpleasant experience in which the dead come, unbidden, to the living (Bennett 1987). In this experience, it is the dead, not the living, who seem to exert agency (Hallam *et al.* 1999:156–158; Valentine 2008:130–133) – displaying some similarities to spirit possession where the spirit has increased agency and the medium or shaman has reduced agency (Endres & Lauser 2011:8–12). This kind of empirical evidence does not support anthropologist Panagiotopoulos's view (forthcoming) that in the modern West dialogues with the dead have been replaced by monologues in which 'the living *represent* the dead because the latter are not there to *present* themselves'. In guiding and appearing to the living, today's dead do indeed present themselves.

No: There are, however, some marked differences between traditional and contemporary interactions with family ancestors. First, though both the living and the dead may today appear to exert agency in relation to the other (Valentine 2008). Today this is not governed by norms of reciprocity, by an *expectation* of exchange. As in traditional ancestor veneration, we care for the dead and they guide us, but when they guide us, there is nothing we *need* do in return. And when we care for their grave, there is nothing they *need* do for us in return.

Second, today's Western dead have little or no power to meddle in the lives of the living. Consequently, survivors' relationships with them are entirely positive (Goss & Klass 2005), motivated by loneliness and loss rather than by any practical services that the dead can offer (Emmons 2003b). The troublesome dead are simply ignored, left behind, forgotten, at least by those psychologically able so to do.

Third, relationships with the dead are governed by personal feeling and personally chosen actions rather than prescribed ritual – there is no accepted ritual for managing the interaction (Klass & Walter 2001). Though grief can, for a while, drive us mad, and though the dead can appear without invitation, contemporary Westerners nevertheless like to see themselves as autonomous self-governing individuals who choose their relationships, in mourning as in the rest of life. Today's 'ancestors' with whom survivors interact can be any deceased family member, irrespective of age or gender, or indeed someone outside the family. Though most 'ancestors' today are family members, choosing them is the task of the individual, so authority shifts from family to individual – a trend found even in Japan (Morioka 1986; Smith 2002; Suzuki 1998, 2013).

Perhaps we may conclude that contemporary practices and imaginings do constitute ancestor veneration, but a veneration transformed by the processes of individualism and secularisation as people increasingly devise their afterlife imaginings from personal experience of bereavement rather than from religious teaching.

Terror, finitude and immortality

Followers of Ernest Becker (1973), most notably proponents of Terror Management Theory (TMT) (see Lifshin *et al.*'s chapter in this volume; Cave

2012), argue that a universal but largely repressed fear of personal extinction motivates humans to construct symbolic immortalities, which in turn drives not only religion, but also culture and civilisation. Sociologist Zygmunt Bauman argues on similar lines (see Jacobsen's chapter in this volume). TMT has now been tested in about 500 social psychology experiments in a number of countries.

I think there may be something in this theory, but only if placed in historical context. Certainly, all humans, unlike other animals, are aware of their finitude, but we cannot know whether or how much this has bothered all humans. Arguably, fear of extinction and the desire to live forever are not inherent in the human condition; Allan Kellehear's (2007) survey of death in Stone Age society finds more evidence of acceptance than repression, as indeed does Talcott Parsons and Victor Lidz (1963) in twentieth-century USA. In their view, anticipation of death, not denial, is what drives society and culture. And this chapter has presented evidence of an ancient and widespread view that the dead become not immortal but temporary ancestors. The origins of ancestor veneration are as likely to lie in the social dynamics of family, land, gender and power as in any universal fear of extinction or desire for immortality.

Contrary to TMT, I have argued that fears of extinction and desires for immortality have been generated, or at least massively amplified, by three historic cultural formations. The first came two or three millennia ago with religions' offer of immortality. Here I side with Radcliffe-Brown (1939) that religious rites and beliefs generate anxiety, against Malinowski's (1931) argument that religion relieves the anxieties inherent in being a mortal human. Michael Leming's finding (2003) that in 1970s USA it was the moderately religious who were most frightened of death supports my argument – religion's offer of immortality comforts the true believer, but merely serves to make the moderately religious person anxious.

The second cultural formation concerns time and the individual. When time is imagined as cyclical, as in many hunter-gatherer and agricultural societies (Eliade 1971), and people find identity in the group, the individual may not find their own death so terrifying. When time is imagined as linear, as it has been in the West for at least two millennia, and especially when identity is found in the individual as it increasingly has been for the past five or more centuries, death becomes more problematic for the individual. If my identity lies ultimately within my individual body and mind, rather than in the group that survives my bodily death, then personal finitude becomes more problematic, and immortality more necessary (Ariès 1981; Burckhardt 1860/1960). Third, and finally, when individualistic cultures become secularised, religious hope fades but leaves finitude as a problem.

Immortality is therefore not, or not only, a response to awareness of finitude; rather, awareness, even terror, of finitude is what humans are left with when linear time comes to dominate over cyclical time, when individualism takes over from collectivism and then when secularisation erodes religions' offer of immortality. It is perhaps not surprising that TMT arose at the end of the twentieth century in the USA – a society devoted to individual achievement within linear time, convinced of human progress, and among modern nations almost uniquely very religious yet undergoing considerable secularisation. These are ideal conditions for generating personal anxiety about finitude and consequent attempts at symbolic immortality.

In some more secular European countries, however, religions' offer of immortality has receded so far from most people's awareness that it fails to inculcate the death anxiety experienced by moderately religious Americans. In affluent countries that, unlike the United States, have well-developed welfare states and/or low levels of economic inequality, many citizens' lives become not only long, but also healthy, materially secure and suffused with general well-being (Wilkinson & Pickett 2009). In such conditions, this life may prove sufficient for personal contentment (Inglehart *et al.* 2008). Thus Danes and Swedes display rather little fear of death and are content to find meaning in more proximate things: family, a bike ride through the forest, the company of friends (Zuckerman 2008). Japan, 'with its lack of monotheism and comparatively widespread acceptance of death with nothing beyond, except for the groups one has been committed to that live on beyond oneself', likewise suggests widespread death anxiety to be not universal but the result of very specific socio-historic formations (Mathews 2013:46). Even many Americans, but noticeably more in affluent California than economically insecure Detroit, have embraced Abraham Maslow's ideal of self-actualisation – in this life. More recently British philosopher Stephen Cave (2012) has promoted the ancient Epicurean wisdom that death cannot be experienced and therefore is not to be feared; rather, awareness of mortality can motivate individuals towards the virtues of living gratefully in the moment and caring for others.

Sociological theorists Berger and Luckmann (1966:120–121) wrote that culture, or what they term a society's symbolic universe, 'links men with their predecessors and their successors in a meaningful totality, serving to transcend the finitude of individual existence and bestowing meaning upon the individual's death'. Symbolic universes and symbolic immortalities can be constructed not only by the not-yet-dead but also by those who survive them, and the balance between the two depends on the society concerned. As *thy* death becomes a more pressing concern than *my* death, how the dead survive depends less on their own pre-mortem fears, beliefs and actions than on those of their survivors. Immortality is constructed from bereavement and other concerns of survivors as much as from pre-mortem fear of personal extinction – which may possibly turn out to have been a two- or three-millennia historical oddity that did indeed shape Western civilisation, but not all cultures and quite possibly not future cultures.

Conclusion

This chapter has suggested that finitude and the search for immortality may not be as primal as some scholars suppose; more primal, perhaps, has been

Table 1.1 Typology of ancestor, immortality and memory

Form of survival	Funerals create	Community of the living
Ancestor	Ancestors	Family
Immortality	Immortality	Religion
Memory	Memories	Individual/various groups

the ritual construction of ancestors. Ancestors, however, have been challenged over the past two to three millennia by world religions' offer of immortality. This in turn has been transformed, paradoxically by Protestantism and definitively by secularism, into the dead surviving only in memory. Yet today, a mutation of ancestor veneration is arguably re-emerging from the soil of Romanticism and post-Protestant secularism. In sketching these trends, I have noted a shift in focus from family to religion to more diverse groups, a tension between monotheism and ancestors, bereavement as a generator of afterlife beliefs, and the possibility that the desire to live forever did not cause but is caused by religions' offer of immortality.

There has been no space to pay proper attention to the immense variety of meanings of traditional ancestors (Barraud *et al.* 1994) that may represent groups much larger than the family (Parker Pearson 2013), not least in Africa (Jindra & Noret 2011; Vansina 1985). I have considered immortal souls but not resurrected bodies, only touched on world religions other than Christianity, and not considered reincarnation. And my account of the contemporary world focuses on the West.

Nevertheless, it may be illuminating to summarise my argument in the following global typology. The typology is a sociological 'ideal type' – a simplified schema, whose components are never found in pure form in the real world yet draw attention to and illuminate conflict, change and messiness in the real world. Each type – ancestor, immortality, memory – if found in its purity would be unstable: family ancestors are vulnerable to large-scale social forces, religious immortality is vulnerable to family love, and secular memory ends up producing ancestors. The typology outlined in Table 1.1 depicts how each form of survival depends on different prerequisites, and aligns with particular kinds of funeral and particular constructions of the social universe inhabited by the living.

The second column indicates that the explicit function of funeral and subsequent rituals depends on how the dead are believed to exist. Thus funerals can create ancestors, they can assist the deceased on the path to immortality or – as in the contemporary Western life-centred celebratory funeral – they can solidify memory for the benefit of survivors.

The third column indicates that how the dead survive correlates with particular constructions of the social world of the living. Thus in ancestral cultures, the family is central. Immortality, by contrast, is rooted in a wider religious understanding of the community of God's children, God's creatures or the people of God – though, as we have seen, heaven for many is populated by close kin. Memories, by contrast, are constructed by the individual, in shared conversation in families and in the practices of all manner of groups; in that memory becomes the dominant way to engage with the dead in a secular society, humankind rather than family or religious community constitutes the potential population of significant dead. Humankind, of course, cannot remember; only individuals and groups can. Yet, survival is not guaranteed to all: only those of some status become ancestors, religions exclude unbelievers, and not everyone can be sure of being remembered. What forms of survival may find an affinity with new notions of being human, such as the cyborg (Haraway 1991), remains to be seen.

This analysis and typology implies that 'continuing bonds' with the dead, conceptualised in North America in the 1990s (Klass *et al.* 1996), can be detected in numerous cultures across millennia. It is highly variable, however, how such bonds have been culturally framed – for example, as filial respect, as a dangerous liaison with spirits, or in terms of romantic love – which presumably could influence how people experience such bonds with the dead, who encourages or discourages them, and why (Klass & Steffen 2017).

Throughout the chapter, I have suggested that analysis of how humans imagine their dead survive needs to consider not only the not-yet-dead's anxiety about their own finitude but also the concerns and activities of mourners. Probably only humans know they will die,[8] but several other species – not only elephants – have been observed to mourn the deaths of kin, so *thy* death, concern at the death of the other, is surely very deeply wired into human brains (Archer 1999). For hunter-gatherers, who over tens of millennia shaped human evolution more than have more recent and shorter-lived cultures, death came suddenly, so the journey to the next life had to be stage-managed by mourners, not by the pre-deceased; only with settled farming and the rise of infections did humans have much warning of impending death and thus the possibility of spiritual preparation (Kellehear 2007). Consider also children. Though, as TMT notes, children come in due course to realise their own mortality, experiencing loss of the other comes far earlier: the little infant's greatest terror is experiencing its mother's (it does not realise, temporary) absence. Psychoanalysts may consider that the infant experiences this as death of self, but the unadorned fact is that sheer terror at the other's absence precedes any conscious anticipation of one's own extinction. For these reasons, as well as the historical, sociological and anthropological evidence adduced in this chapter, it seems promising to consider the role of *thy* death as well as *my* death in generating notions of post-mortem survival, both universally and specifically in contemporary societies.[9]

Notes

1 In memory of two sociological ancestors, Michael C. Kearl and Chang-Won Park, whose ideas survive through the ritual interaction between living and dead scholars that publications like this comprise – I hope I have treated them with the care

they deserve. Among the living, I acknowledge Ashley Rudolf and Nikki Salkeld for inviting me to Falmouth University to test part of the argument; and Marion Bowman, Sam Carr, Stephen Cave, Karina Croucher, Dennis Klass and Dorothea Lüddeckens for their helpful comments.

2 See note 4 for justification of this term.
3 Elsewhere (Walter 2015), I suggest some connections between different forms of survival and different communication technologies.
4 The term 'world religions' is currently in disfavour within religious studies, as its focus on formal theology and institutional religion detracts attention from everyday lived experiences of religion. In this chapter, however, I argue that it was precisely the formal, priestly, doctrinal aspects of institutional religion that challenged ancestor veneration, and the global power of institutional religions' deity revealed the more limited powers of family ancestors. In this chapter, 'world religion' is therefore the appropriate term.
5 In Judaism, what is immortal is not the individual, but God's collective covenant with His people.
6 Mormon posthumous conversion is the only exception to this in 'Protestant' theology.
7 The shift here to 'we' is intentional, for Western funerals and mourning, even – perhaps especially – in their secular form, are profoundly influenced by Protestantism.
8 Kellehear (2007) questions this.
9 TMT experiments typically increase 'mortality salience' – awareness of their own mortality – in subjects and then correlate this with various attitudinal changes. It could be productive to develop a measure of 'bereavement salience' – awareness of loved ones' mortality – and measure its effects.

References

Archer, John (1999): *The Nature of Grief: The Evolution and Psychology of Reactions to Loss*. London: Routledge.
Ariès, Philippe (1981): *The Hour of Our Death*. London: Allen Lane.
Árnason, Arnar (2012): 'Individuals and Relationships: On the Possibilities and Impossibilities of Presence', in Douglas J. Davies & Chang-Won Park (eds): *Emotion, Identity and Death*. Aldershot: Ashgate Publishing.
Assmann, Aleida (2008): 'Canon and Archive', in Astrid Erll & Ansgar Nünning (eds): *Cultural Memory Studies*. Berlin: de Gruyter, pp. 97–107.
Barraud, Cécile, Daniel de Coppet, André Iteanu & Raymond Jamous (1994): *Of Relations and the Dead: Four Societies Viewed from the Angle of Their Exchanges*. London: Bloomsbury.
Baudrillard, Jean (1993): *Symbolic Exchange and Death*. London: Sage Publications.
Becker, Ernest (1973): *The Denial of Death*. New York: Free Press.
Bennett, Gillian (1987): *Traditions of Belief: Women, Folklore and the Supernatural Today*. London: Penguin Books.
Berger, Peter L. & Thomas Luckmann (1966): *The Social Construction of Reality*. London: Allen Lane.
Bowker, John (1991): *The Meanings of Death*. Cambridge: Cambridge University Press.
Brown, Guy (2007): *The Living End: The Future of Death, Aging and Immortality*. London: Macmillan.
Bryant, Clifton D. (2003): 'Hosts and Ghosts: The Dead as Visitors in Cross-Cultural Perspective', in Clifton D. Bryant (ed.): *Handbook of Death and Dying, Volume 1*. Thousand Oaks, CA: Sage Publications.

Burckhardt, Jacob (1860/1960): *The Civilization of the Renaissance*. New York: Mentor.

Butler, Judith (2004): *Precarious Life: The Powers of Mourning and Violence*. London: Verso.

Calhoun, C. J. (1980): 'The Authority of Ancestors'. *Man*, 15 (2):304–319.

Cannell, Fenella (2011): 'English Ancestors: The Moral Possibilities of Popular Genealogy'. *Journal of the Royal Anthropological Institute*, 17 (3):462–480.

Cave, Stephen (2012): *Immortality: The Quest to Live Forever and How It Drives Civilisation*. London: Biteback.

Chidester, David (2002): *Patterns of Transcendence: Religion, Death and Dying*. Belmont, CA: Wadsworth.

Davies, Douglas J. (1993): 'The Dead at the Eucharist'. *Modern Churchman*, 34 (3):26–32.

Day, Abby (2012): 'Extraordinary Relationality: Ancestor Veneration in Late Euro-American Society'. *Nordic Journal of Religion and Society*, 25 (2):169–181.

Doka, Kenneth J. (ed.) (2002): *Disenfranchised Grief*. Champaign, IL: Research Press.

Douglas, Mary (2004): *Jacob's Tears*. Oxford: Oxford University Press.

Duffy, Eamon (1992): *The Stripping of the Altars: Traditional Religion in England, 1400–1580*. New Haven, CT: Yale University Press.

Eliade, Mircea (1971): *The Myth of the Eternal Return*. Princeton, NJ: Princeton University Press.

Emmons, Charles F. (2003a): 'Ghosts: The Dead Among Us', in Clifton D. Bryant (ed.): *Handbook of Death and Dying, Volume 1*. Thousand Oaks, CA: Sage Publications.

Emmons, Charles F. (2003b): 'The Spiritualist Movement: Bringing the Dead Back', in Clifton D. Bryant (ed.): *Handbook of Death and Dying, Volume 1*. Thousand Oaks, CA: Sage Publications.

Endres, Kirsten W. & Andrea Lauser (eds) (2011): *Engaging the Spirit World: Popular Beliefs and Practices in Modern Southeast Asia*. Oxford: Berghahn.

Espírito Santo, Diana & Ruy Blanes (eds) (2013): *The Social life of Spirits*. Chicago: University of Chicago Press.

Fortes, Meyer (1965): 'Some Reflections on Ancestor Worship in Africa', in Meyer Fortes & Germaine Dieterlen (eds): *African Systems of Thought*. Oxford: Oxford University Press.

Francis, Doris, Leonie Kellaher & Georgina Neophytou (2005): *The Secret Cemetery*. Oxford: Berg.

Gittings, Clare (1984): *Death, Burial and the Individual in Early Modern England*. London: Croom Helm.

Goss, Robert E. & Dennis Klass (2005): *Dead but Not Lost: Grief Narratives in Religious Traditions*. Walnut Creek, CA: AltaMira.

Hallam, Elizabeth, Jenny Hockey & Glennys Howarth (1999): *Beyond the Body*. London: Routledge.

Hamilton, Malcolm (1998): *Sociology and the World's Religions*. Basingstoke: Macmillan.

Haraway, Donna (1991): 'A Cyborg Manifesto', in Donna Haraway (ed.): *Simians, Cyborgs and Women*. New York: Routledge.

Hauenstein, Hans (2009): *Lost Souls? Presence and Identity of the Dead in Sociological and Theological Perspectives*. Unpublished master's thesis, University of Bath.

Horstmann, Alexander (2011): 'Reconfiguring *Manora Rongkru*: Ancestor Worship and Spirit Possession in Southern Thailand', in Kirsten Endres & Andrea Lauser (eds): *Engaging the Spirit World*. Oxford: Berghahn.

Howarth, Glennys (2000): 'Dismantling the Boundaries between Life and Death'. *Mortality*, 5 (2):127–138.

Inglehart, Ronald, Roberto Foa, Christopher Peterson & Christian Welzel (2008): 'Development, Freedom, and Rising Happiness: A Global Perspective (1981–2007)'. *Perspectives on Psychological Science*, 3 (4):264–285.

Jacobi, Keith P. (2003): 'The Malevolent "Undead": Cross-Cultural Perspectives', in Clifton D. Bryant (ed.): *Handbook of Death and Dying, Volume 1*. Thousand Oaks, CA: Sage Publications.

Jindra, Michael & Joël Noret (eds) (2011): *Funerals in Africa*. Oxford: Berghahn.

Jonsson, Annika (2015): 'Post-Mortem Social Death'. *Contemporary Social Science*, 10 (3):284–295.

Kearl, Michael C. & Anoel Rinaldi (1983): 'The Political Uses of the Dead as Symbols in Contemporary Civil Religions'. *Social Forces*, 61:693–708.

Keinänen, Marja-Liisa (2014): 'Feeding the Dead: Women "Doing" Religion and Kinship in Traditional Russian Orthodox Karelia', in Terhi Utriainen & Päivi Salmesvuori (eds): *Finnish Women Making Religion: Between Ancestors and Angels*. Basingstoke: Palgrave/Macmillan.

Kellehear, Allan (2007): *A Social History of Dying*. Cambridge: Cambridge University Press.

Kete, Mary L. (2000): *Sentimental Collaborations: Mourning and Middle-Class Identity in Nineteenth-Century America*. Durham, NC: Duke University Press.

Klass, Dennis & Tony Walter (2001): 'Processes of Grieving: How Bonds Are Continued', in Margaret S. Stroebe, Robert O. Hansson, Wolfgang Stroebe & Henk Schut (eds): *Handbook of Bereavement Research: Consequences, Coping and Care*. Washington, DC: American Psychological Association.

Klass, Dennis & Edith Steffen (eds) (2017): *Continuing Bonds in Bereavement: New Directions for Research and Practice.* New York: Routledge.

Klass, Dennis, Phyllis R. Silverman & Steven L. Nickman (eds) (1996): *Continuing Bonds*. Bristol, PA: Taylor & Francis.

Klein, Kerwin L. (2000): 'On the Emergence of Memory in Historical Discourse'. *Representations*, 69:127–150.

Kopytoff, Igor (1971): 'Ancestors as Elders in Africa'. *Africa*, 41 (2):129–142.

Ladwig, Patrice (2011): 'Can Things Reach the Dead?', in Kirsten Endres & Andrea Lauser (eds): *Engaging the Spirit*. Oxford: Berghahn.

Lambek, Michael (2007): 'The Cares of Alice Alder: Recuperating Kinship and History in Switzerland', in Janet Carsten (ed.): *Ghosts of Memory: Essays on Remembrance and Relatedness*. Oxford: Blackwell.

Laqueur, Thomas W. (2015): *The Work of the Dead: A Cultural History of Mortal Remains*. Princeton, NJ: Princeton University Press.

Lehmann, Arthur C. & James E. Myers (1985): 'Ghosts, Souls, Ancestors', in Arthur Lehmann & James Myers (eds): *Magic, Witchcraft and Religion*. Palo Alto, CA: Mayfield.

Leming, Michael (2003): 'Religion and the Mediation of Death Fear', in Clifton D. Bryant (ed.): *Handbook of Death and Dying, Volume 1*. Thousand Oaks, CA: Sage Publications.

Lofland, Lynn (1985): 'The Social Shaping of Emotion: The Case of Grief'. *Symbolic Interaction*, 8 (2):171–190.

McDannell, Colleen & Bernhard Lang (2001): *Heaven: A History*. New Haven, CT: Yale University Press.

Malefijt, Annemarie de Waal (1968): *Religion and Culture*. New York: Macmillan.

Malinowski, Bronislaw (1931): 'Culture', in *Encyclopaedia of the Social Sciences, Volume IV*. New York: Macmillan.

Marwit, Samuel J. & Dennis Klass (1995): 'Grief and the Role of the Inner Representation of the Deceased'. *Omega,* 30:283–298.

Mathews, Gordon (2013): 'Death and "The Pursuit of a Life Worth Living" in Japan', in Hikaru Suzuki (ed.): *Death and Dying in Contemporary Japan*. London: Routledge.

Mbiti, John S. (1970): *African Religions and Philosophies*. Garden City, NY: Doubleday.

Meillassoux, Claude (1972): 'From Reproduction to Production: A Marxist Approach to Economic Anthropology'. *Economy and Society*, 1 (1):93–105.

Mills, Antonia (2001): 'Sacred Land and Coming Back: How Gitxsan and Witsuwit'en Reincarnation Stretches Western Boundaries'. *Canadian Journal of Native Studies*, 21:309–331.

Misztal, Barbara A. (2004): 'The Sacralization of Memory'. *European Journal of Cultural Studies*, 7 (1):67–84.

Morioka, Kiyomi (1986): 'Ancestor Worship in Contemporary Japan: Continuity and Change', in George A. DeVos & Takao Sofue (eds): *Religion and the Family in S.E. Asia*. Berkeley, CA: University of California Press.

Moss, Miriam S. & Sidney Z. Moss (1984): 'Some Aspects of the Elderly Widow(er)'s Persistent Tie with the Deceased Spouse'. *Omega*, 15 (3):196–206.

Mount, Ferdinand (1982): *The Subversive Family*. London: Cape.

Ochoa, Todd Ramón (2010): *Society of the Dead: Quita Manaquita and Palo Praise in Cuba*. Berkeley, CA: University of California Press.

Panagiotopoulos, Anastasios (forthcoming): 'Introduction', in Anastasios Panagiotopoulos & Diana Espírito Santo (eds): *Articulate Necrographies: Comparative Perspectives on the Voices and Silences of the Dead*. Bloomington: Indiana University Press.

Panagiotopoulos, Anastasios & Diana Espírito Santo (eds) (forthcoming): *Articulate Necrographies: Comparative Perspectives on the Voices and Silences of the Dead*. Bloomington: Indiana University Press.

Park, Chang-Won (2009): 'Confucian Beliefs and Traditions', in Clifton D. Bryant & Dennis L. Peck (eds): *Encyclopedia of Death and the Human Experience, Volume I*. London: Sage Publications.

Park, Chang-Won (2010): 'Between God and Ancestors: Ancestral Practice in Korean Protestantism'. *International Journal for the Study of the Christian Church*, 10 (4):257–273.

Parker Pearson, Mike (1999): *The Archaeology of Death and Burial*. Stroud: Sutton Publishing.

Parker Pearson, Mike (2013): 'Researching Stonehenge: Theories Past and Present'. *Archaeology International*, 16:72–83.

Parsons, Talcott & Victor M. Lidz (1963): 'Death in American Society', in Edwin Shneidman (ed.): *Essays in Self-Destruction*. New York: Science House.

Quartier, Thomas (2011): 'A Place for the Dead: "Angels" and "Heaven" in Personalised Eschatology', in Marius Rotar & Adriana Teodorescu (eds): *Dying and Death in 18th–21st Century Europe.* Newcastle-upon-Tyne: Cambridge Scholars.

Radcliffe-Brown, Alfred R. (1939): *Taboo*. Cambridge: Cambridge University Press.

Scott, Janet L. (2007): *For Gods, Ghosts and Ancestors: The Chinese Tradition of Paper Offering*. Seattle: University of Washington Press.

Smart, Ninian (1996): *The Religious Experience*. Upper Saddle River, NJ: Prentice Hall.

Smith, Robert J. (1974): *Ancestor Worship in Contemporary Japan*. Stanford, CA: Stanford University Press.

Smith, Robert J. (2002): 'The Living and the Dead in Japanese Popular Religion', in Susan Orpett Long (ed.): *Lives in Motion*. Ithaca, NY: Cornell East Asia Series.

Steadman, Lyle B., Craig T. Palmer & Christopher F. Tilley (1996): 'The Universality of Ancestor Worship'. *Ethnology*, 35 (1):63–76.

Straight, Belinda (2006): 'Becoming Dead: The Entangled Agencies of the Dearly Departed'. *Anthropology & Humanism*, 31 (2):101–110.

Stroebe, Margaret S., Kenneth J. Gergen & Wolfgang Stroebe (1992): 'Broken Hearts or Broken Bonds: Love and Death in Historical Perspective'. *American Psychologist*, 47:1205–1212.

Suzuki, Hikaru (1998): 'Japanese Death Rituals in Transit: From Household Ancestors to Beloved Antecendents'. *Journal of Contemporary Religion*, 13 (2):171–188.

Suzuki, Hikaru (ed.) (2013): *Death and Dying in Contemporary Japan*. London: Routledge.

Unruh, David (1983): 'Death and Personal History: Strategies of Identity Preservation'. *Social Problems*, 30 (3):340–351.

Valentine, Christine (2008): *Bereavement Narratives: Continuing Bonds in the Twenty-First Century*. London: Routledge.

Vansina, Jan (1985): *Oral Tradition as History*. Madison: University of Wisconsin Press.

Vitebsky, Piers (1992): *Dialogues with the Dead: The Discussion of Mortality Among the Sora of Eastern India*. New Delhi: Cambridge University Press.

Vitebsky, Piers (2008): 'Loving and Forgetting: Moments of Inarticulacy in Tribal India'. *Journal of the Royal Anthropological Institute (New Series)*, 14:243–261.

Walter, Tony (1996): *The Eclipse of Eternity: A Sociology of the Afterlife*. Basingstoke: Macmillan.

Walter, Tony (2015): 'Communication Media and the Dead: From the Stone Age to Facebook'. *Mortality*, 20 (3):215–232.

Walter, Tony (2016): 'The Angelic Dead: Bereavement and Vernacular Religion in the 21st Century'. *Omega*, 73 (1):3–28.

Walter, Tony (forthcoming): 'Has Western Modernity Removed the Dead from the World of the Living?', in Anastasios Panagiotopoulos & Diana Espírito Santo (eds): *Articulate Necrographies: Comparative Perspectives on the Voices and Silences of the Dead*. Bloomington: Indiana University Press.

Watson, James L. & Evelyn S. Rawski (eds) (1988): *Death Ritual in Late Imperial and Modern China*. Berkeley, CA: University of California Press.

Watson, Rubie S. (1988): 'Remembering the Dead: Graves and Politics in Southeastern China', in James L. Watson and Evelyn S. Rawski (eds): *Death Ritual in Late Imperial and Modern China*. Berkeley, CA: University of California Press.

Whitley, James (2002): 'Too Many Ancestors?'. *Antiquity*, 76 (291):119–126.

Wilkinson, Richard & Kate Pickett (2009): *The Spirit Level: Why Equality Is Better for Everyone*. London: Allen Lane.

Zuckerman, Phil (2008): *Society without God: What the Least Religious Nations Can Tell Us about Contentment*. New York: New York University Press.

2 The future of death and the four pathways to immortality

Guy Brown

Introduction

Throughout history, people have sought survival or immortality in four main ways. First, by staying alive as long as possible – this is the realm of magic and medicine. Second, by surviving death in some attenuated spirit form – this is the realm of spiritualism and religion. Third, by surviving through our children and children's children – this is the realm of genetics and family. Fourth, by our works and deeds, embedded in memory and society – this is the realm of memetics and culture. These four drives, for survival of the body, mind, genes and memes respectively, have been and continue to be central motivators of all we do in life. I have suggested (Brown 2007), and Stephen Cave (2013) has given a much more compelling and comprehensive argument, that the history of civilization has been shaped and continues to be moulded by these four central drives for survival. I am not going to retell that story here, but rather assess where we have got to and where we are heading in humanity's quest for immortality. I am a professor at the University of Cambridge, doing research on the diseases of ageing, and so I am interested in what science can tell us about immortality.

Over the last 200 years, average lifespan has more than doubled, but the rate of ageing has not changed, so that we currently experience much more ageing, age-related disease, disability and dementia before we die. This degenerative end to life is resulting in a fragmentation of the self and death itself. I argue here that: ageing is not natural, was not selected by natural selection and will not be removed by medicine – ageing is our future. Therefore, survival by pathway 1 above, i.e. bodily survival, will inevitably lead to the Tithonus scenario of endless ageing. Path I can be updated by preventing this ageing. Pathway 2, survival of the mind, can be updated by reproducing the objective aspects of mind in a robot/computer. Pathway 3, survival of the genes, can be enhanced by biological cloning. And pathway 4, survival of the memes, is being accelerated and transformed by electronic cloning of memes. But will these methods result in survival? It depends on whether we regard partial survival of parts of the self as survival at all. And this depends on whether we regard the self as a unitary soul or as the sum of its changing components. And this in turn depends on what we identify with: for example, whether we think of our ideas, or our children, or our future selves as part of ourselves now.

> The great wild bull is lying down, never to rise again,
> the lord Gilgamesh is lying down, never to rise again,
> he is lying on his death bed, never to rise again,
> he is lying on a bed of woe, never to rise again.
> He is not capable of standing, he is not capable of sitting, he can
>   only groan,
> he is not capable of eating, he is not capable of drinking, he can
>   only groan,
> the lock of Namtar holds him fast, he is not capable of rising.
> Namtar who has no hands, who has no feet, who snatches a man
>   by night,
> Namtar, who gores, has hold of the lord Gilgamesh.
>
> (George 2000)

Namtar is Death, and this is one of the oldest known accounts of an individual's death. It is a fragment of the Epic of Gilgamesh, of which the core was probably composed at the Sumerian court of King Shulgi in the twenty-first century BC, and was elaborated over a thousand years of storytelling into the greatest epic of the pre-classical era (George 2000). It tells of a semi-mythical hero, Gilgamesh, King of Uruk (in modern Iraq), some time between 2800 and 2500 BC. Gilgamesh is a lover of life, but the death of a friend sends him off on a quest for immortality, which ultimately leads to his own death. But on the way he learns about the four traditional routes to immortality.

We are going to follow Gilgamesh in trying to understand how practical the four aforementioned routes to immortality are. However, we are also going to take some detours on the way, including: why death exists, and why our survival is so important to us, but why the truth about survival is not essential to what we believe. And I am going to point out some of the misconceptions that continue to lead us down blind alleys in our quest. So that hopefully in the end we are looking for types of immortality that are both achievable and worth having.

Pathway to immortality 1: survival of the body

The most direct route to immortality is to not die. But, despite a multitude of people trying in myriad ways, no one in the history of the world has yet succeeded. However, thinking about the problem this way is an example of digital thinking – i.e. conceiving of something in terms of just two states, in this case: mortal or immortal – rather than analogue thinking – i.e. conceiving of something in terms of a continuum, in this case: degrees of mortality/ immortality or just how long we live. Most people are trying to live longer, not to live forever. And if we look at it this way, there is no doubt that mortality is in retreat. Average lifespan in the world has increased between two- and threefold in the last 200 years (Riley 2001). Life expectancy at birth continues to increase at the astonishing rate of about 2.5 years per decade (six hours per day), and there is absolutely no sign of this rate increasing or decreasing (Oeppen & Vaupel 2002). Average life expectancy in the United Kingdom today is about 80 years, which is roughly the average age at which people are dying. But if life expectancy continues to increase at the current rate, someone born today would be expected to live 100 years on average, because by the time they reached 80 years of age, life expectancy would have increased by almost 20 years.

Lifespan has increased largely because society as a whole has focused on removing or reducing causes of death (Riley 2001). The main causes of death used to be extrinsic: starvation, violence and infection. But extrinsic causes of death have been picked off one-by-one by social, political and economic change, sanitation, education, science, medicine and technology. Thus, nowadays the main causes of death are intrinsic to the body and driven by ageing: cancer, stroke and heart diseases account for about 50 per cent of all deaths. However, these intrinsic causes are also being reduced rapidly: for example, death rates due to stroke and heart attack at any particular age have fallen dramatically over the last 30 years. Why? Because if something becomes a major cause of death, it also becomes a major medical, scientific and political target. Why? Because to survive is the most basic biological goal of humans. Evolution by natural selection selects those individuals that survive and/or reproduce more than others, so survival and reproduction are the fundamental design principles of all organisms on earth including humans. Thus, we want to survive.

There is no doubt that we are living longer and are likely to continue to live longer. That's the good news. The bad news is that the rate of ageing does not appear to have changed over the last 200 years, and possibly the last 2,000 years (Kirkwood & Austad 2000). The rate of ageing is how much we age over some period, for example a decade or the first 50 years of life. However, ageing appears to increase exponentially with years of age, i.e. the rate of ageing speeds up as we get older. So, because we are living two or three times as long as we did two centuries ago, but the rate of ageing has not changed, the unhappy consequence is that we are living long enough to age much more before we die. Hence we are an ageing society (Brown 2015).

Increasing lifespan without decreasing the rate of ageing results in the Tithonus scenario. Tithonus was a hero of Greek myth, who was granted immortality by Zeus at the request of Tithonus's lover Eos, goddess of the dawn. However, Eos had forgotten to also request eternal youth, so that Tithonus aged to an extreme extent and shrivelled up into a cicada, living forever, but begging for death. Unfortunately that is where we are all headed, perhaps not as cicadas, but extreme ageing is inevitable if we continue to increase lifespan without altering the rate of ageing. The consequences are all around us: pensions crisis, care crisis, health system crisis, epidemics of Alzheimer's and other diseases of ageing.

Age-related spending by EU governments was €3.1 trillion in 2010, equivalent to 25% of GDP (including 11% on pensions, 7% on health care and 2% on long-term care of the old). And this expenditure is projected to rise to 30% of GDP in 2060, but is thought by the EU to be economically unsustainable (European Commission 2012). The direct and indirect costs of dementia alone were €130 billion in 2009 in the EU (European Commission 2012). The 2010 health care costs of the EU population older than 65 years were €900 billion. We simply cannot continue to reduce death rates without reducing the rate of ageing, because the economy cannot sustain this (Brown 2015).

The prevalence of dementia and many other diseases of ageing increases exponentially with age, thus a linear increase in average lifespan of 2.5 years per decade is causing a rapid increase in dementia, disability and disease at the end of life (Brayne 2007). Currently about a quarter of people get dementia before they die, but this may increase to half by the end of the century, i.e. when our children will be dying. Even in the absence of dementia, disability and disease, extreme ageing results in an irreversible decline in life functions, including loss of sight, hearing, taste, reproduction, mobility, memory and cognition. We are currently faced with a degenerative end to life, with death preceded by up to a decade of increasing ill health and extreme ageing (Xie *et al.* 2008). How did we get into this mess? For the last century we have focused on surviving, removing causes of death, without reducing ageing or the diseases of ageing proportionately. The lesson we need to learn from the Tithonus scenario is that immortality has economic, social and personal costs, and it may not be worth those costs, unless we remove ageing.

Death in the past used to be more or less digital, i.e. we switched rapidly at death from being fully alive to fully dead. That is because people used to die young or in their prime, and they died relatively rapidly from infection, violence or starvation. Life in the past has been described as nasty, brutish and short, but this is also a good description of death in the past. However, death is no longer an event terminating a short life; it has become a process over years at the end of a long life. Death has become an analogue process, like a dimmer switch mediating a 'fading of the light', rather than an on–off switch (Brown 2007). Death has broken up into multiple processes occurring at different rates: death of reproductive life, death of sexual life, death of work life, death of social life, death of ambition, loss of different senses and part of the body and mind. Life itself is no longer digital – it is no longer fully off or on – when we are suffering from extreme ageing and/or dementia, we are no longer fully alive. We used to think that life started digitally – switched from fully off to fully on – at the point of conception or birth, but we now accept that we gradually grow into life, i.e. that life is an analogue process. In the future, we will have to accept that we also grow out of life gradually over a period of years, and we eventually reach the terminal event after a degenerative end to life.

The death of Gilgamesh described in the quote above was a typical death of the past, probably from an infection, causing a fever lasting six days. He died in his prime from a death that was nasty, brutish and short. But at least he was spared the indignities of a modern death: waiting endlessly for the terminal event in the ruins of the former body and mind, slowly crushed by extreme ageing and ushered away by morphine.

Gilgamesh begins the Assyrian version of the epic as the young, virile, warmongering King of Uruk, lording it over his people:

> Gilgamesh sounds the alarm bell for his own amusement, his arrogance has no bounds by day or night. No son is left with his father, for Gilgamesh takes them all, even the children; yet the king should be shepherd to his people. His lust leaves no virgin to her lover, neither the warrior's daughter nor the wife of the noble; yet this is the shepherd of the city, wise, comely, and resolute.
>
> (George 2000)

The gods give Gilgamesh a passionate 'wild-man' friend to distract him from wreaking havoc on the city. But the untimely death of this friend, Enkidu, leaves Gilgamesh in a mid-life crisis. Gilgamesh abandons everything, and sets out alone for the ends of the earth in a doomed quest for immortality. He follows the nightly path of the sun under the earth to the gardens of Paradise, and from thence he is ferried across the waters of death to the end of the world. There, at the end of his quest, he meets Utnapishtim, the one-and-only mortal to whom the gods have granted immortality. Utnapishtim reveals the secret of a plant that restores lost youth. Gilgamesh is triumphant, and at last heads home, but on the way he loses the secret of everlasting youth down a well. Oops! Gilgamesh is distraught and has to face his fate, to return home empty-handed and await his death.

The modern version of staying alive by magic is staying alive by medicine. But as we have seen, there is no point staying alive unless ageing is reduced. So how can we prevent ageing?

Unfortunately, ageing is not like another disease that we might hope to cure; rather it is *all* age-related diseases, including cancer, cardiovascular diseases and neurodegenerative diseases, plus *all* age-related dysfunction, including loss of sight, mobility and memory, plus *everything else* that might go wrong with the body and mind with age if life were further extended (Kirkwood & Austad 2000). And ageing is not one thing or process, but dozens, possibly hundreds, of different things. Ageing is all the possible ways that our body and brains can go wrong with age, driven by the almost infinite number of ways that the millions of components in our bodies can interact when not selected by evolution. Thus, ageing is not digital (all-or-nothing), so it cannot be turned off or on. Ageing is not going to be removed by some magic bullet.

However, that does not mean that ageing is intractable, it just means that each component of ageing will have to be knocked off one at a time to reduce the rate or impact of ageing.

There are ten known causes or 'hallmarks' of ageing, so by eliminating these we can make a start on slowing ageing (López-Otín *et al.* 2013). These hallmarks are: (1) DNA damage, (2) telomere shortening (damage to the ends of our chromosomes), (3) epigenetic changes (faulty regulation of DNA), (4) damage to proteins, (5) defective sensing of nutrients, (6) damage to mitochondria (dysfunctional energy generation), (7) cellular senescence (cells stop dividing and lose function), (8) stem cell depletion (cells no longer capable of replacing other cells), (9) chronic inflammation (the system protecting us from occasional infection and damage is stuck on), and (10) hormones or other signals in the blood are too high or too low. So, for example, our DNA becomes increasingly damaged with age, due to oxidants, defective repair or excessive replication of the DNA. And this can cause our cells to 'senesce', i.e. stop dividing and lose function. And this can be particularly problematic for our stem cells, whose function is to divide and replace our other cells. And senescence can result in inflammation, which contributes to age-related diseases in part by damaging proteins. And high nutrient levels promote ageing via a variety of signalling pathways, which can become defective with age: for example, a defective response to the hormone insulin cause diabetes (López-Otín *et al.* 2013).

What are the prospects that interfering with these and other factors will reduce ageing in the future? Well, there is evidence that interfering with these factors can affect lifespan or aspects of ageing in mice or rats (López-Otín *et al.* 2013). However, mice and rats live only two or three years, so it is difficult to know whether ageing in rodents can be extrapolated to human ageing. Also, the treatments or interventions used in rodents, such as genetic engineering or starvation, are not easily applicable to humans. And testing potential treatments for ageing in old humans is difficult because of the length of time, expense and potential side effects involved. All of these factors mean that progress in reducing ageing is likely to be slow – but important!

Some have argued that research on ageing is a bad thing because eliminating ageing might cause a variety of problems for society and individuals. However, ageing is not a digital process that can be switched off, so arguments about whether eliminating ageing is good have little bearing on whether reducing ageing is good. We would not argue that medicine is bad because immortality is bad, so it makes no sense to argue that reducing ageing is bad because immortality is bad.

Some have argued that reducing ageing is bad because ageing is natural. However, ageing is not natural, as it does not occur in nature and was not 'designed' by evolution. Rather ageing is an unintentional side effect of civilization removing extrinsic causes of death, allowing us to live long enough to age significantly. There is little or no ageing of animals in the wild, because they die from starvation, infection or predation before they age. And humans

before civilization lived 20 or 30 years, and therefore died before ageing significantly. Furthermore, ageing does not result from evolution by natural selection; rather it results from the absence of natural selection of aged individuals
in the past as they did not exist (Kirkwood & Austad 2000). Ageing results
from accumulating damage to our biochemical machinery (López-Otín *et al.*
2013), and evolution by natural selection could not eliminate this ageing in
the past because it did not exist until civilization revealed it by preventing
extrinsic causes of death. So ageing is not 'natural', but rather a by-product
of our culture.

Pathway to immortality 2: survival of the mind

The next best thing to staying alive is: the body dying but the mind staying
alive. Throughout history, people have believed it possible to survive death
in some attenuated mental form as ghosts or spirits. And they have invested
enormous energy and time in attempts to achieve this through religion or
magic. Of course, this was a colossal mistake and blind alley based on the
false belief that the mind can exist independent of the body. The belief in
minds independent of bodies was part of a wider belief system that saw all
movement and change as caused by some form of mind in matter (Russell
1945). If something moved or had behaviour, for example a rock falling or
wind blowing, then it may be inhabited by some kind of spirit or be animated
at a distance by some spirit, mind or god. This was a reasonable belief based
on the evidence available at the time. And it remains an attractive belief now,
if we ignore the fact that there is no evidence of minds independent of bodies,
and our current understanding of how minds depend on brains.

The motivation for belief in immortality is important here. From a scientific perspective, it may seem illogical to believe in what is not true. But from
the perspectives of psychology, truth is not an end in itself, but rather a means
to achieve happiness (Franken 2007). Happiness (or contentment, pleasure,
absence of pain, etc.) is the only direct goal and motivation of life. Thus,
from this perspective, it is illogical to believe something true if it makes you
unhappy in the short and long term. And so it may be reasonable to believe
whatever makes you happy about life-after-death, irrespective of whether it is
true or not. If so – and I believe it is both logical and true – we need to be care-
ful about judging someone stupid for believing something untrue or illogical!

According to the Epic of Gilgamesh, death is the oblivion of never-ending sleep, only broken by the nightmares of a shadow-world, where people's
attenuated spirits survive as birds eating dust and clay in eternal darkness.
The dead were regarded with dread, and it was important that they should
not return from their shadow-world to plague the living. In the Sumerian
version of the story, the fate of Gilgamesh is decided by an assembly of the
gods: 'Let Gilgamesh as a ghost, below among the dead, be the governor
of the nether world. Let him be pre-eminent among the ghosts, so that he
will pass judgments and render verdicts' (George 2000). So Gilgamesh, who

sought immortality in life, is instead granted a tenuous immortality in death. The gods make Gilgamesh a minor god of the Underworld, and indeed there was a Sumerian cult that worshiped Gilgamesh as an Underworld god in third millennium BC (George 2000). Does this count as immortality? Well, nowadays we would count this as survival by pathway 4 (culture) rather than pathway 2 (mind without body), because most of us believe that mind cannot survive without bodies.

Is there, then, any viable, modern version of this route to immortality via survival of the mind? The most direct analogue is the concept of somehow uploading the mind to a computer, Internet or robot. If the mind/brain is an information-processing machine that processes incoming information from the senses etc. via electrical signals, memory and brain software, and outputs to muscles controlling speech and actions, then the same information processing should be able to be modelled on a computer. And if it could be successfully modelled, then connecting this model to similar sensory input devices and similar motor output devices should result in something that behaved in a similar way to the original mind.

An analogous concept arises from brain–electronic interface devices that monitor the electrical activity of multiple neurons in the brain and/or directly stimulate the electrical activity of neurons in the brain. Such devices have been used, for example, to directly connect the brain to a computer, so that a computer cursor can be controlled directly by a person's mind. If the mind can be directly connected to a computer and in principle to the Internet, then one can imagine that the mind could be downloaded somehow. Alternatively, one can imagine replacing each neuron (or set of neurons) in the brain by a computer chip with the same input–output functions, so that if all neurons are so substituted, then in theory this electronic brain should have exactly the same behaviour as the original biological brain.

If my brain could be accurately simulated by computer software or electronic hardware, would this count as a version of me, and would it help me survive death? Well, first one should say that it would be impossible to do either of these things today, as we do not know how and do not understand the brain sufficiently. But if we ignore this practical problem, then there is the even more knotty problem that we do not understand what consciousness is, and therefore would not know whether such a device had a similar consciousness to me. If we made a device that replicated all my behaviours exactly, we would still want to know what it felt like from the inside, i.e. what experiences the devices would have subjectively.

There are three main meanings of the word 'consciousness': (1) awareness, as in 'I am aware/conscious of a dog or a headache'; (2) thought, in particular the internal speech that is at the centre of the stream of consciousness; and (3) subjective experience, i.e. the sensory experiences that arise in the brain/mind as a result of external sensation (vision, hearing, smell, taste, touch, pain) or internally via memory, imagining, dreams and internal speech. Awareness and thought can be defined functionally if we ignore the subjective experiences associated with them: for example, awareness is the detection and correct categorization of something, so that both awareness and thought could be replaced by a software and hardware device that did the same thing. However, the 'hard problem' is subjective experience, such as the experience of a headache or patch of blue, as it cannot be defined functionally, and it is probably a thing, rather than a process (Chalmers 2010). For example, subjective experience may be the substance of the brain, e.g. the electric fields, i.e. an intrinsic property of all matter, but its form would be shaped by brain activity. If so, then although a device might simulate my awareness and thought, it would not thereby accurately simulate my subjective experience. It may have some subjective experience, but likely of a radically different kind, because the substance would be different. Such a device could be made to be more like the brain in substance, but the logical extrapolation of this is to simply duplicate the brain, rather than download the functional aspects of the mind to a computer. Downloading the functional aspects of my brain to a machine/computer/Internet, without trying to make the subjective experience the same, is like generating a zombie version of me – minus the taste for human flesh, hopefully!

In conclusion, we know too little about the brain/mind to gain immortality by downloading the mind to a computer, and even if we could download the functional (information-processing) aspects of the mind, this is unlikely to result in a similar type of subjective experience, i.e. it is unlikely to feel the same from the inside. However, copying the functional aspects of mind reproduces a central aspect of who we are. But does this count as survival? We will have to leave that discussion until we have acquainted ourselves with genetic and memetic survival.

Pathway to immortality 3: survival of the genes

Throughout history people have sought some aspect of immortality through their children and children's children (Cave 2013). People have felt that something is passed to them by their parents and then passed on to their children. What that something is has been ill-defined: a name, a legacy, blood, an inheritance, the family. Psychologically this may correspond to identification with the family and motivation to benefit the family. We have multiple identities, for example I may identify as a human, as male, as an Englishman, as a Bristol Rovers supporter, etc., etc., but one of my central identities is with my family. Family identities are strong, almost as strong as self-identity, such that some people are prepared to kill or die for the family, in particular for their children.

From a biological perspective, the origin of this psychological identification and motivation to benefit the family is that we share genes, and the ill-defined something that links our ancestors and descendants is those shared genes. We know that this biology is important, because most animals on earth promote the survival of their offspring or others with whom they share genes. And evolution by natural selection, and therefore the design of all organisms, is driven by the survival of the genes and nothing else. From the evolutionary perspective we are 'gene machines' designed to spread our genes (Dawkins 1976). However, during the evolution of some animals it has been found beneficial for the spread of their genes to endow individual gene machines with personal minds containing selves, models of the world, motivations, desires and emotions. These minds enabled animals to figure out what to do in any particular situation based on all current and past experience, rather than fixed responses programmed before birth (Dawkins 1976). This made animals such as ourselves vastly more adaptable, but also gave us some independence of evolution as we could change the world and our models of the world.

The central motivations that evolved in animals were to survive and to reproduce, as only animals with such motivations written into their DNA were likely to survive and pass on their DNA long term. Survival of the individual was promoted by motivating individuals to survive: for example, to fear death, to avoid predation, to hunger for food, etc. Reproduction was promoted in part by motivating animals to have sex a lot, but also by the motivation to promote the survival and welfare of their progeny, experienced as love, bonding and identification with the progeny and co-parent. This enhanced the spread of their genes, and by these genes spread the motivation. Thus evolution has endowed us with the desire to survive, bond, reproduce and promote the welfare of our children and other family members.

Then why do we die? If evolution by natural selection works by selecting genotypes that survive, i.e. die less, why do organism still die at enormous rates? If natural selection only selected by death, then death should have been eliminated long ago. But natural selection also selects by reproduction, i.e. genotypes that reproduce more, and if reproduction and preventing death compete for resources, then genotypes that devote all their resources to preventing death will have none left for reproduction, and thus the genes for this will not spread. The genes that will spread best will be those that allocate resources optimally between reproduction and preventing death. Also, once an individual has reproduced, there is a much reduced selection pressure on the genes to prevent death, because the genes have already been passed on. Thus, in a sense, death is a price we pay for reproduction.

In the epic of Gilgamesh, there is a central preoccupation with the survival of the individual's name, preserved either by descendants, by society or by writing. This may relate to the ancient belief that the representation of something (whether in image or name) was magically connected to the thing represented. Thus survival of someone's image, child or name enabled some form of survival of the individual. The final stanza of the old Sumerian story concludes:

> Men, as many are given names,
> their funerary statues have been fashioned since days of old,
> and stationed in chapels in the temples of the gods:
> how their names are pronounced will never be forgotten!

The goddess Aruru, elder sister of Enlil,
for the sake of his name gave men offspring:
their statues have been fashioned since days of old,
and their names still spoken in the land.

(George 2000)

Men, who were mortal, could not escape becoming shades in the Underworld, but they could survive in partial form through the collective memory of their names, either through their offspring, or images and prayers in the temples, or their renown, causing their names to live on in other people's minds and to live again on other people's lips.

Is there a modern version of survival via our genes? Having children dilutes our genes by 50 per cent, as our children get 50 per cent of their genes from one parent and 50 per cent from the other parent. This results in rapid dilution of our genes over the generations. Cloning would enable us to pass 100 per cent of our genes to our derivative clone. Cloning is currently illegal in humans, but has been done successfully in other mammals, and almost certainly could be done in humans if there was sufficient motivation. Cloning can be done, for example, by removing a live cell from your skin and fusing it with a human egg cell from which the nucleus has been removed, and then putting this egg into a receptive woman to bring to term. The resulting baby would be genetically identical to you (in the same way as an identical twin), but of course it would be younger than you, and would acquire different experience than you. So when the clone grew up it would look like you at the same age, and behave the same way to the extent that this is genetically determined, but obviously differ to the extent that this is determined by non-genetic factors.

Would having a clone count as survival? It would certainly count as genetic survival, and it would be much more similar to you than a normal child. But it would be missing your life experiences, ideas, skills and memories, things that we consider in the next section. So we will leave it until the last section to discuss the deeper issues of whether a clone or clone plus my mind would count as survival.

Pathway to immortality 4: survival of the memes

In reality a family passes on more than just genes to the next generation, it also passes on memories, ways of doing things, attitudes, skills, ideas, ways of talking, sayings, songs, jokes, knowledge, false beliefs, etc., etc. These types of things are learnt by children actively or passively from their parents to a greater or lesser extent. This is known as cultural transmission, and it does not just occur in families, it also occurs in schools and universities, in churches, workplaces and clubs, and via books, magazines, television and the Internet. It is occurring anywhere and everywhere, where one component of the mind or behaviour is passed from one person to another. This cultural transmission may be direct, as when one person teaches some knowledge or skill to another person, or indirect, as when someone writes a book or blog, or draws something, or composes some music, or designs a house, or does something else that is then experienced by someone else, affecting their mind. The transmission may be of more or less fidelity, i.e. a skill or idea or song may be transmitted from one person to another so that it is exactly the same in the second person as in the original, or it may be changed in a variety of ways and to different extents.

A unit of cultural inheritance has been called a 'meme' in analogy with a gene as the unit of genetic inheritance (Dawkins 1976). A phrase, a song, a behaviour might be a 'meme', the definition is loose. Memes are stored as memories in the brain – in a sense memories are memes. But memes can also be stored outside the brain in books, works of art, etc., which can then go into memory when experienced. Human culture has evolved much more rapidly than human genetics, because memes are transmitted and changed much more rapidly than genes. Memes are like bits of software that can pass from brain to brain, altering the behaviour of humans. And in our digital age, memes can reproduce very rapidly: for example, a tweet, a YouTube video, a rumour.

Survival via memes (pathway 4) overlaps somewhat with survival of the mind (pathway 2), but they are distinguishable because minds are containers while memes are content, analogous to hardware and software, or bodies and genes. And minds can contain things other than memes, and memes can exist outside minds. But we could regard survival of the memes as survival of a component of minds – just as we could regard the survival of genes as survival of a component of bodies.

Throughout history people have sought a form of immortality by doing things that will be remembered by others, and therefore live on after their death within other people or imbedded in our culture (Cave 2013). This could be as simple as being kind to people, so that they remember you, or as grand as creating a scientific theory that changes the world. What survives may be a memory in living people, or something in the world that affects living people such as a book or song or idea that may affect many people when experienced. We call this type of survival memetic and what survives memes, i.e. transmission of something from one mind to another that is recognizably the same in the two minds, for instance, an idea or skill. However, we could include in this type of survival anything that someone did that had an effect on other people after they died, and this might include things that were not strictly memetic. For example, someone being kind (or horrible) to others may cause them to be remembered after their death (and therefore survive in the memory of others), but this is not strictly memetic unless it leads the living person to be kind (or horrible) to others.

People have done things and continue to do things, because by doing them they benefit other people and/or contribute to human culture. This is one of the central reasons people do things other than to survive or reproduce the body. And part of the reason for doing this may be to survive or reproduce part of the mind. We create ideas, theories, books, songs, tweets, etc. so that they can be reproduced in other minds. We are continually receiving memes from other people and media, etc., into our brains, where they either die out, or are passed on to others, or mutated or combined with other memes to produce new memes that are passed on. We can look at this from the perspective of the memes/culture rather than the individual, and see the flow of memes from brain to brain, some reproducing rapidly, some dying out, some evolving into new memes (Dawkins 1976). From this perspective, we could view our minds as a collection of memes (behaviours, skills, beliefs, ideas, etc.), some changing, some staying the same, some active, some hidden away.

Information technology has provided powerful ways of promoting cultural/memetic survival and proliferation in the modern world. Tweeting provides a means of spreading a thought rapidly through thousands of brains. YouTube provides a more visual version. Life blogging enables a life to be recorded and reproduced in tedious detail. The Internet is the ideal medium for the rapid spread of memes of all varieties. Media has become global and instantaneous, such that if anything happens anywhere of sufficient interest it can be reproduced across the planet in minutes. Of course, rapid information spread can lead to short attention spans, and short survival. But information technology and the Internet also provide massive information storage and powerful means of searching and retrieving that information. It has never been such a great time to be a meme!

Gilgamesh complains:

> In my city people are dying, and hearts are full of distress. People are lost, which fills me with dismay. I reach my neck over the city wall, and see corpses in the water making the river almost overflow. This will happen to me too – that is the way of things. No one is tall enough to reach heaven; no one can reach wide enough to stretch over the mountains. Since a man cannot pass beyond the final end of life, I want to set off into the mountains, to establish my renown there. Where my renown can be established, I will establish my name; and where my renown cannot be established, I shall establish the renown of the gods.
>
> (Faculty of Oriental Studies 2006)

The Assyrian version of the epic ends with Gilgamesh at last reaching home, and consoling himself by contemplating the walls of Uruk, the walls that he rebuilt, the testament that he believes will survive after his death to preserve his name, stamped into the bricks, his little piece of immortality. It is these walls, the walls of Uruk, that were uncovered by modern archaeologists to reveal the remains of the oldest known city in the world.

But ultimately Gilgamesh's name obtained immortality through the story, the Epic of Gilgamesh. That story was famous for a thousand years throughout Mesopotamia, the cradle of civilization. So the story was copied and adapted many times on myriad clay tablets. The story was then lost for another 2,000 years, before the first fragments were dug up in the nineteenth century from the ruins of Nineveh, where they had lain for 25 centuries. The Epic of Gilgamesh lies as a gigantic fragmented jigsaw puzzle (or puzzles) under the deserts of Iraq, of which we have a few pieces that can be put together in multiple ways. And every few years a new version incorporating the latest fragments is published. The name of Gilgamesh lives again!

What counts as survival?

Is memetic survival a type of survival worth having? It depends partly on whether we think of our self as digital and unified, or analogue and composed of parts such as memes. If we believe that the self/soul is unitary and the core self unchanging throughout life, then we are likely to believe that learnt behaviours, beliefs, ideas, etc. are peripheral to the self, and not a vehicle for survival after death. However, if we believe that the self is composed of learnt behaviours, beliefs, ideas, etc., that change throughout life, then we may be open to the idea that parts of the self are transferred or reproduced via cultural transmission.

Part of the issue here is whether partial survival counts as survival at all. If we believe that the mind/self is unitary, we may not believe that partial transmission/survival of the mind/self counts at all. And we may want to survive intact or not at all. At the other end of the spectrum, we may be quite happy for little bits of ourselves (memes) to be floating around in other people's minds. Similarly, we may think that survival through our children does not count, because our children are not the same as us. But if they are partially the same as us, because many of our genes and memes survive in them, then whether we count this as survival depends on our concept of self. Some would say that the self changes throughout life, so that little of the baby survives in the old man, while others would assert that the core self remains the same. But these different views may be looking at different parts of the self, i.e. the experience-dependent part that changes, and the genetically programmed part that remains the same.

However, an even deeper issue arises if we could generate someone identical to us to replace us when we die. Surely this would count as survival? This issue was explored via a thought experiment of Derek Parfit (1984), retold in slightly different form here. An astronaut blasts off into space, but crash-lands on Mars. Fortunately, the astronaut finds an emergency telephone box on Mars, but when she enters, it is not of the usual type. The instructions say that when the astronaut presses the big, green button, lasers will scan her to locate the coordinates of every molecule in her body. This will destroy her, but the coordinates will be sent to a similar box on earth, where the data will be used to assemble an exact copy of herself from a box full of spare molecules. So, taking a deep breath, she presses the big, green button, and is beamed back to Earth for a happy reunion with family and friends.

There the story should have come to a happy ending, but unfortunately five years later the astronaut crash-lands on Mars again! She kicks herself, but rapidly makes her way to the phone box for transmission back to Earth. However, the phone box has been upgraded, and the instructions now proudly announce that the scanning process has been improved such that when determining the location of each molecule in her body, these molecules will not be destroyed or even damaged. So that if and when she presses the big, green button, she will be scanned and copied to Earth, but the original will remain on Mars.

Her dilemma is: to press or not to press? If she presses, she may either go home to Earth, or be left on Mars while her 'copy' goes home to her husband and kids. Where will her 'consciousness' go? And what happened five years ago? Is she the copy, of which the original was destroyed in the box five years ago? Or would it be better to think that when the button is pressed, the original is destroyed and two copies made, one remaining on Mars and the other sent to Earth? Can we think of ourselves as dying every night when we go to sleep, and a copy of us reboots in the morning? Our consciousness disappears during dreamless sleep, while the memories and propensity to act, behave and think in certain ways are retained in the physical structure of the brain overnight to reboot our consciousness in the morning. Perhaps this type of consciousness, the stream of consciousness, only exists in the present. If so, then whether I identify with myself yesterday or tomorrow is not a question of fact, but rather a question of choice and culture. If so, the result of the astronaut pressing the big, green button will be two (initially identical) consciousnesses – but whether the consciousness existing prior to pressing the button should identify with one or other subsequent bits of consciousness is a question of identity, not fact. My consciousness in the present cannot choose to be another piece of consciousness in my past or future or someone else's consciousness. My consciousness can only be my consciousness now. But I can choose to identify with a piece of 'my' consciousness in the past or future, by thinking of it as mine. Similarly, I can choose to identify with the consciousness of my children or others sharing my genes and memes in the future. An analogous thought experiment is to imagine a clone of myself identical in body and mind. Would such a clone ensure my survival if I died? Well, it depends what I identify with: my genes, my memes, my body, my mind, my consciousness, or all of the above?

This question of identity may seem abstruse, but it is central to what we mean by survival. What do we mean by survival? A baby may survive to be a 100-year-old man, with causal continuity and the same DNA, but the baby and old man will not look or behave the same, and they will have different matter and consciousness. Whether the old man thinks of himself as the same person as the baby is therefore a question of how he thinks of himself – and that is up to him or his culture. And if you could survive to be 1,000 years old, would the 1,000-year-old identify with you now, or should you identify the potential 1,000-year-old as the same person? I do not think we can say whether someone should identify with something or not, any more than we should say whether someone should feel something or not. Whether we feel that we are surviving by having children or clones or ideas is a question of identity, that is, whether we feel that those children or clones or ideas are part of the wider me or not. So whether surviving via our bodies or minds or genes or memes counts as 'really' surviving depends on whether we 'really' think of those surviving entities as ours, and whether we 'really' feel that it counts as survival, not whether 'in reality' we survive by these means.

Of course, we do not normally consciously choose what we identify with. The default is for our identity to be unconsciously determined by our genes and culture. And this defines what we regard as 'us', and therefore what counts as survival. But as rational beings, we can reprogram our identity – at least to some extent.

Conclusions

To summarize this chapter, people have sought immortality in four main ways, via survival of the body, mind, genes or memes. Over the last two centuries, global efforts to increase survival of the body have been successful, so that average lifespan has more than doubled. However, because the rate of ageing has not changed, the cost of increased lifespan has been increased ageing, diseases of ageing, dementia, disability and a degenerative end to life. The solution should be to reduce the rate of ageing, but ageing is not like another disease that can be cured. It is *all* age-related diseases, disabilities and dysfunctions. Ageing did not evolve by natural selection, therefore it is not natural, but rather an unfortunate side effect of extending lifespan beyond ages that were selected in our evolutionary past. Ageing will never be eliminated, but it can and should be reduced. Otherwise, further extending lifespan will result in the Tithonus scenario, and survival of the body will be bought at the expensive of the mind.

In the past, it was thought that the mind could survive death of the body, but we now know that mind cannot survive without matter. We can update this pathway to immortality by trying to replicate the functional aspects of the mind in a computer or robot, but this will leave out the subjective aspects of mind, i.e. what it feels like to be a person/mind. And unfortunately we have no idea how to engineer subjective experience directly.

We were designed over four billion years of evolution by natural selection to promote the survival of our genes. Evolution has not eliminated death, probably because this would require resources to be taken away from reproduction. Evolution by natural selection has given us our fear of death, and our will to survive via our selves, our children and others with whom we share genes. We can update this pathway by cloning to ensure survival of all genes. However, human evolution has also given us individual minds, populated by memes and culture that evolve much more rapidly than genes. And we can update survival of our memes by electronic storage and dispersal via the Internet, Twitter, etc.

Whether we identify with our body, mind, genes or memes at other times than now is a question of identity, i.e. what we feel counts as ours. And in particular whether we can identify with partial versions of ourselves, such as our children or our memes in other people. We also have to bear in mind that what we believe in (and identify with) is not just determined by what is true, but also more directly by what makes us happy.

References

Brayne, Carol (2007): 'The Elephant in the Room: Healthy Brains in Later Life, Epidemiology and Public Health'. *Nature Reviews Neuroscience*, 8 (3):233–239.

Brown, Guy (2007): *The Living End: The Future of Death, Ageing and Immortality*. London: Macmillan.

Brown, Guy (2015): 'Living Too Long: The Current Focus of Medical Research on Increasing the Quantity, Rather Than the Quality, of Life Is Damaging Our Health and Harming the Economy'. *EMBO Reports*, 16 (2):137–141.

Cave, Stephen (2013): *Immortality: The Quest to Live Forever and How It Drives Civilization*. London: Biteback Publishing.

Chalmers, David (2010): *The Character of Consciousness*. Oxford: Oxford University Press.

Dawkins, Richard (1976): *The Selfish Gene*. Oxford: Oxford University Press.

European Commission (2012): *The 2012 Ageing Report: Economic and Budgetary Projections for the EU27 Member States (2010–2060)*. Brussels: European Commission.

Faculty of Oriental Studies (2006): *The Electronic Text Corpus of Sumerian Literature*. Oxford: University of Oxford.

Franken, Robert E. (2007): *Human Motivation* (6th edn). Calgary: University of Calgary.

George, Andrew (2000): *The Epic of Gilgamesh* (translated from the Sumerian). London: Penguin Classics.

Kirkwood, Thomas B. & Steven N. Austad (2000): 'Why Do We Age?'. *Nature*, 408 (6809):233–238.

López-Otín, Carlos, Maria A. Blasco, Linda Partridge, Manuel Serrano & Guido Kroemer (2013): 'The Hallmarks of Ageing'. *Cell*, 153 (6):1194–1217.

Oeppen, Jim & James W. Vaupel (2002): 'Broken Limits to Life Expectancy'. *Science*, 296 (5570):1029–1031.

Parfit, Derek (1984): *Reasons and Persons*. Oxford: Oxford University Press.

Riley, James C. (2001): *Rising Life Expectancy: A Global History*. Cambridge: Cambridge University Press.

Russell, Bertrand (1945): *A History of Western Philosophy*. London: George Allen & Unwin Ltd.

Xie, Jing, Fiona E. Matthews, Carol Jagger, John Bond & Carol Brayne (2008): 'The Oldest Old in England and Wales: A Descriptive Analysis Based on the MRC Cognitive Function and Ageing Study'. *Age and Ageing*, 37 (4):396–402.

3 Individualised immortality in liquid-modern times

Teasing out the topic of symbolic immortality in the sociology of Zygmunt Bauman

Michael Hviid Jacobsen

Introduction

It has recently been suggested that the 'topic of death, often monopolized by theology, philosophy and even psychology through its studies of grief and bereavement, has rarely been treated as a signature of sociological theorizing' (Blum 2015:24–25). This is indeed true. Moreover, the companion topic of death – that of immortality – has conventionally not been seen as an obvious theme for most sociology books or in sociological theorising. In fact, the discipline (perhaps besides the sub-disciplines of the 'sociology of religion' and 'the sociology of death and dying') cannot pride itself on having paid much attention at all to making sense of this important domain of human and social life. The few sociologists who have taken an interest in studying death and dying, or immortality for that matter, have not made a name or career for themselves due to their interest in these – in the eyes of their discipline relatively obscure – topics. Most often, their work has been relegated to the margins of a discipline much more concerned with studying social structure, social stratification, social organisation and similar traditional sociological themes.

However, one of the few prominent sociologists who have taken the topic of immortality seriously is Polish social theorist, Zygmunt Bauman. He has written some quite extraordinary texts dissecting our culture's ingenious yet often unacknowledged attempts to make sense of death and our death anxieties through different immortality strategies. But even Bauman's significant contribution to understanding and theorising death and immortality has gone relatively unnoticed as compared to the popularity of his acclaimed study of the Holocaust and its modern origins, his position as one of the primary 'prophets of postmodernity' or his important coining of the metaphor of 'liquid modernity'. I therefore agree with the recent observation that 'despite his prominence, Bauman's long-term writing on the role of culture in coping with death-anxieties is largely neglected in the sociological and thanatological literature of death and dying, particularly in the United States' (Higo 2012/

2013:222). Despite the centrality of the topics in his work, Bauman's long-standing interest in death and immortality has also been largely overlooked by some of his most insightful and influential interpreters in their introductions to his work (see, e.g., Blackshaw 2005; Davis 2008; Smith 1998; Tester 2004). Most often, critics and commentators, students and researchers focus on his important and inspirational work on the Holocaust, postmodernity, morality, consumerism or liquid modernity – and for good reason. This is indeed a treasure trove for anyone trying to come to grips with some of the main changes in modernity and some of the major challenges confronting contemporary society. But just as Bauman was among the first to deal in-depth sociologically with overlooked topics such as freedom (Bauman 1988), the Holocaust (Bauman 1989) and morality (Bauman 1993), so he was also one of the first to try to develop a substantial sociological account of death and immortality in the book *Mortality, Immortality and Other Life Strategies* (1992b). So contrary to what is often debated or found interesting in socio-logical circles, the topics of death and immortality occupy a central position in the work of Bauman (see, e.g., Jacobsen 2011).

In this chapter, we will explore in some detail the ideas of death and immortality in the writings of Zygmunt Bauman – primarily relying on his magisterial book *Mortality, Immortality and Other Life Strategies* (1992b) – as part of his more comprehensive analysis of the transformation of modern society and its most recent postmodern and liquid-modern incarnations. We shall look into the different ways in which society, according to Bauman, con-tinuously constructs and entertains changing understandings and visions of immortality that are intimately linked to how society understands and seeks to make sense of life and death.

Mortality, Immortality and Other Life Strategies: a 'radical book'

My own first encounter with the work of Zygmunt Bauman was actually due to my youthful infatuation with the topics of death and immortality, and ever since my student days in the mid-1990s, these topics and the work of Bauman have been inextricably linked concerns in large parts of my own writings (see, e.g., Jacobsen 1997, 2013, 2016a). I still vividly remember discussing the find-ings of my master's thesis with him during those days and receiving generous and encouraging comments via fax. There is no doubt that death and immor-tality are topics close to Bauman's heart. According to Peter Beilharz, one of the most prominent Bauman interpreters, Bauman's own favourite among his many published books – revealed in conversation without hesitation – perhaps even his 'unloved child', is *Mortality, Immortality and Other Life Strategies* (Beilharz 2000:146). It was written when Bauman was in his mid-sixties and had just retired from the University of Leeds. I am sure the idea behind the book had been cooking long before this. To many who had followed the devel-opment of his writings, the book must have come as a surprise or even a shock – it was published in the slipstream of his incisive theoretical analysis of the changing role of intellectuals in the transition from modernity to postmodernity (Bauman 1987), his discussion of the idea of freedom (Bauman 1988), his critically acclaimed study of the Holocaust as a thoroughly modern phenomenon (Bauman 1989), his in-depth analysis of the modern war against and social production of ambivalence (Bauman 1991) and his initial flirtation with the idea of postmodernity (Bauman 1992a). However, *Mortality, Immortality and Other Life Strategies* (1992b) was perhaps not as surprising after all as it followed up on, substantiated and concretised the general analytical template used in other books from around this time of 'premodernity' giving way to 'modernity' (later to be labelled 'solid modernity'), which was again superseded by 'postmodernity' (later relabelled 'liquid modernity'). Already at the beginning of the book, Bauman admitted that this chronology was in no way a historically correct fact but more of an abstract idealisation and a heuristic device intended to show how changes in life, death and immortality could be approached and captured analytically. He stated that people, after all, do not live first in a premodern, then in a modern and then again in a postmodern world, but that all these different and consecutive 'worlds' are merely abstract intellectual idealisations of one single, yet complex and incoherent, life process that the sociologist – just as everybody else – tries so desperately to make understandable and coherent (Bauman 1992b:11). Nevertheless, as an analytical schema this template, as we shall see later, worked well in highlighting some of the fundamental changes in our cultural comprehension of death and immortality.

Mortality, Immortality and Other Life Strategies is, in the apt words of Robert Bocock in his review of the book, a 'radical book' because it goes to the very heart and root of our most fundamental human problem with existence – the fact that we must die (Bocock 1993:123). It is also a radical book because, as mentioned, it tangles with topics conventionally not pursued by sociologists. According to Peter Beilharz, it is also a 'peculiar book' as it, according to him, is more of 'a corridor that leads nowhere in particular than it is a bridge or a door' (Beilharz 2000:145). Actually, I rather see the book as in many ways an archetypal Bauman book, because it struggles to understand and capture that which has otherwise been neglected by sociologists, namely death and immortality. In this way, the book harks back to Bauman's pattern of trying to shed light on heretofore overlooked themes such as culture, utopia, the Holocaust, freedom and morality. In fact, Bauman's magnum opus *Modernity and the Holocaust* (1989) also investigated – more generally, however – how modern society perpetuated a culture of industrialised and bureaucratised mass death here directed specifically against the Jews. One may surmise that this book may have led him onto the track of his later study of death and immortality as topics in their own right. At the time when *Mortality, Immortality and Other Life Strategies* was published in the early 1990s, Bauman was in fact among the few key sociologists – together with Peter L. Berger, Norbert Elias and Jean Baudrillard – to take the topics of death and immortality seriously in their own right. However, at the beginning of the book Bauman stated that he did not regard his ideas as a contribution to the emerging sub-field of 'the sociology of death and dying', which investigates how we treat people about to die or commemorate those already dead. Neither was his book about the historically changing visions and images of death and its aftermath held by members of society – such as in the classic studies by French historian Philippe Ariès (1974, 1981). Finally, the book was not about the so-called 'death mentalities' and the accompanying practices relating to death in a given society. Rather, according to Bauman, 'the immodest intention' of his book was to unpack and analytically unravel the way death is present in human institutions, beliefs and rituals (Bauman 1992b:1–2). He also insisted that his 'method' of investigating death and immortality is that of a 'psychoanalysis' of the 'collective unconscious' that was concealed in, but which could also be analytically recovered from, culturally created and culturally sustained life (Bauman 1992b:8). Bauman's work can thus be seen as a study of death and immortality through the lens of so-called human/cultural 'life strategies' (or what will later be called 'symbolic immortality'), and simultaneously as an eye-opener to a death-defying culture and the immortality-ignoring discipline of sociology.

Death: the destroyer and creator of meaning

Death is an aporia to humans. It does not really make much sense to us. It is incomprehensible, because it is the 'unknown' incarnate, it is 'non-being', all negation, emptiness and 'absolute nothing' (Bauman 1992b:2). Existence without ourselves in it is actually quite unimaginable to us. Death describes 'absence' – thus any definition of death will always point backwards to that which has been and was before, but which is no more. In itself, death has no past and no future, but at the same time, as Bauman states, death *is*, it is *real*, and the problem is that we know it (Bauman 1992b:14). Death detracts from life: it destroys meaning, it wrecks relationships, it robs our lives of loved ones, it defies permanence, it decimates our dreams and desires and it defiantly annuls all our desperate attempts to stay alive. Death is indeed a problem – and it is a problem compared to which all of our other problems, no matter how serious, seem to pale. As Norbert Elias once observed:

> Death is the problem of the living. Dead people have no problems. Of the many creatures on this earth that die, it is human beings alone for whom dying is a problem … They alone of all living beings know that they shall die; they alone can anticipate their own end … It is not actually death, but the *knowledge of death*, that creates problems for human beings.
>
> (Elias 1985/2001:3–5, my emphasis)

According to Bauman, humans are the only creatures who not only know that they will die. They also know that they know. Add to this the fact that they also know that they fear death. Death, in Bauman's view, is therefore the primary source of our fears. We fear death because, contrary to all our other problems and sources of fear, it is for all practical intents and purposes irreparable, irreversible, irredeemable, insuperable, irremediable, irrevocable, beyond recall or remedy, the point of no return, the final, the ultimate, the end of everything (Bauman 2006:29). Moreover, death cannot be wished away – it stubbornly remains even despite our most persistent efforts at eradicating or forgetting about it. As once captured by Eugène Ionesco, 'death is our main problem and others are less important. It is the wall and the limit. It is the only inescapable alienation; it gives us a sense of our limits' (Ionesco quoted in Porter 1986). Maybe humans do not so much fear death 'as such', but rather the gnawing *awareness of death*, so 'whenever I am, I am in the company of my *awareness* that sooner or later death *must* put an end to my being here' (Bauman 2006:30). It is indeed terrifying to live with this awareness day after day throughout life. As Ernest Becker stated in *The Denial of Death* (1973), humans are conscious animals who are aware of their own mortality – hence they can only try to flee or nullify this awareness, and therefore the history of humanity is also the history of humanity's continuous attempts to deal with the problem of death. Thus, world history, as G. W. F. Hegel once insisted, is all about what man does with death (Whaley 1981:1).

Because death cannot remain a secret or a non-existing entity for long without awakening our awareness, people instead try to suspend the knowledge of death, to fight death or to imagine that death is not definitive. Throughout history, humankind in various – at times quite primitive, at other times rather ingenious – ways have sought to reconcile themselves with the reality of death through different immortality-imitating practices (see, e.g., Toynbee 1980). In this way, phenomena such as 'transcendence', 'survival' and 'immortality' are all integral to human existence, and it is exactly our ineradicable knowledge and awareness of mortality that in the end seem to spur our incessant quest for immortality. Since immortality by and large is an 'unnatural condition, which won't come by itself unless cajoled or forced into being', immortality is made into a 'task' for humans to perform (Bauman 1999b:242). As Bauman on different occasions has thus observed:

> Knowing of one's mortality means at the same time knowing of *the possibility of immortality* … To be aware of mortality means to imagine immortality; to dream of immortality; to work towards immortality.
>
> (Bauman 1997:153, original emphasis)

> Our human way of being-in-the-world consists in imagining, designing, experimenting with, putting to a test ever-new stratagems of living meaningfully with the meaninglessness – that is living with the awareness of mortality.
>
> (Bauman in Jacobsen & Kearl 2014:316)

In his compelling book, *How to Live Forever or Die Trying*, Bryan Appleyard testified that 'everybody dies. Therefore I must die. This being inconceivable, we invent immortality and these inventions are civilisation' (Appleyard 2007:15). Substitute the word 'civilisation' with 'culture', and then you basically have Bauman's point of view. To him, culture is the bulwark against the potentially paralysing reality of death – it is an invention intended to keep death at bay. In his words, 'all human cultures can be decoded as ingenious contraptions calculated to make life with the awareness of mortality liveable' (Bauman 2006:31). Culture ascribes meaning to human life, because it consists of and points to things past, present and future that outlive the – compared to the infinity of time – rather short lifespan of the individual human being (Bauman 1992b:8). Culture is all about transcending and surviving the life of the individual mortal human being – hence one of the main purposes of culture is preservation and permanence (Bauman 1992b:9). At the end of the day, culture is about suspending and annulling the gruesome reality of death. Not just culture, however, but also society, social organisation and all the shared symbols we use and many of the ideas we collectively entertain are, in Bauman's view, seen as important ways to counter or contest the inevitability of human mortality. In this rather bizarre way, death makes life meaningful (Bauman 1992b:9). It is only because humans necessarily will and must die that death makes any sense. It is because of death that culture acquires its meaning. And it is only because humans will and must die that the prospect of or hope for immortality continues to be such a tantalising promise.

What Bauman is writing about in *Mortality, Immortality and Other Life Strategies* and elsewhere when dealing with the topics of death and immortality, without him ever specifically using this phrase to characterise his own ideas, may then be summarised by the notion of 'symbolic immortality'. Originally coined by Robert J. Lifton (1973), the concept of 'symbolic immortality' spells out how – since there is incontrovertible evidence that humans will and must necessarily die – people nevertheless still pursue and uphold beliefs in something more lasting than their own mortal lives through, for example, their biological offspring, religious beliefs, being an integral part of 'nature', or in the continuity of their identity beyond death through creative and artistic productions (see, e.g., Vigilant & Williamson 2003). Symbolic immortality is not the same as 'actual' or 'literal' immortality – symbolic immortality is rather 'immortality-by-proxy'. It is not something that is ever really achieved, it does not destroy death or remove it from life, but it is indeed something that may give us the impression that death is not meaningless and that a life lived in the shadow of inevitable death is somehow meaningful. Let us now look into how society or culture – first modern, then postmodern – according to Bauman has pursued different paths to symbolic immortality.

The modern deconstruction of death

Man has always struggled to find some meaning in death. This has perhaps especially been the case with the coming of modern, increasingly secularised and technologically advanced society (Choron 1973). In such a society, any metaphysical or religious recipes for eternal life are viewed with widespread suspicion, whereas medical prescriptions for prolonged living or technological gadgets for suspended animation seem to be in high demand. Bauman's book *Mortality, Immortality and Other Life Strategies* (1992b) provides a comprehensive and thought-provoking account of how humans have tried to deal with, defy and defeat death. As he reveals from the outset, during the modern and postmodern periods primarily two strategies have been used in order to diminish the power and presence of death in human life. As Bauman states, the first strategy, the 'modern' variant called the 'deconstruction of mortality', wanted to 'dissolve the issue of the struggle in an ever growing and never exhausted set of battles against particular diseases and other threats to life', whereas the latter strategy, the 'postmodern' type called the 'deconstruction of immortality', strove to 'substitute notoriety for historical memory, and disappearance for final – irreversible – death, and to transform life into an unstoppable, daily rehearsal of universal "mortality" of things and the effacement of opposition between the transient and the durable' (Bauman 1992b:10). Let us first look into the modern deconstruction strategy before then dealing with its postmodern counterpart.

With the advent of modern society, death – previously a powerful, natural and unavoidable presence in the everyday life of the local community – was gradually transformed. It now became the concern of medical experts and specialists, whereas in the premodern period (described by Philippe Ariès 1981 as a 'tamed death') it had primarily belonged to the realms of religion and magic. Modernity, Bauman writes, was a drive to mastery (Bauman 1992b:132): mastery over nature as well as second nature, mastery over life as well as death – it was a drive full of ambition, confidence and hope. Life was to be emancipated from the unfreedom, defeat and necessity associated with death. Human mastery over life and death was to replace mystery, rituals, traditions and communal practices of the Dark Ages. As observantly noted by Bauman, once death ceased to be 'tame', it instead became a guilty secret, quite literally like a skeleton in the cupboard that was left in the orderly, neat, functional and beautiful home that modern society had promised to build (Bauman 1992b:134). Modernity did everything in its power to keep death in the cupboard and to prevent the skeletons from ever being discovered. In the process, modernity turned 'tamed death' into 'forbidden death' (Ariès 1981).

With the gradual advancement of modernity, this development became ever more pronounced – death was now an enemy to be battled on all fronts and to be eliminated from the face of the earth. In a world increasingly relying on the self-professed ideas of order, reason and enlightenment, death became a leftover, an anomaly and an embarrassment. In Bauman's words, death became the scandal of reason and the ultimate humiliation of modern rationality (Bauman 1992b:15). The problem, however, was that the self-same modern society that declared war on death was first and foremost unable to deliver what it promised, and second, it was unable to substitute the belief systems of yore, now deemed backward and uncivilised, for anything more meaningful. Death – previously seen as a necessary gateway to the next world and an entry-point into another sphere of existence – now became a brutal stop sign, and death – previously a public affair attended by the local community – now became a thoroughly privatised ending to the equally privatised affair called 'human life' (Bauman 1992b:130). In this way, death was the defiant antithesis of everything modernity stood for – its ambitions, aspirations and dreams. Death became pathological, associated with disease and old age. Processes of medicalisation, institution-alisation and professionalisation of death were set in motion, resulting in the gradual sequestration of death and with it also of ageing and dying (Elias 1985/ 2001). To all practical intents and purposes, death was moved behind the scenes of society and far away from public view – it was now something to take place and be handled behind closed curtains and sealed doors. In the middle of the twentieth century, British sociologist Geoffrey Gorer (1955) thus described this tendency as the 'pornography of death', in which death and mourning were shrouded in prudery and relegated to the realm of the unpleasant and problem-atic. Death – like sexuality – was surrounded by taboo, denial, secrecy, privacy, silence and social distance, meaning that the dying, the dead and the bereaved were left to professionals trained in treatment, therapy and the 'managing' and 'processing' of the dead body. Moreover, so-called 'closed awareness contexts' ensured that the dying would be kept in the dark about their terminal situation and imminent death, thus making any uncomfortable talk about death unlikely and also making sure that death did not disrupt the lives of those not yet about to die (Glaser & Strauss 1965).

In modern society, to put it shortly, death is 'adiaphorized', to use one of Bauman's powerful concepts – it is merely a task to be dealt with, and emptied of any moral meaning death has now become a technical problem to be solved. If enough efforts are put into the project, death will eventually be defeated. Meanwhile, the process of dying is cut into pieces, and, as Ariès admirably put it,

> death in the hospital is no longer the occasion of a ritual ceremony, over which the dying person presides amidst his assembled relatives and friends ... Death has been dissected, cut to bits by a series of little steps, which finally makes it impossible to know which step was the real death.
> (Ariès 1974:88)

Modernity's omnipotent strategy of instituting a medical mastery over death is also evident in the development of the science of cryonics, which is but one bizarre example of a particularly modern mentality hoping that 'Faust's head can now be transplanted onto the cadaver of Frankenstein's monster' (Beilharz 2000:149). Bauman's description of the modern deconstructing strategy of mortality, trying to make it into something to be dealt with, man-aged, cured and solved and hence made 'safe', testifies to the grand illusion and wilful intervention of a modern society that felt increasingly uncomfort-able with the awareness of death.

The postmodern deconstruction of immortality

Whereas modern society and modern medicine, as we saw above, declared an all-out war on death, trying desperately to kill it off by way of scientific advances and a sequestration and institutionalisation of the dying and the dead (thereby making them to all practical intents and purposes socially invisible to a death-denying culture), the situation in postmodernity is somewhat different. Not that medical science has altogether surrendered the fight, but now the modern deconstruction of mortality is matched and supplemented by what Bauman calls the 'postmodern deconstruction of immortality'. Therefore, the postmodern deconstruction of immortality does not mean the total disappearance of its modern counterpart aimed at deconstructing mortality through medicine and technology. Rather, another dimension is now added to the continuous fight against death.

If modernity, according to Bauman, was all about creating stability, order, durability, predictability and permanence, then postmodernity (later in his writings labelled 'liquid modernity') is instead characterised by the episodic, the constantly changing and the unpredictable. If modern society was populated by 'pilgrims', each knowing and planning which route in life to follow in order to arrive at the desired destination, postmodern society is inhabited by 'nomads' and 'sensation seekers' searching here and there for some purpose, meaning and pleasure in life. In their zigzagging routes through life, they have neither itinerary nor end goal. Moreover, postmodernity inaugurates a heretofore unseen process of individualisation or privatisation that not only liberates but also puts pressure on the individual to make sense of it all by himself or herself. Accompanying this postmodern privatisation of life is a corresponding postmodern privatisation of death, meaning that it is now up to the solitary individual to fight off death and to try to counter the many different causes of death. As Bauman has stated, all deaths have causes and people do not die from mortality but from specific and individual causes such as lung cancer, blood clot, kidney failure, cardiac arrest or internal bleeding. Our society is obsessed with finding the causes of death, as if this would in the end prevent people from dying altogether. People are led to believe that if they stop smoking, if they refrain from eating unhealthy food, if they exercise and if they look after their bodies, then they will be able to defeat most of the causes of death. So although fighting death, terrible and incomprehensible death, is meaningless, fighting the numerous specific and individual causes of death turns into the very purpose of life (Bauman 1992c:5–7). So whereas death previously came at the end of life, the concern with death now fills every single living second and informs every decision made about health, exercise, eating habits, diet and so on. The postmodern world, as we shall see later, is obsessed with bodily immortality and health matters (what Bauman captures with the notions of 'self-care', 'health' and 'fitness'), which means that the battle against the multiple *causes of death* becomes a permanent and time-consuming – yet nevertheless ultimately unwinnable – state of war waged against the mortal body.

Besides this individualisation and privatisation of the fight against death, and particularly the fight against the causes of death, postmodernity also deconstructs immortality claims in another way. Whereas modern society relied on a unilinear conception of time in which 'time was an arrow with a pointer' (Bauman 1992b:162), postmodernity dissolves time – and with it also conceptions of death and immortality – into apparently disconnected moments each in their own way holding the potential for immortal bliss. In the process, the boundary between life, death and immortality is blurred. Not immortality *tomorrow* – rather, immortality *today*; immortality *now*:

> If modernity deconstructed death into a bagful of unpleasant, but tameable illnesses ... in the society that emerged at the far end of the modern era it is the majestic yet distant immortal bliss that is being deconstructed into a sackful of bigger or smaller, but always within-reach, satisfactions, so that in the ecstasy of enjoyment the likeness of the ultimate perfection may dissolve and vanish from view ... Each moment, or no moment, is immortal. Immortality is here – but not here to stay. Immortality is as transient and evanescent as the rest of things.
>
> (Bauman 1992b:164)

This postmodern deconstruction effort means that immortality, previously conceived of as the promise of a paradisiacal life lurking *after* the earthly one, is now replaced by a constant process of endless repetition, of disappearance and reappearance, coming and going, decaying and regenerating. The fundamentally episodic nature of postmodern life, with no obvious connecting points between past, present and future, supports this deconstruction of immortality and its decomposition of eternity. Immortality is no longer defined as a state or a destination to be finally arrived at – rather, it is part of death's daily dress rehearsal, in which the evanescence, ephemerality, transience and replaceability of everything ensures that death is de-dramatised and loses some of its deadly sting. This is also the main reason why notoriety and celebrity culture thrive in contemporary postmodern society. Instead of the past's reliance on achievement-based memorialisation (for kings, warlords, popes and poets) and an accompanying acceptance of the delay of gratification, everybody (even nobodies) now instantaneously wants their 15 minutes of immortal fame instead of waiting, quite possibly in vain, to discover that there is nothing to be gained or obtained after death – something to which we return later.

In such a postmodern world, it is, in a strange and roundabout way, now immortality itself that becomes mortal (Bauman 1992b:173), and in postmodern society, fighting death by reinventing immortality, as Bauman concludes, now becomes the very meaning of life, something to be worked at constantly – an endless toil unlikely ever to end, until it eventually will, despite all the efforts. Such a life lived in the shadow of death is also a life forgetful of death, because nothing lasts forever and nothing seems to disappear forever. As Bauman observed, 'the impact of death is at its most powerful (and creative)' exactly 'when death *does not appear under its own name*; in areas and times not dedicated to it' (Bauman 1992b:7, original emphasis). This is indeed an apt summary of the paradoxical postmodern approach to death and immortality.

Life strategies and survival policies

Man is, perhaps first and foremost, a *homo immortalis* – an immortality-striving creature (Jacobsen 1997). Bauman quotes Elias Canetti's insight that man is a survivor and that 'the most elementary and obvious form of success is to remain alive' (Canetti in Bauman 1992b:33). In a piece published the same year as *Mortality, Immortality and Other Life Strategies*, perhaps a spin-off from the book, Bauman elaborated in a bit more detail on the notions of 'life strategies' and 'survival policies' (Bauman 1992c). In the text entitled 'Survival as a Social Construct', he proposed an interesting typology of four types of 'life strategies' or 'policies of survival' pursued by people throughout time, all of which are also examples of different ways to obtain 'symbolic immortality'. If actual immortality is not regarded as a realistic option, the idea that people can live *forever*, then the pursuit of survival – living longer than others – becomes a viable and alluring strategy.

As the first survival policy, Bauman suggests that the notions of 'God' or 'Religion' are perhaps the oldest and most conventional form of human investment in immortality. It is a kind of immortality resting on the idea that it is through religious thoughts and deeds that transcendence, the road to true immortality, may be achieved (Bauman 1992c:13). Anyone believing in divine providence, salvation, redemption and in a heavenly paradise awaiting those who live pious lives, pray and otherwise abide by the rules of any given religion is in principle capable of obtaining this kind of immortality. Contrariwise, those not believing are destined for damnation and suffering in the sulphurous fumes of Purgatory or hell. To all practical intents and purposes, however, the ultimate proof of success of this survival strategy/policy is securely located well beyond human earthly experience. It is therefore immune to testing. This is simultaneously the main attraction as well as the Achilles heel of this survival policy – you will never know, until it is too late, whether your investment – your deeds, thoughts and indulgences – actually paid off. In times of so-called 'secularisation' (at least in the Western world), this strategy still survives but without the same attraction and widespread support as in its heyday in premodern society.

The second survival policy is called 'common cause', which collectivises any claim to immortality, while downplaying the importance of the individual's bodily/physical death. When you die, you do it for the Party, the State, the Nation or the Führer – or anyone possessing that wonderful charismatic quality of which Max Weber wrote. Bauman states that this survival policy has always been the trademark of nationalistic and totalitarian ideologies willingly sacrificing its foot soldiers as cannon fodder in trenches or on the battlefield by promising them the possibility of living on in the memory and eternal gratitude of the community. For example, the annual Nazi rally in Nuremberg ritualised the eerie reading aloud of the names of those who died in the failed beer cellar putsch in 1923. However, as Bauman emphasises, this kind of immortality is vested in causes and collectivities, not in individuals (Bauman 1992c:15). The willingness to self-sacrifice, to kill or to be killed, is exactly what fuels this survival policy. A lot of inhuman atrocities – from the Nazi Holocaust to contemporary Islamic terrorism – have been committed in the name of some higher or nobler cause that legitimises sacrificing other people. Although particularly prominent during what Eric Hobsbawm once called 'the age of extremes' in the twentieth century, this survival policy is and will remain evident in any kind of collectivist ideology promising salvation and immortalisation for the price of one's life. However, as Weber also pinpointed, charismatic leaders as well as political ideologies come and go. Hence there is really no solid guarantee that one's ultimate sacrifice will be eternally commemorated, as forgetfulness and amnesia is part and parcel of most known cultures.

As already observed by Erich Fromm in *Escape from Freedom* (1941), there are primarily two paths people may follow when trying to escape the unbearable burden of human freedom and loneliness and in order to experience some sense of security: totalitarianism on the one hand and spontaneous involvement in love relationships on the other. The third survival policy of Bauman's is exactly that of 'love', and 'love takes over where God and the Despot-with-a-mission left off' (Bauman 1992c:16). Quoting Otto Rank, Bauman states that 'bereaved by God and His secular emulators, the modern person needs *somebody*, some individual ideology of justification, to replace the declining collective ideologies' (Bauman 1992c:16). In what Bauman beautifully calls the 'trans-individual universe of two', immortality is sought in romantic and/or sexual relationships in which one experiences a sense of eternity through apparently undying love and lasting affection. In the end, however, nothing lasts forever. The success of this strategy may therefore turn out to be rather short-lived, because the 'stakes in immortality have been invested in another mortal creature, and this brute fact cannot be concealed for long by even the most passionate deification of the partner' (Bauman 1992c:17). Even sexual intimacy and excitement cannot for long bear such overblown hopes (Bauman 1992c:18). Thus, finding a 'younger model' may be one way of trying – however futilely – to keep this illusion of the immortality of love alive, but in the end it is as flawed as all the other strategies.

Finally, the policy of 'self-care', 'health' and 'fitness', which are the interchangeable terms Bauman reserves for the contemporary ultra-individualistic and body-focused survival cult. As he suggests, if achieving immortality – that is, the hope to live 'forever' – cannot be made into a realistic and realisable goal, then health can (Bauman 1992c:19). Eschatology is now transformed into technology. This survival strategy is first and foremost concerned with the body – keeping it healthy, strong, beautiful, youthful and most importantly alive. It is about longevity and about fighting old age and the bodily ravages of time. In this strategy, the gym's treadmill, a self-imposed puritan lifestyle regime and plastic surgery is substituted for the stairway leading to the pearly gates of heaven, for the bravery of death on the battlefield and for the passionate intimacy of inter-human love. Bauman states that through self-care, health and fitness, the impossible task of escaping the mortality of the human body is never confronted in its awesome totality, because it is being split into a never-ending series of concrete challenges. The big and ultimately unwinnable war is transformed into winnable battles (Bauman 1992c:18). This defence of health, this constant concern with self-care, now becomes a lifelong regime for its followers: death is battled on a daily basis through diets, exercise schemes, weight watching and functional foods – no skipping fitness class, always carefully study the listing of E-numbers and make sure to pay the doctor a regular visit. Outliving others becomes the main, nay, the only sign of one's success, and, as Bauman emphatically observes, 'survival needs constant reassurance: and the only convincing reassurance is the death of others; *not me*' (Bauman 1992c:11, original emphasis). So although self-care is supposedly an individualistic strategy, at the end of the day it still relies on the fact that others fail in their bid for survival and in this paradoxical way it is, as most other survival strategies, ultimately dependent on others.

Bauman's thought-provoking text on the 'social construction of survival' shows how the fantasies, strategies, policies and practices associated with our quest to survive and to live long lives are culturally inscribed and changing conceptions that each in their own way say a lot about the way we, in general, conduct and understand our lives in the shadow of death. Although Bauman is not intending to provide an ironclad historical chronology of the coming and going of different survival strategies, he is, nevertheless, implying that we have experienced a shift in the emphasis on and attraction of the different policies when stating that the present, postmodern habitat seems to be particularly hospitable to the promotion of the policy of self-care (Bauman 1992c:21). As Bauman shows, all these strategies and policies contain their potentials and strengths as well as their problems and weak spots. Moreover, they can be either prosocial or anti-social, making people join hands or turning them against each other and into deadly adversaries and competitors. He is especially critical of the postmodern self-care strategy, and he states that the postmodern-style strategy of survivalism is anti-social – it is a downright refusal of solidarity (Bauman 1992c:31). Bauman's piece also reads as a biting critique of the equally Faustian and Freudian idea of *causa sui* – the desperate project of Man becoming God, becoming the master of his own destiny – in order to obtain immortality (Bauman 1992c:12). And so there is very little likelihood that the incessant human quest for immortality is ever going to die out – but this does not mean that it stays the same.

The liquid-modern individualisation of the inroads to immortality

Bauman's piece on the different life strategies and survival policies ends with a brief discussion of survivalism as a stratifying factor. Survival – just as freedom – is for Bauman a social construction and a social relation, and in order for some to be able to access it, others must necessarily be denied that same right (Bauman 1992c:26–27). Bids for immortality are not – and never have been – equally distributed in society (Bauman 1992b:65). The chance of being immortalised or memorised in posterity increases quite drastically with one's social status and economic resources. The rich, powerful and the well-educated not only live longer – as a rule, they are also remembered and revered for a longer period of time after their death. Whereas previously this possibility was almost exclusively a right reserved for people belonging to the upper rungs of the social ladder (the societal elite of royalty, aristocracy and clerisy), it has now become something craved and at times also success-fully obtained by other groups as well. There is ample evidence to support the idea of a historical shift in what Norbert Elias (1987) once termed the 'We–I Balance' from the former (the 'We') towards the latter (the 'I'). The pendu-lum, as Elias proposed, has gradually swung from collectivity/community towards the individual, which is an illustrative way of explicating the process of so-called 'individualisation'. This also changes our conceptions of death and immortality. As already observed by Joseph Pieper, 'the more consciously man lives as an individual, the less he is capable of ignoring death' (Pieper 1969 quoted in Appleyard 2007:110). In an increasingly individualised world like our liquid-modern society, in which everybody is concerned with creat-ing their own self-identities and life trajectories as unique individuals, and in which they are interpellated by society as individuals (Bauman 2001), death becomes a terrible and unimaginable personal affront – something that we, qua individuals, must try to confront.

In his book *In Search of Politics* (1999a) – after leaving the topic of immortality behind for several years after the publication of *Mortality, Immortality and Other Life Strategies* – Bauman once again revisited and expanded upon it (see also Bauman 1998a, 1998b, 1999b). Drawing on the terminology of Greek-French philosopher Cornelius Castoriadis, Bauman here proposed that immortality stakes can be pursued through, respec-tively, 'heteronomous', 'heteronomous/autonomous' and 'autonomous' strategies. Elsewhere, Bauman has also labelled these different strategies 'depersonalised', 'impersonalised' and 'personalised' types of immortal-ity (Bauman 2006:36–37). Whereas the first strategy refers to, for exam-ple, the religious promise of transcendental or otherworldly salvation, the second points to the previously described collectivised 'common cause' of nationalism and totalitarianism (but also the family), and the last one describes much more individualised forms of immortality – such as the aforementioned 'self-care' strategy and the rush towards celebrity status.

Bids for immortality are no longer predominantly otherworldly or located in overarching collectivities and totalities; they are instead fast becoming thisworldly, individualised and very concrete. According to Bauman, particularly the autonomous/personalised versions today seem to be in high demand. It is now more about trying out the 'immortality experience' than about actual immortality. He thus stated that we are now witnessing an overcrowding of the bridges leading to immortality. What we see is nothing less than a 'democratisation of immortality', in which even ordinary people now start to dream of, crave and expect immortal experience and status (see Bauman 1999a:31–44; see also McKenzie n.d.). However, when everybody wants to become or feel immortal, nobody really seems to succeed in their endeavour; when everybody can lay claim to immortality, the illusion is irreparably broken and no one really becomes immortal – at least not for long. Thus, the destratification of immortality in the end seems to undermine itself.

As Bauman has noted on several occasions, today fame has been replaced by notoriety as the most promising and rewarding way to obtain the status of celebrity/immortality. Whereas previously, belonging to the select group of 'chosen ones' – the great men of history, warriors, nobilities and writers – would guarantee symbolic immortality in the shape of cultural and collective recollection in posterity, today bidding for immortality has become public property and has been thoroughly democratised – from Hollywood celebrities, sports stars and reality television participants trickling down to quite ordinary people with their thousands of posted 'selfies' on Instagram, Snapchat or Facebook, everybody is now laying claim to their 15 minutes of fame and to being 'noticed'. 'Post it online or perish' seems to be the new mantra. Publishing one's memoirs or novels is no longer reserved for truly famous or capable writers. Everybody now wants their story to be told and read. In our world of democratised immortality, so-called 'immortality brokers' (such as advertisers, marketing companies, critics, gallery owners, publishers, television programmers and talk-show hosts as well as editors of the press) are all instrumental in creating a sense of 'immortality-by-proxy' before death as well as posthumously for those not-so-known celebrities (the by now endless ranks of wannabe-celebrities but nevertheless quite ordinary people participating in the numerous television game shows and reality programmes), whom we might otherwise quickly forget all about: 'It is not the great deeds which are immortalized; the deeds become great the moment they are "immortalized" by having been forced – for a brief, elusive, but never fully erasable moment – into the centre of public attention' (Bauman 1992b:172).

Fads and fashions come and go – the same goes for wannabe-celebrities, whose images and identities are invented and groomed by an ever-expanding immortality-investment industry. One major consequence of this is that demands for immortality, now understood as a craving for 'public attention', are counter-productive and create an overload of images and identities, resulting in an overcrowding of the narrow bridges leading to immortality. We simply cannot celebrate, commemorate and remember *everybody*. As mentioned, when everybody suddenly aspires to become immortal, nobody (or only very few) will actually achieve it, since our limited collective attention and memory simply cannot cater for the endless amount of aspirations for fame, remembrance or notoriety. In this way, today's democratised immortality is more of a curse than a blessing – it is like a snake insatiably chewing away on its own tail.

Immortality, utopia and morality

As mentioned earlier, throughout his writings Bauman has always concerned himself with various unconventional topics that only rarely preoccupy other sociologists. Death and immortality have surely been some of them. Freedom is another. The Holocaust has perhaps been the most publicised. Morality is yet another, and utopia is also one of the recurring relatively obscure themes appearing in his writings (see Jacobsen 2004, 2012, 2016b).

Ever since the mid-1970s, Bauman has been writing about utopia on and off, and his book *Socialism: The Active Utopia* (1976) was an impressive attempt to salvage the reality-shattering and reality-transcending potential of utopian ideas from their often totalitarian and project-oriented connotations. Even though Bauman has written extensively about utopia, he has never ventured into presenting a vision of an actual or perfected utopian society. Inspired by the critical utopian phenomenology of Ernst Bloch, Bauman's utopia has always remained a utopia of possibility – utopia as an impulse – something not-yet-existing, and in fact something never to be put into existence for the danger of it turning into often deadly experiments in social engineering and planning (Aidnik & Jacobsen 2016). The same goes for his understanding of immortality. Immortality is *not* something to be actually achieved or realised – it is a hopeful horizon towards which humans may travel. So in many ways, Bauman's description of the twists and turns of immortality claims resembles his depiction of the historical convulsions and transformations of utopia. Most modern – or what Bauman has more specifically called 'solid-modern' – conceptions of utopia left very little room for the individual. They were primarily concerned with utopia as a collective phenomenon – for example, blueprints of an ideal island state, a radiant city, a national/ethnic enclave or a tightly knit community of equal-minded people (see, e.g., Jones & Ellis 2015). As such, solid-modern utopias were very little concerned with the individual's dreams or choices, whether they pertained to life, death or immortality.

Quite to the contrary with 'liquid modernity' (Bauman's term from the 2000 book bearing the same name now substituting the previously preferred notion of 'postmodernity'), which, as we saw above, inaugurates a heretofore unseen individualisation of human life chances and life choices (Bauman 2000, 2001). Now anything slightly associated with 'the social' or 'the collective' is regarded with ill-concealed suspicion. Liquid modernity is not concerned with creating lasting social arrangements, with grandiose collective projects or with the delay of gratification. Rather, it is all about the short term: immediate satisfaction, maximal impact and instant obsolescence are the mantras of liquid-modern life. It is about taking the waiting out of the wanting – everything must now be instantaneous. Moreover, liquid-modern society is a conspicuous consumer society populated by so-called 'sensation seekers' and consumers who spend their whole lives consuming. In liquid-modern society, in Bauman's gloomy words, we end up consuming life (Bauman 2007a). Bauman has poignantly labelled this liquid-modern utopia a 'hunting utopia' in which insatiable 'hunters' constantly search for new prey to provide their lives with meaning, prosperity and happiness (Bauman 2007b). Although admittedly a bizarre utopia

> measured by orthodox standards ... a utopia all the same, promising the same unattainable prize brandished by all utopias, namely an ultimate and radical solution to human problems past, present and future, and an ultimate and radical cure for the sorrows and pains of the human condition.
>
> (Bauman 2007b:108)

Immortality transformed or deconstructed from a destination presumably waiting somewhere on the 'other side', at the end of life, into one's daily doings now means that immortality as utopia is all of a sudden – and perhaps for the first time in history – within human reach. It is a utopia lived *in* rather than a utopia dreamed of or lived *towards*. Immortality is not just 'closer than you think' (Shostak 2003) – in Bauman's view, it is here *now*, up for grabs. However, living *inside utopia* means *living immortality every day*, which puts a lot of pressure on immortality that now has to be continuously reignited and reinvented, tried and tested. So instead of promising future reward, redemption or salvation, immortal hunting utopia may, Bauman seems to suggest, instead turn out to be something of a living hell. In his brilliant short story 'The Immortal', Argentinian writer Jorge Luis Borges (1970) once showed the dreadful repetitive character of living inside immortal utopia in which nobody dies and in which nothing can only happen once, and thus every act, every occurrence, every spoken word is just another echo of what has gone before so many times. Nothing, in Borges's words, is 'preciously precarious' as in mortal life. This is perhaps an apt characterisation of our liquid-modern immortal hunting utopia.

Our concern with death has not diminished in liquid-modern society with its instant immortal utopia – rather, according to Bauman, it now perhaps fills more than ever before: 'the memory of death is an integral part of any of life's functions. It is accorded high, perhaps the foremost authority whenever a choice is to be made in a life made of choices' (Bauman 2006:41). Liquid-modern immortal utopia inaugurates individualisation and self-concern that threatens the increasingly fragile and fissiparous human bonds and the weakened responsibility for others. And so there is, as always in Bauman's writings, also an unmistakable moral edge to his sociology of immortality. He thus unsurprisingly ended *Mortality, Immortality and Other Life Strategies* by discussing the notion of 'dying for the Other' – something anticipating his later postmodern moral writings in the mid-1990s (for more, see, e.g., Bauman 1993). In Bauman's view, the willingness to die for another person – even for a total stranger – epitomises morality. He forcefully, principally and beautifully stated the following:

> No principle or norm can claim to be moral as long as it justifies the death of anOther, let alone the murder of anOther – in the same way as no principle or norm can claim to be moral, if it implies that my responsibility for the Other stops short of the gift of my life.
>
> (Bauman 1992b:210)

In this way, sacrificing one's own life for the Other – to relinquish one's own claims to life, to prosperity, to pleasure, to happiness, to fame, to survival and not least to immortality – is seen by Bauman as the constitutive act of individuality and as the ultimate act of morality. Living a moral life is not just about 'being-with' or 'being-beside' the Other, it is about 'being-for' and even 'dying-for' an Other. Even though one's own life is indeed precious, and should never be taken or given up easily, one's responsibility for the Other, according to Bauman (who is here closely following the moral philosophy of Emmanuel Lévinas), is utterly unequivocal, unquenchable and decidedly one-sided. Thus, striving for one's own success in obtaining survival or immortality can never justify abdicating the responsibility for the Other's well-being or survival. Particularly because self-sacrifice is not on the top of the agenda in liquid-modern society (but rather 'self-care' seems to be), it is for Bauman important to stress the potential dangers – to society, to responsibility and to morality – of us now living inside a thoroughly individualised liquid-modern utopia of immortality.

Conclusion

This chapter has explored the topics of death and symbolic immortality in the writings of Zygmunt Bauman. Even though immortality is conventionally not a theme studied closely by sociologists, Bauman has shown how an understanding of immortality and so-called 'life strategies' and 'survival policies' may provide more general insights into the workings of society and into the human condition. According to Bauman, as we saw, we have passed from a solid-modern deconstruction of death in which we desperately fought all the different causes of death and relied on medical expertise to save us from mortality, to a postmodern/liquid-modern deconstruction of immortality in which we constantly rehearse and redefine the boundaries between life, death and transcendence. Nothing now seems to disappear forever and everything may be endlessly recycled and repeated.

As Bauman has insisted, his ideas do not necessarily provide a 'histori-cally correct' or exhaustive account of understandings of immortality. It is rather an attempt to sociologise and theorise the topic of immortality – to deconstruct how we conventionally imagine immortality. True, Bauman pri-marily presents a rather simplified Westernised image of how death is tack-led and immortality imagined, thereby neglecting the bountiful information on cultural practices and beliefs from other cultural contexts. Thus, it has been claimed that 'Bauman has contributed to perpetuating the dominant, Christian-centric Western discourse on our attitudes toward death and dying' (Higo 2012/2013:223). It is, however, important to appreciate that although Bauman's examples are indeed exclusively taken from an affluent contem-porary Western context, they nevertheless still point to how cultures – per-haps even every culture – each in their own way seek to deconstruct death and remove its sting from social life through various immortality-imitating practices. Obviously, Bauman is not telling the *whole* story about death and immortality, but he is showing us how they are intricately woven into many things and doings in life that we do *not* normally associate with death and immortality.

Moreover, Zygmunt Bauman's sociology has contributed greatly to under-standing some significant transformations in the way we – as a society and as individuals – conceive of and practise immortality. Although he does not directly claim any historical continuity in the various types of proposed life strategies (such as religion, common cause, love and fitness), he nevertheless insists that in contemporary liquid-modern society, immortality – like any-thing else – has been individualised. From the religious faith in a heavenly afterlife reserved for the 'righteous' and the 'chosen ones' and the 'common cause' of totalitarian or nationalist ideologies to our contemporary preoc-cupation with bodily optimisation and fitness, immortality has been trans-formed almost beyond recognition. During the process, immortality has turned from something waiting at the end of life into something to be pursued and practised – as an endless toil – on a daily basis. Just as utopia has been thoroughly individualised, so has also immortality. According to Bauman, concerns with immortality have changed from promising redemption and resolution at the end of life to now consuming every waking moment of the denizens of liquid modernity. Maybe this is a bizarre form of immortality measured by conventional standards, but nevertheless it is still immortality as it promises, however unfulfilled, to release humans from their anxieties relat-ing to the inevitability of death. In this way, immortality is never finalised or completed – it is part and parcel of a constant process of living life. Thus, immortality is not something we live towards but something we rehearse on a daily basis. Immortality is not the finishing line or a destination to be finally arrived at – it is rather the very essence of the way we live and organise our everyday lives in liquid-modern society. In this admittedly peculiar way we are now all immortal until the opposite is proven. As Bauman often quotes Robert Louis Stevenson's famous maxim: 'to travel hopefully is a better thing than to arrive' (Bauman 2004:116). Immortality, like utopia, is thus an integral part of our human-being-in-the-world. Without it, we would be unable to live meaningful lives and to carry on living with the annoying and gnawing awareness of death. A world without such immortal hopes would indeed be almost impossible to imagine.[1]

Note

1 After the completion of this chapter, Zygmunt Bauman passed away on January 9th 2017. According to newspaper reports, Bauman's second wife, Aleksandra Jasinska-Kania, in informing friends in Poland of his demise, stated that he has now gone to 'liquid eternity'. (*Daily Mail Online*, January 9 2017)

References

Aidnik, Martin & Michael Hviid Jacobsen (2016): 'Not Yet: Probing the Potentials and Problems in the Utopian Understandings of Ernst Bloch and Zygmunt Bauman', in Michael Hviid Jacobsen (ed.): *Beyond Bauman: Critical Engagements and Creative Excursions*. London: Routledge, pp. 136–162.

Appleyard, Bryan (2007): *How to Live Forever or Die Trying: On the New Immortality*. New York: Simon & Schuster.

Ariès, Philippe (1974): *Western Attitudes Toward Death from the Middle Ages to the Present*. Baltimore: Johns Hopkins University Press.

Ariès, Philippe (1981): *The Hour of Our Death*. London: Allen Lane.

Bauman, Zygmunt (1976): *Socialism: The Active Utopia*. London: Hutchinson.

Bauman, Zygmunt (1987): *Legislators and Interpreters*. Cambridge: Polity Press.

Bauman, Zygmunt (1988): *Freedom*. Milton Keynes: Open University Press.

Bauman, Zygmunt (1989): *Modernity and the Holocaust*. Cambridge: Polity Press.

Bauman, Zygmunt (1991): *Modernity and Ambivalence*. Cambridge: Polity Press.

Bauman, Zygmunt (1992a): *Intimations of Postmodernity*. London: Routledge.

Bauman, Zygmunt (1992b): *Mortality, Immortality and Other Life Strategies*. Cambridge: Polity Press.

Bauman, Zygmunt (1992c): 'Survival as a Social Construct'. *Theory, Culture & Society*, 9:1–36.

Bauman, Zygmunt (1993): *Postmodern Ethics*. Oxford: Blackwell.

Bauman, Zygmunt (1997): 'Immortality, Postmodern Version', in *Postmodernity and Its Discontents*. Cambridge: Polity Press, pp. 152–164.

Bauman, Zygmunt (1998a): 'Postmodern Adventures of Life and Death', in Graham Scrambler & Paul Higgs (eds): *Modernity, Medicine and Health: Medical Sociology Towards 2000*. London: Routledge, pp. 216–231.

Bauman, Zygmunt (1998b): 'On Art, Death and Postmodernity: And What They Do to Each Other', in Miku Hannula (ed.): *Stopping the Process? Contemporary Views on Art and Exhibition*. Helsinki: Nordic Institute for Contemporary Art, pp. 21–34.

Bauman, Zygmunt (1999a): *In Search of Politics*. Cambridge: Polity Press.

Bauman, Zygmunt (1999b): 'Immortality, Biology and Computers', in Diederik Aerts, Jan Broekaert & Ernest Mathiss (eds): *Einstein Meets Magritte: An Interdisciplinary Reflection*. Dordrecht: Kluwer Academic Publishing, pp. 241–252.

Bauman, Zygmunt (2000): *Liquid Modernity*. Cambridge: Polity Press.

Bauman, Zygmunt (2001): *The Individualized Society*. Cambridge: Polity Press.

Bauman, Zygmunt (2004): *Wasted Lives: Modernity and Its Outcasts*. Cambridge: Polity Press.

Bauman, Zygmunt (2006): 'Dread of Death', in *Liquid Fear*. Cambridge: Polity Press, pp. 22–53.

Bauman, Zygmunt (2007a): *Consuming Life*. Cambridge: Polity Press.

Bauman, Zygmunt (2007b): 'Utopia in an Age of Uncertainty', in *Liquid Times: Living in an Age of Uncertainty*. Cambridge: Polity Press, pp. 94–110.

Becker, Ernest (1973): *The Denial of Death*. New York: Free Press.

Beilharz, Peter (2000): *Dialectic of Modernity*. London: Sage Publications.

Blackshaw, Tony (2005): *Zygmunt Bauman*. London: Routledge.

Blum, Alan (2015): 'Death, Happiness and the Meaning of Life: The View from Sociology'. *Journal of Classical Sociology*, 15 (1):24–38.

Bocock, Robert (1993): 'Review of *Mortality, Immortality and Other Life Strategies*'. *History of the Human Sciences*, 6 (4):117–123.

Borges, Jorge Luis (1970): 'The Immortal', in Donald A. Yates & James E. Irby (eds): *Labyrinths: Selected Stories and Other Writings*. Harmondsworth: Penguin Books, pp. 135–149.

Choron, Jacques (1973): *Death and Modern Man*. New York: Collier Books.

Davis, Mark (2008): *Freedom and Consumerism: A Critique of Zygmunt Bauman's Sociology*. Farnham: Ashgate Publishing.

Elias, Norbert (1985/2001): *The Loneliness of the Dying*. London: Continuum.

Elias, Norbert (1987): *The Society of Individuals*. Oxford: Blackwell.

Fromm, Erich (1941): *Escape from Freedom*. New York: Farrar & Rinehart.

Glaser, Barney G. & Anselm L. Strauss (1965): *Awareness of Dying*. Chicago: Aldine.

Gorer, Geoffrey (1955): 'The Pornography of Death'. *Encounter*, October, pp. 49–52.

Higo, Masa (2012/2013): 'Surviving Death-Anxieties in Liquid Modern Times: Examining Zygmunt Bauman's Theory of Death and Dying'. *Omega: Journal of Death and Dying*, 65 (3):221–238.

Jacobsen, Michael Hviid (1997): *The Myth of Homo Immortalis: Contours of a Thanatology of Radicalized Modernity*. Unpublished Master's Thesis, Aalborg University.

Jacobsen, Michael Hviid (2004): 'From Solid Modern Utopia to Liquid Modern Anti-Utopia? Tracing the Utopian Strand in the Sociology of Zygmunt Bauman'. *Utopian Studies*, 15 (1):63–87.

Jacobsen, Michael Hviid (2011): 'Sociology, Mortality and Solidarity: An Interview with Zygmunt Bauman on Death, Dying and Immortality'. *Mortality*, 16 (4):380–393.

Jacobsen, Michael Hviid (2012): 'Liquid Modern "Utopia": Zygmunt Bauman on the Transformation of Utopia', in Michael Hviid Jacobsen & Keith Tester (eds): *Utopia: Social Theory and the Future*. Aldershot: Ashgate Publishing, pp. 69–98.

Jacobsen, Michael Hviid (ed.) (2013): *Deconstructing Death: Changing Cultures of Death, Dying, Bereavement and Care in the Nordic Countries*. Odense: University Press of Southern Denmark.

Jacobsen, Michael Hviid (2016a): ' "Spectacular Death": Proposing a New Fifth Phase to Philippe Ariès's Admirable History of Death'. *Humanities*, 5 (19). Available online at: www.mdpi.com/2076-0787/5/2/19.

Jacobsen, Michael Hviid (2016b): 'Zygmunt Bauman: An Ambivalent Utopian'. *Revue Internationale de Philosophie*, 70 (277/3):347–364.

Jacobsen, Michael Hviid & Michael C. Kearl (2014): 'Liquid Immortality: An Interview with Zygmunt Bauman'. *Mortality*, 19 (3):303–317.

Jones, Clint & Cameron Ellis (eds) (2015): *Utopia and the Individual: A Multidisciplinary Study of Humanity and Perfection*. London: Routledge.

Lifton, Robert J. (1973): 'The Sense of Immortality: On Death and the Continuity of Life'. *American Journal of Psychoanalysis*, 33:3–15.

McKenzie, Jordan (n.d.): *The Democratization of Immortality and the Problem of History: Zygmunt Bauman and Facebook*. Unpublished manuscript, available online at: www.tasa.org.au/wp-content/uploads/2008/12/McKenzie-Jordan.pdf.

Pieper, Joseph (1969): *Death and Immortality*. London: Burns & Oates.

Porter, Melinda C. (1986): *Through Parisian Eyes: Reflections on Contemporary French Arts and Culture*. Oxford: Oxford University Press.

Shostak, Stanley (2003): 'Immortality: Closer Than You Think', in Arthur B. Shostak (ed.): *Viable Utopian Ideas: Shaping a Better World*. London: M. E. Sharpe.

Smith, Dennis (1998): *Zygmunt Bauman: Prophet of Postmodernity*. Cambridge: Polity Press.

Tester, Keith (2004): *The Social Thought of Zygmunt Bauman*. London: Palgrave/Macmillan.

Toynbee, Arnold (1980): 'Various Ways in Which Human Beings Have Sought to Reconcile Themselves to the Fact of Death', in Edwin S. Shneidman (ed.): *Death: Current Perspectives*. Palo Alto, CA: Mayfield, pp. 11–34.

Vigilant, Lee G. & John B. Williamson (2003): 'Symbolic Immortality and Social Theory: The Relevance of an Underutilized Concept', in Clifton D. Bryant (ed.): *Handbook of Death and Dying, Volume 1: The Presence of Death*. Thousand Oaks, CA: Sage Publications, pp. 173–182.

Whaley, Joachim (ed.) (1981): *Mirrors of Mortality*. London: Macmillan.

4   Terror management theory

Surviving the awareness of death one way or another

Uri Lifshin, Peter J. Helm and Jeff Greenberg

Introduction

To survive is to not die. Most living organisms seem to be biologically pre-disposed to survive, by avoiding as much as possible that which could kill them. One animal, however, the human being, knows full well that it will die, sooner or later, no matter what. This means that temporary measures to avert death are not sufficient. Rather we humans must solve the problem of inevitable death by seeking ways to feel immortal. We do this largely by creating a symbolic representation of reality called *culture* that ultimately convinces us that we may somehow continue to exist after death – either literally (e.g., in heaven or through reincarnation) or symbolically (e.g., in the memory of others, through lasting impact on the world or via identification with one's social group). In this chapter, we present a psychological theory, called 'Terror Management Theory' (TMT) (see Greenberg *et al.* 1986), which describes how human beings strive to transcend death by adhering to *cultural worldviews* that provide them with hopes for symbolic and sometimes literal immortality. As this chapter unfolds, we will see how this motivation manifests itself in modern times and how it sometimes serves physical survival but in many instances may work against it. According to TMT, in order to enjoy the literal or symbolic immortality that their cultures offer, people are motivated to maintain a sense of *self-esteem* – the feeling that they are valuable members of a meaningful universe, who are living up to the standards of their cultural worldviews. Thus self-esteem embeds us psychologically in a symbolic reality in which physical death is not the end of us. TMT also describes how, in order to gain a protective sense of death transcendence, people are motivated to maintain *close relationships* that help perpetuate their symbolic (and genetic) legacy, and to *deny their creature-like nature* in order to feel superior to and different from all the other (meaningless and mortal) animals.

We begin by briefly presenting the existential and psychodynamic roots of TMT and its basic premises. We then review empirical evidence from the TMT literature exemplifying the different ways in which humans attempt to gain a sense of immortality, and how these efforts shape fundamental aspects of human social behavior. Finally, we consider how although sometimes TMT strategies may promote human survival, by fostering positive values, norms and positive social relationships, they might often undermine it and actually promote death and destruction.

The roots of Terror Management Theory

Terror Management Theory (Greenberg *et al.* 1986) is based on the writings of American cultural anthropologist Ernest Becker (1971, 1973, 1975). In his works, Becker attempted to create a synthesis of the 'science of man', while leaning heavily on both psychodynamic theory and existential philosophy. Becker argued that human beings are hunted by the fear of death like no other animal. Because unlike most (if not all) other animals, humans are aware of themselves, and also have the cognitive ability to realize that they are *mortal* and that they are going to die in the future. To cope with this situation, humans subscribe to beliefs and associate themselves with socio-cultural structures that convince them that they may last beyond death. They become a part of a nation, a religion, a group, something larger and more powerful than themselves. They adhere to cultural worldviews that give them a sense of meaning and value and help them feel like they transcend their limited, creature-like, mortal selves.

Becker (e.g., 1971) points out that unlike most other animals, human beings are born as completely helpless and dependent beings. When babies are alone or in danger, they experience anxiety and cry out to their parents for help. The love from their caregivers soothes this anxiety and grants them feelings of security. As the children grow older, they learn that in order to get this sense of protection from their parents, they sometimes need to behave in ways that match their parents' expectations: they need to be good boys and girls. This, according to Becker, is the source of self-esteem. 'Am I a good boy/girl?' 'Do I deserve the protection of my (omnipotent) parent?' When children grow up, and their cognitive ability develops, they come to realize that both they and their parents are *mortal* and that they are going to die. Now they need something greater than their parents for psychological protection. They need something that is not subjected to the reality of death, like deities, leaders or nations. But, in order to gain protection from these cultural structures, children now need to live up to new expectations, norms and values; they need to be good citizens or devoted religious followers. They need to live up to the standards of their cultural worldviews; they need to feel like the heroes in the drama of their life; they need to have self-esteem.

Thus, unlike Sigmund Freud (e.g., 1924/1961), who argued that the development of the superego and the socialization process are responses to forbidden desires to have sex with their opposite-sex parent (i.e., the resolution of the Oedipus complex), Becker points out that children's socialization and the development of a superego are actually responses to the development of the awareness of danger and death. They learn that by living up to internalized standards of value, they are loved and protected. In this way, self-esteem serves as a buffer against anxiety.

Empirical support for Terror Management Theory

Building on Becker's insights, TMT asserts that much of human behavior is aimed at 'solving' the problem of mortality. TMT researchers argued that Becker's analysis provides the most compelling explanation of *why people need self-esteem* and *why people from different cultures have a hard time coexisting peacefully*. According to TMT, to avoid the potentially threatening awareness of mortality, people construct and maintain *cultural worldviews*, which buffer against anxiety by 'providing standards of value that are derived from that meaningful conception of reality and by promising protection and death transcendence to those who meet those standards of value' (Greenberg *et al*. 1997:65). Self-esteem is the degree to which one lives up to the standards of one's cultural worldviews and is therefore worthy of the literal or symbolic sense of immortality that the worldview offers. For example, if one believes in the Christian worldview, then one must be a devoted Christian to actually gain God's protection and ultimately to get to heaven. At its core, self-esteem is the sense that one is a person of enduring value in a meaningful world, rather than a mere material creature fated only to perish upon death.

Being experimental social psychologists, Jeff Greenberg, Sheldon Solomon and Tom Pyszczynski began testing their theory empirically. In the following pages we describe the main hypotheses testing TMT, and focus on the different ways in which people attempt to transcend death and feel immortal.

The mortality salience hypothesis

The first test of TMT was the mortality salience (MS) hypothesis, which states that 'if a psychological structure provides protection against the potential for terror engendered by knowledge of mortality, then reminding people of their mortality should increase their need for protection provided by that structure' (Greenberg *et al*. 1997:72). In the first test of this hypothesis, Abram Rosenblatt *et al*. (1989) reminded participants of their mortality (or not) and then measured how much they uphold their cultural worldviews. In one study, municipal judges who were reminded of death set a much higher bail to a worldview-violating target – a prostitute. In another study, this effect was replicated only among those who found prostitution to be immoral. The MS hypothesis was further supported in hundreds of experiments from countries across the globe (for integrative reviews, see Greenberg *et al*. 2014; Solomon *et al*. 2015). These studies show that after MS, participants are more likely to defend and uphold their cultural worldviews (e.g., Greenberg *et al*. 1990; Greenberg *et al*. 1995); behave aggressively towards those who hold conflicting worldviews (e.g., McGregor *et al*. 1998; Pyszczynski *et al*. 2006); strive toward enhancing their self-esteem by living up to standards of cultural worldviews, like donating money to charity (e.g., Hirschberger *et al*. 2008; Jonas *et al*. 2002); or attempt to directly establish their symbolic immortality by attaining fame or having offspring (e.g., Greenberg *et al*. 2010; Wisman & Goldenberg 2005).

The fact that the MS hypothesis received wide empirical support suggests that *death*-related concerns motivate people to uphold and defend their cultural worldviews and enhance their self-esteem. Many studies continually use the MS hypothesis to test whether different domains of human thought and behavior are related to terror management needs. Although the 'classic' MS prime asked participants to consciously think about their mortality, MS can be induced in a variety of ways, including subliminal or subtle priming of death-related words; exposure to T-shirts, flyers or banners that include death-related images like skulls; footage of death, terrorism or natural disasters; proximity to cemeteries, and more (e.g., Greenberg *et al.* 2014; Pyszczynski *et al.* 2003). Studies have also found that experiencing the death of others can also increase terror management responses in the form of ingroup identification (e.g., Lifshin, Helm *et al.* 2015a). Importantly, in the vast majority of published studies these effects have been found to be unique to thinking about death, rather than other negative control topics, such as thinking about experiencing intense and uncontrollable pain, life being meaninglessness, an exam failure, temporal discontinuity, general anxieties, experiencing uncertainty, public speaking, expectancy violations, social exclusion, and more (e.g., Greenberg *et al.* 2014; Pyszczynski, Greenberg *et al.* 2006).

The anxiety buffer hypothesis

The second hypothesis, which tested TMT and its formulation of self-esteem, is the anxiety buffer hypothesis. This hypothesis states that 'if a psychological structure [e.g., self-esteem and cultural worldviews] provides protection against anxiety, then augmenting that structure should reduce anxiety in response to subsequent threat' (Greenberg *et al.* 1997:72). If self-esteem acts as a buffer against death-related concerns, people with high (or elevated) self-esteem should be protected from the typical MS responses. In support for this hypothesis, Greenberg *et al.* (1992) found that experimentally elevating participants' sense of self-esteem, by giving bogus personality feedback that was very positive (compared to neutral), reduced subsequent self-reported anxiety and physiological arousal in response to viewing highly disturbing death-related footage or to anticipating painful electric shocks. Furthermore, subsequent studies showed that enhancing participants' self-esteem or validating their cultural worldviews can reduce MS-related defensiveness like cultural worldview defense or self-esteem striving (e.g., Dechesne *et al.* 2003; Harmon-Jones *et al.* 1997).

The death thought accessibility hypothesis

The third hypothesis testing TMT is the death thought accessibility (DTA) hypothesis, according to which, if psychological structures (e.g., self-esteem and cultural worldviews) provide protection against the thought of death, then undermining them should increase the accessibility of death-related thoughts (e.g., Schimel *et al.* 2007). In support of this hypothesis, studies have found that threatening people's sense of self-esteem or undermining the validity of their cultural worldviews increases the accessibility of death-related thoughts in consciousness (Hayes *et al.* 2008; Schimel *et al.* 2007; for a review, see Hayes *et al.* 2010).

Terror management strategies for immortality

Although TMT explains very complex socio-cultural dynamics, it could also be boiled down to a more simple equation: to cope with the problem of death, people convince themselves that they are somehow immortal. This immortality can take a variety of shapes. Some forms of immortality are defined as *literal immortality beliefs*: for example, the belief that one would continue to exist in heaven or be reincarnated as a different person. Other forms of belief are considered *symbolic immortality beliefs*. These include being remembered by future generations or being a part of a culture that persists after death (e.g., Lifton 1979). Most if not all of these ideas are generated from the cultural worldviews, although some are more concerned with personal relationships. In the next section we present research in the framework of TMT, which demonstrates the ways in which cultural worldviews, personal relationships and disassociation from animals can grant people a sense of immortality.

Immortality via cultural self-enhancement

Perhaps the most obvious source of both literal and symbolic immortality beliefs is through cultural self-enhancement. All human cultures promise their followers some form of immortality: religious beliefs offer people literal immortality beliefs, and nationalism provides them with symbolic immortality beliefs (e.g., Lifton 1968). Studies using the anxiety buffer hypothesis found that high investment in both types of immortality beliefs helps to reduce death-related concerns. For example, Eva Jonas and Peter Fischer (2006) showed that participants who are high on intrinsic religiosity exhibit less defensiveness after MS primes. Victor Florian and Mario Mikulincer (1998) found that people with a high sense of symbolic immortality report less fear of death, as well as less defensiveness after a MS prime.

One problem with cultural self-enhancement, however, is that often different cultural worldviews are incompatible with one another. If one person believes that there is only one God, who created the universe in seven days, and another person believes that the universe was created not by God but by some random turn of events, then they cannot both be right. Because these beliefs serve as anxiety buffers, maintaining their validity is of critical importance. Thus each person is highly motivated to defend their own cultural beliefs, especially when death is salient, and people need to bring these beliefs online to feel secure. Oftentimes, validating one's worldview requires eliminating competing worldviews, even at the cost of violence and aggression. Studies in the framework of TMT have directly supported this analysis by showing that after MS people are more likely to aggress against those with different cultural worldviews. Holly McGregor *et al.* (1998) showed that after thinking about death, liberal and conservative participants gave twice the amount of hot sauce to a participant with a different political worldview compared to the amount of hot sauce allocated by participants who did not think about death. Pyszczynski *et al.* (2006) found that conservative American participants thinking about death were more likely to support extreme military actions against terrorists compared to participants who did not think about death, even if many innocent civilians would be killed. In another experiment, Iranian students thinking about death were more supportive toward martyr-dom attacks on American targets, compared to Iranian students who were not thinking about death. This evidence demonstrates that many of the instances of prejudice and intercultural violence that continually occur throughout human history are in fact related to the need to suppress the terror of death.

Despite the rather pessimistic reality of wars and conflict, studies have also demonstrated that more tolerant and peaceful cultural values and norms may reverse this effect and promote more peaceful attitudes in response to MS (Greenberg, Simon *et al.* 1992; Jonas *et al.* 2008; Pyszczynski, Abdollahi *et al.* 2006). Furthermore, perceiving people of different cultures as more similar by thinking about shared human experiences (Motyl *et al.* 2011), or by focusing on common threats like global warming, may reduce intercultural conflicts and promote peace (Pyszczynski *et al.* 2012).

Some types of cultural self-enhancement may depend less on specific cul-tural beliefs that may vary across cultures. People can gain a sense of self-esteem through being prosocial (e.g., Jonas *et al.* 2002), becoming famous (e.g., Greenberg *et al.* 2010), investing in their work (Yaakobi 2015), in art (e.g., Landau *et al.* 2010) or in sports (Zestcott *et al.* 2016). Uri Lifshin, Peter Helm, Melissa Soenke and Jeff Greenberg (2015c) showed that people can even get a sense of symbolic immortality through creating symbolic representations of themselves online in a type of 'digital immortality' (e.g., via Facebook). These researchers hypothesized that since Facebook accounts can remain active after people die, it may provide people with a sense of symbolic immortality and help terror management. In support of this idea, the researchers found that experiencing the death of close others or just thinking about death can cause more positive attitudes toward Facebook, and that threatening Facebook's ability to provide symbolic continuity after death (by telling participants that all inactive accounts would be deleted) enhances DTA.

Immortality via inter-personal relationships

Another way in which people can get a sense of symbolic immortality is through close personal relationships (romantic and non-romantic) and feel-ings of attachment security (e.g., Hart *et al.* 2005; Mikulincer *et al.* 2003).

Personal relationships can grant people a sense of security and immortality in a number of ways. They can provide people a sense of meaning, attachment security, belonging, self-esteem and the sense that they have a generative effect on others.

Much of the research focusing on the capacity of close relationships to buffer against existential concerns has focused on the role of romantic and peer relationships. Victor Florian *et al.* (2002) found that participants who thought about death reported higher levels of romantic commitment compared to participants in control conditions. In a second experiment, thinking about romantic commitment reduced the effects of MS on judgments of worldview violators. In a third experiment, priming relational insecurity via separation primes increased DTA, compared to priming academic hardship or priming a neutral control condition. These studies demonstrate how committed romantic relationships can help people feel secure in the shadow of death. Other studies have built on these insights to further understand dynamics in romantic relationships. For example, studies found that thinking about death causes participants to have exaggerated perceptions of how positively their partners view them (Cox & Arndt 2012), fosters forgiveness in response to a partner's unkindness (Van Tongeren *et al.* 2013) and causes greater partner jealously and distress after reading vignettes describing physical and emotional infidelity (Hackathorn & Cornell 2015).

There is also evidence that parental attachment figures play a role in managing existential concerns in adulthood. Studies found that death-related primes increase accessibility of attachment constructs, which indicates that attachment needs serve a defensive function against mortality-related concerns (Mikulincer *et al.* 2002). Cathy Cox *et al.* (2008) tested this idea by asking participants to recall instances of their parents after MS and found that DTA and worldview defense decreased while feelings of self-worth increased. Further, MS inductions resulted in greater ease of recalling positive interactions with parents and increased desire for proximity to parents among insecure individuals. Interestingly, for secure individuals, MS led to greater desire for proximity to romantic partners, suggesting that when attachment needs are adequately met, one is able to successfully transfer one's relational needs from parents to peer relationships.

Aside from granting feelings of belonging, self-esteem and attachment security (e.g., Mikulincer *et al.* 2003), romantic relationships also offer a path to immortality through one's progeny. Studies in the framework of TMT found death reminders increase desire for offspring and objections to birth control strategies (Wisman & Goldenberg 2005; Zhou *et al.* 2009). By producing children, parental legacy and genetic material may transcend individual existence. Furthermore, studies also demonstrated how parenting can help cope with death-related concerns. Erez Yaakobi *et al.* (2014) found that MS increased accessibility of parental cognitions relative to control primes and that activating parenthood-related cognitions reduced DTA after MS. They also found that highlighting obstacles to parenthood leads to an increase in DTA, suggesting that the possibility of achieving immortality via children and parenthood serves terror management functions.

Immortality via disassociation from the body and from animals

While human beings attempt to create their different routes to immortality, they are always pulled back down by the facts of life: humans, like all other animals, live in a *body* that gets old, dies and decays. Thus, to feel truly emancipated from death-related concerns people need to be able to disassociate themselves from the rest of the animals, as well as from their own creature-like body (e.g., Becker 1971, 1975; Goldenberg *et al.* 2000). In one of the first empirical tests for this idea, Goldenberg *et al.* (2001) found that after thinking about death, participants reported more disgust toward animals and examples of human creatureliness (e.g., human body products), and preferred essays that depict humans as distinctly different from animals over essays that portray humans as similar to animals. Goldenberg *et al.* (2002) found that priming human–animal similarity and thinking about the physical (but not romantic) aspects of sex increase DTA in consciousness, and that after priming human–animal similarity (compared to human–animal differences) MS led participants to be less attracted to the physical aspects of sex. Goldenberg *et al.* (2006) found that thinking about death led participants high in neuroticism to withdraw from physical sensation and spend less time in a foot-massager. After thinking about death, humans are motivated to disassociate for their physical animal-like bodies, by disassociation as well as by objectification (for a review, see Goldenberg 2012).

But humans do not just want to disassociate from animals. To convince ourselves that we do not share the same mortal fate as animals, we humans need to feel that we are *better* than other animals (e.g., Becker 1975; Marino & Mountain 2015). In support of this idea, studies conducted in the framework of TMT show that death primes cause more negative attitudes toward animals (Beatson & Halloran 2007), and even lead participants to be more supportive of the killing of animals (Lifshin, Greenberg, Zestcott & Sullivan 2016). These studies and others found that these effects are not moderated by the participants' gender, pre-existing attitudes toward the cause of animal rights or other religious or political worldviews. In another demonstration of the human need to feel superior to animals, Soenke *et al.* (in press) found that after MS people tend to disagree more with the idea that dolphins could be smarter than humans, and that thinking that dolphins are more intelligent than humans increases DTA. By maintaining our superiority over other animals we can delude ourselves that we will not eventually become food for worms, as they do.

Studies in the framework of TMT have also extended this reasoning to understand people's environmental concerns. If nature can remind us of our mortality (as opposed to human enterprise), then thinking about death should make people dislike wild environments. In support of this idea, studies found that thinking about death makes people view natural wilderness more negatively than a cultivated garden (Koole & Van den Berg 2005). Other studies have shown that this effect can extend to environmental concerns: for people who were initially low on environmental concerns, thinking about death can enhance negative attitudes toward nature and reduce environmental concerns, while the opposite effect can occur for people highly invested in pro-environmental values (Fritsche *et al.* 2010; Vess & Arndt 2008). Thus, at least in the case of environmental concerns, existential concerns may be beneficial, depending on the person's values, as well as the momentary salience of specific pro-self or prosocial norms (e.g., Jonas *et al.* 2008).

Survival versus immortality

Terror management trajectories may often be good for life and can promote survival by promoting close relationships (e.g., Mikulincer *et al.* 2003) and increasing ingroup cohesiveness (e.g., Castano 2004) or prosocial behavior (e.g., Hirschberger *et al.* 2008; Jonas *et al.* 2002; for a review of the positive side of terror management, see Vail *et al.* 2012). Ironically, however, oftentimes people's attempts to avoid death could in fact promote the death of themselves and of people around them (e.g., Becker 1975; Pyszczynski *et al.* 2008).

The most obvious example of this is the finding that in order to defend their cultural worldviews, after thinking about death people are more willing to go to war and die for their cause (e.g., Pyszczynski *et al.* 2006), even when they are fighting for a lost cause (e.g., Hirschberger & Ein-Dor 2006). In a recent study demonstrating this, Gilad Hirschberger *et al.* (2015) found that in the context of intercultural conflicts, MS primes lead participants to prefer a justice-oriented mindset over a cost–benefit utility mindset, and the justice mindset was associated with more support for military violence. In Study 1, Israeli participants assigned to an MS or a control condition read about a Hamas attack on Israel with either no casualties or many casualties. Then the researchers measured justice and utility motivations and support for military violence against the Hamas. As hypothesized, the effect of MS on support for political violence was mediated by a desire for justice, but not by a cost–benefit utility mindset. In a subsequent study, the researchers replicated these results in regard to support for a pre-emptive military strike on Iran's nuclear facilities. These findings suggest that when existential concerns are salient, people may support violent solutions to political conflicts for emotional rather than rational reasons. Indeed, studies in the framework of TMT show that thinking about death and terrorism makes people support charismatic leaders who use 'us or them' rhetoric and promise justice and the defeat of all evil (e.g., Landau *et al.* 2004).

Another instance where striving for immortality conflicts with survival is when people deny themselves medical treatment, either because it directly conflicts with their cultural worldviews (e.g., in the case of people believing that only God can or should cure them), or because they want to deny (at least implicitly) the fact that their bodies are fragile. Matthew Vess *et al.* (2009)

found that after thinking about death, individuals high on religious fundamentalism were more supportive of using prayer than medical-based intervention, and were more likely to refuse medical treatment based on religious
beliefs in order to cure diseases. Thus, a person's desire to achieve a sense of
literal immortality and need to uphold religious beliefs may directly conflict
with actions that may increase survival. One rather extreme example of this is
the mass murder-suicide committed by hundreds of members of the Peoples
Temple in the 1978 'Jonestown Massacre', as cult members killed themselves
and their children because they believed Reverend Jim Jones's promise of literal immortality.

In a related vein, we have conducted studies investigating people's support for developing technologies that would slow down the aging process
and eventually enable indefinite life extension (ILE). Some scientists and
scholars are attempting to promote this possibility by harnessing advances
in cellular biology and cybernetics to supplement the human body (e.g., de
Grey & Rae 2007). ILE technologies could also be helpful in curing many
kinds of diseases. However, many people object to the mere idea of ILE,
since it may conflict with religious beliefs and the idea of an afterlife. If people believe that they are going to reunite with their families in heaven, they
might not want to extend their life here on earth. To test this idea we (Lifshin,
Greenberg, Soenke *et al.* in press) had participants who were high and low in
religiosity think about death or about an aversive control topic and then read
a bogus scientific article claiming either that ILE is possible in our lifetime
(at least for our 19-year-old participants), or that ILE is not possible within
our lifetime. We then measured the degree to which participants believed in
the afterlife, and subsequently their support for ILE (all these materials were
presented as part of an elaborate cover story so that participants would not
be aware of our hypothesis). The results showed that for participants who
were low in religiosity, reading that ILE is possible and thinking about death
both caused a decrease in belief in the afterlife, and this decrease in afterlife
belief was related to more positive attitudes toward ILE. Thus people would
only support these technologies if they do not conflict with their afterlife
beliefs. In another correlational study we (Lifshin, Helm *et al.* 2015b) found
in three large samples that while men believe in the afterlife less than women,
they have more positive attitudes toward ILE than women do.

Terror management needs might also directly steer individuals away from
making healthy decisions in a more implicit way. According to the terror management health model (Goldenberg & Arndt 2008), while consciously thinking about death can promote more healthy behavior, after a delay period,
when thoughts of death become subconscious, people might prefer behaviors
that increase self-esteem over behaviors that keep the corporal body salient
and promote actual survival (for a discussion of the dual process of terror
management, in terms of proximal and distal responses to thinking about
death, see Pyszczynski *et al.* 1999). In support of this model, Routledge *et al.*
(2004) found that when concerns about death were the focus of attention,

participants reported more intentions to protect themselves from sun exposure (e.g., by using sunscreen). In contrast, when thoughts about death were outside the focus of attention, participants who valued being tanned showed decreased interest in sun protection. In another experiment, after MS, participants led to associate a tan with attractiveness increased interest in tanning products and services. In yet another set of studies, Jamie Goldenberg *et al.* (2008) found that after MS, reminders of human creatureliness (our similarity to other animals) reduced women's intentions to conduct breast cancer self-examinations, and that thinking about human creatureliness caused women to perform shorter self-examinations compared to when human uniqueness (disassociation from animals) was primed.

Understanding this dynamic can help promote more healthy behaviors. Jamie Arndt *et al.* (2003) found that thinking about death can make participants value fitness more if they also perceive fitness as a source of self-esteem. Cox *et al.* (2009) found that after thinking about death, female college students who were led to think that tanning is more fashionable reported higher intentions to tan, while participants who were led to think that tanning is not fashionable reported lower intentions to tan. In a second study, after MS, female beach-goers preferred higher sun protection sunscreen after reading an article about the attractiveness of paler skin tones.

The human need to transcend death can also manifest itself in other dangerous or risky behaviors, which may promote people's sense of self-esteem or alleviate their existential concerns. Orit Taubman-Ben-Ari *et al.* (1999) found that thinking about death causes men to engage in more reckless driving if they value driving as a source of self-esteem. Other studies show that thinking about death can cause people to engage in more risky decision making in gambling (Hart *et al.* 2010), to consume more psychoactive drugs like alcohol or cannabis (Ein-Dor *et al.* 2014; Nagar & Rabinovitz 2015) or to smoke more tobacco (e.g., Arndt *et al.* 2013).

Conclusion

Based on the interdisciplinary writing of Ernest Becker (e.g., 1973), Terror Management Theory (TMT) suggests that much of human behavior stems from the need to avoid the potentially anxiety-provoking awareness of mortality. The theory suggests that part of the reason that humans create, maintain, defend and adhere to cultural worldviews is to gain a sense of protection from death, by feeling as if they are valuable members in a meaningful universe that may transcend death either literally or symbolically. The theory has been widely supported by a variety of complementary hypotheses (e.g., the MS, the anxiety buffer and the DTA hypotheses) that show that thinking about death motivates people to protect their cultural worldviews and to try to attain self-esteem by living up to their standards. Having valid cultural worldviews, self-esteem and close relationships allow people to gain a sense of death transcendence and gain psychological security. TMT helps explain the psychological functions of self-esteem and cultural worldviews.

As we have shown in this chapter many findings, in the framework of TMT suggest that thinking about death can eventually promote human survival: for example, when it promotes prosocial behavior (e.g., Jonas *et al.* 2002) or close relationships (e.g., Florian *et al.* 2002). Furthermore, maintaining a sense of self-esteem and hopes for immortality are sometimes necessary for our normal and anxiety-free functioning (e.g., Pyszczynski & Kesebir 2011). However, oftentimes people's need to attain a sense of immortality can lead to negative consequences for themselves and for others who are different from them (e.g., Goldenberg *et al.* 2008; Pyszczynski *et al.* 2006; Taubman-Ben-Ari *et al.* 1999; Vess *et al.* 2009), jeopardizing current and future human survival. As Becker put it in his final book *Escape from Evil*:

> The thing that makes man the most devastating animal that has ever stuck his neck up into the sky is that he wants a stature and destiny that is impossible for an animal; He wants an earth that is not an earth but a heaven, and the price for this kind of fantastic ambition is to make the earth an even more eager graveyard than it naturally is.

(Becker 1975:96)

Following Becker, TMT provides a realistic view of the human condition. By better understanding the human condition, we could perhaps steer somewhat away from attempting to achieve a sense of immortality, and instead focus our limited lifetime on promoting the actual survival and well-being of ourselves and our fellow animals. Although future technological developments may eventually enhance human survivalism in different ways, and perhaps bring humans that much closer to achieving actual biological immortality, until that happens, perhaps the best we can do is to make sure that we promote our *actual* survival, and not spill the glass that is already half full.

References

Arndt, Jamie, Jeff Schimel & Jamie Goldenberg (2003): 'Death Can Be Good for Your Health: Fitness Intentions as a Proximal and Distal Defense against Mortality Salience'. *Journal of Applied Social Psychology*, 33 (8):1726–1746.

Arndt, Jamie, Kenneth Vail, Cathy Cox, Jamie Goldenberg, Thomas Piasecki & Frederick Gibbons (2013): 'The Interactive Effect of Mortality Reminders and Tobacco Craving on Smoking Topography'. *Health Psychology*, 32 (5):525–532.

Beatson, Ruth & Michael Halloran (2007): 'Humans Rule! The Effects of Creatureliness Reminders, Mortality Salience and Self-Esteem on Attitudes towards Animals'. *British Journal of Social Psychology*, 46 (3):619–632.

Becker, Ernest (1971): *The Birth and Death of Meaning* (2nd edn). New York: Free Press.

Becker, Ernest (1973): *The Denial of Death*. New York: Free Press.

Becker, Ernest (1975): *Escape from Evil*. New York: Free Press.

Castano, Emanuele (2004): 'In Case of Death, Cling to the Ingroup'. *European Journal of Social Psychology*, 34 (4):375–384.

Cox, Cathy & Jamie Arndt (2012): 'How Sweet It Is to Be Loved by You: The Role of Perceived Regard in the Terror Management of Close Relationships'. *Journal of Personality and Social Psychology*, 102 (3):616–632.

Cox, Cathy, Jamie Arndt, Tom Pyszczynski, Jeff Greenberg, Adbolhossein Abdollahi & Sheldon Solomon (2008): 'Terror Management and Adults' Attachment to Their Parents: The Safe Haven Remains'. *Journal of Personality and Social Psychology*, 94 (4):696–717.

Cox, Cathy, Douglas Cooper, Matthew Vess, Jamie Arndt, Jamie Goldenberg & Clay Routledge (2009): 'Bronze Is Beautiful but Pale Can Be Pretty: The Effects of Appearance Standards and Mortality Salience on Sun-Tanning Outcomes'. *Health Psychology*, 28 (6):746–752.

Dechesne, Mark, Tom Pyszczynski, Jamie Arndt, Sean Ransom, Kennon Sheldon, Ad van Knippenberg & Jaques Janssen (2003): 'Literal and Symbolic Immortality: The Effect of Evidence of Literal Immortality on Self-Esteem Striving in Response to Mortality Salience'. *Journal of Personality and Social Psychology*, 84 (4):722–737.

De Grey, Aubrey & Michael Rae (2007): *Ending Aging: The Rejuvenation Breakthroughs That Could Reverse Aging in Our Lifetime*. New York: St. Martin's Press.

Ein-Dor, Tsachi, Gilad Hirschberger, Adi Perry, Noga Levin, Roi Cohen, Hadar Horesh & Elad Rothschild (2014): 'Implicit Death Primes Increase Alcohol Consumption'. *Health Psychology*, 33 (7):748–751.

Florian, Victor & Mario Mikulincer (1998): 'Symbolic Immortality and the Management of the Terror of Death'. *Journal of Personality and Social Psychology*, 74 (3):725–734.

Florian, Victor, Mario Mikulincer & Gilad Hirschberger (2002): 'The Anxiety-Buffering Function of Close Relationships: Evidence That Relationship Commitment Acts as a Terror Management Mechanism'. *Journal of Personality and Social Psychology*, 82 (4):527–542.

Freud, Sigmund (1924/1961): 'The Dissolution of the Oedipus Complex', in James Strachey (ed.): *The Standard Edition of the Complete Psychological Works of Sigmund Freud, Volume 19*. London: Hogarth Press, pp. 171–180.

Fritsche, Immo, Eva Jonas, Daniela N. Kayser & Nicolas Koranyi (2010): 'Existential Threat and Compliance with Pro-Environmental Norms'. *Journal of Environmental Psychology*, 30 (1):67–79.

Goldenberg, Jamie (2012): 'A Body of Terror: Denial of Death and the Creaturely Body', in Phillip Shaver & Mario Mikulincer (eds): *Meaning, Mortality and Choice: The Social Psychology of Existential Concerns*. Washington, DC: American Psychological Association, pp. 93–110.

Goldenberg, Jamie & Jamie Arndt (2008): 'The Implications of Death for Health: A Terror Management Health Model for Behavioral Health Promotion'. *Psychological Review*, 115 (4):1032–1053.

Goldenberg, Jamie, Jamie Arndt, Joshua Hart & Clay Routledge (2008): 'Uncovering an Existential Barrier to Breast Self-Exam Behavior'. *Journal of Experimental Social Psychology*, 44 (2):260–274.

Goldenberg, Jamie, Cathy Cox, Tom Pyszczynski, Jeff Greenberg & Sheldon Solomon (2002): 'Understanding Human Ambivalence about Sex: The Effects of Stripping Sex of Meaning'. *Journal of Sex Research*, 39 (4):310–320.

Goldenberg, Jamie, Joshua Hart, Tom Pyszczynski, Gwendolyn Warnica, Mark Landau & Lisa Thomas (2006): 'Ambivalence toward the Body: Death, Neuroticism and the Flight from Physical Sensation'. *Personality and Social Psychology Bulletin*, 32 (9):1264–1277.

Goldenberg, Jamie, Tom Pyszczynski, Jeff Greenberg & Sheldon Solomon (2000): 'Fleeing the Body: A Terror Management Perspective on the Problem of Human Corporeality'. *Psychology and Social Psychology Review*, 4 (3):200–218.

Goldenberg, Jamie, Tom Pyszczynski, Jeff Greenberg, Sheldon Solomon, Benjamin Kluck & Robin Cornwell (2001): 'I Am Not an Animal: Mortality Salience, Disgust and the Denial of Human Creatureliness'. *Journal of Experimental Psychology*, 130 (3):427–435.

Greenberg, Jeff, Spee Kosloff, Sheldon Solomon, Florette Cohen & Mark Landau (2010): 'Toward Understanding the Fame Game: The Effect of Mortality Salience on the Appeal of Fame'. *Self and Identity*, 9 (1):1–18.

Greenberg, Jeff, Jonathan Porteus, Linda Simon, Tom Pyszczynski & Sheldon Solomon (1995): 'Evidence of a Terror Management Function of Cultural Icons: The Effects of Mortality Salience on the Inappropriate Use of Cherished Cultural Symbols'. *Personality and Social Psychology Bulletin*, 21 (11):1221–1228.

Greenberg, Jeff, Tom Pyszczynski & Sheldon Solomon (1986): 'The Causes and Consequences of a Need for Self-Esteem: A Terror Management Theory', in Roy F. Baumeister (ed.): *Public Self and Private Self*. New York: Springer, pp. 189–212.

Greenberg, Jeff, Tom Pyszczynski, Sheldon Solomon, Abram Rosenblatt, Mitchell Veeder, Shari Kirkland & Deborah Lyon (1990): 'Evidence for Terror Management Theory II: The Effects of Mortality Salience on Reactions to Those Who Threaten or Bolster the Cultural Worldview'. *Journal of Personality and Social Psychology*, 58 (2):308–318.

Greenberg, Jeff, Tom Pyszczynski & Sheldon Solomon (1997): 'Terror Management Theory of Self-Esteem and Cultural Worldviews: Empirical Assessments and Conceptual Refinements', in Mark P. Zanna (ed.): *Advances in Experimental Social Psychology, Volume 29*. San Diego, CA: Academic Press, pp. 61–141.

Greenberg, Jeff, Linda Simon, Tom Pyszczynski, Sheldon Solomon & Dan Chatel (1992): 'Terror Management and Tolerance: Does Mortality Salience Always Intensify Negative Reactions to Others Who Threaten One's Worldview?'. *Journal of Personality and Social Psychology*, 63 (2):212–220.

Greenberg, Jeff, Sheldon Solomon, Tom Pyszczynski, Abram Rosenblatt, John Burling, Deborah Lyon & Elizabeth Pinel (1992): 'Why Do People Need Self-Esteem? Converging Evidence That Self-Esteem Serves an Anxiety-Buffering Function'. *Journal of Personality and Social Psychology*, 63 (6):913–922.

Greenberg, Jeff, Kenneth Vail & Tom Pyszczynski (2014): 'Terror Management Theory and Research: How the Desire for Death Transcendence Drives Our Strivings for Meaning and Significance', in Andrew J. Elliot (ed.): *Advances in Motivation Science, Volume 1*. Oxford: Elsevier, pp. 85–134.

Hackathorn, Jana, & Kathryn Cornell (2015): 'Terror Management and Evolutionary Theory: Examination of Jealousy Reactions after Mortality Salience'. *Journal of Integrated Social Sciences*, 5 (1):27–39.

Harmon-Jones, Eddie, Linda Simon, Jeff Greenberg, Tom Pyszczynski, Sheldon Solomon & Holly McGregor (1997): 'Terror Management Theory and Self-Esteem: Evidence that Increased Self-Esteem Reduced Mortality Salience Effects'. *Journal of Personality and Social Psychology*, 72 (1):24–36.

Hart, Joshua, James Schwabach & Sheldon Solomon (2010): 'Going for Broke: Mortality Salience Increases Risky Decision Making on the Iowa Gambling Task'. *British Journal of Social Psychology*, 49 (2):425–432.

Hart, Joshua, Phillip Shaver & Jamie Goldenberg (2005): 'Attachment, Self-Esteem, Worldviews and Terror Management: Evidence for a Tripartite Security System'. *Journal of Personality and Social Psychology*, 88 (6):999–1013.

Hayes, Joseph, Jeff Schimel, Jamie Arndt & Erik Faucher (2010): 'A Theoretical and Empirical Review of the Death-Thought Accessibility Concept in Terror Management Research'. *Psychological Bulletin*, 136 (5):699–739.

Hayes, Joseph, Jeff Schimel, Erik Faucher & Todd Williams (2008): 'Evidence for the DTA Hypothesis II: Threatening Self-Esteem Increases Death-Thought Accessibility'. *Journal of Experimental Social Psychology*, 44 (3):600–613.

Hirschberger, Gilad & Tsachi Ein-Dor (2006): 'Defenders of a Lost Cause: Terror Management and Violent Resistance to the Disengagement Plan'. *Personality and Social Psychology Bulletin*, 32 (6):761–769.

Hirschberger, Gilad, Tsachi Ein-Dor & Shaul Almakias (2008): 'The Self-Protective Altruist: Terror Management and the Ambivalent Nature of Prosocial Behavior'. *Personality and Social Psychology Bulletin*, 34 (5):666–678.

Hirschberger, Gilad, Tom Pyszczynski & Tsachi Ein-Dor (2015): 'Why Does Existential Threat Promote Intergroup Violence? Examining the Role of Retributive Justice and Cost-Benefit Utility Motivations'. *Frontiers in Psychology*, 6:1761 (online publication).

Jonas, Eva & Peter Fischer (2006): 'Terror Management and Religion: Evidence That Intrinsic Religiousness Mitigates Worldview Defense Following Mortality Salience'. *Journal of Personality and Social Psychology*, 91 (3):553–567.

Jonas, Eva, Andy Martens, Daniela Niesta Kayser, Immo Fritsche, Daniel Sullivan & Jeff Greenberg (2008): 'Focus Theory of Normative Conduct and Terror Management Theory: The Interactive Impact of Mortality Salience and Norm Salience on Social Judgment'. *Journal of Personality and Social Psychology*, 95 (6):1239–1251.

Jonas, Eva, Jeff Schimel, Jeff Greenberg & Tom Pyszczynski (2002): 'The Scrooge Effect: Evidence That Mortality Salience Increases Prosocial Attitudes and Behavior'. *Personality and Social Psychology Bulletin*, 28 (10):1342–1353.

Koole, Sander & Agnes van den Berg (2005): 'Lost in the Wilderness: Terror Management, Action Orientation and Nature Evaluation'. *Journal of Personality and Social Psychology*, 88 (6):1014–1028.

Landau, Mark, Sheldon Solomon, Jeff Greenberg, Florette Cohen, Tom Pyszczynski, Jamie Arndt, Claude Miller, Daniel Ogilvie & Alison Cook (2004): 'Deliver Us from Evil: The Effects of Mortality Salience and Reminders of 9/11 on Support for President George W. Bush'. *Personality and Social Psychology Bulletin*, 30 (9):1136–1150.

Landau, Mark, Daniel Sullivan & Sheldon Solomon (2010): 'On Graves and Graven Images: A Terror Management Analysis of the Psychological Functions of Art'. *European Review of Social Psychology*, 21 (1):114–154.

Lifshin, Uri, Jeff Greenberg, Melissa Soenke, Alex Darrel & Tom Pyszczynski (in press): 'Mortality Salience, Religiosity and Indefinite Life Extension: Evidence of a Reciprocal Relationship between Afterlife Beliefs and Support for Forestalling Death'. *Religion Brain and Behavior*.

Lifshin, Uri, Jeff Greenberg, Colin Zestcott & Daniel Sullivan (2016): 'The Evil Animal: A Terror Management Theory Perspective on the Human Tendency to Kill Animals'. *Personality and Social Psychology Bulletin* (Manuscript under review).

Lifshin, Uri, Peter Helm, Jeff Greenberg, Melissa Soenke, Dev Ashish & Daniel Sullivan (2015a): 'Evidence of Higher Ingroup Identity in Young Adults Who Have Experienced the Death of a Close Other'. *Self and Identity* (Manuscript under review).

Lifshin, Uri, Peter Helm, Jeff Greenberg, Melissa Soenke, Alex Darrel & Tom Pyszczynski (2015b): 'Women Want the Heavens, Men Want the Earth: Gender Differences in Support for Life Extension Technologies'. Unpublished manuscript, University of Arizona.

Lifshin, Uri, Peter Helm, Melissa Soenke & Jeff Greenberg (2015): 'Digital Immortality: Terror Management Online via Facebook'. Unpublished manuscript, University of Arizona.

Lifton, Robert J. (1968): *Revolutionary Immortality: Mao Tse-tung and the Chinese Cultural Revolution*. New York: Random House.

Lifton, Robert J. (1979): *The Broken Connection: On Death and the Continuity of Life*. New York: Basic Books.

McGregor, Holly, Joel Lieberman, Jeff Greenberg, Sheldon Solomon, Jamie Arndt, Linda Simon & Tom Pyszczynski (1998): 'Terror Management and Aggression: Evidence that Mortality Salience Promotes Aggression against Worldview-Threatening Individuals'. *Journal of Personality and Social Psychology*, 74 (3):590–605.

Marino, Lori & Michael Mountain (2015): 'Denial of Death and the Relationship between Humans and Other Animals'. *Anthrozoös*, 28 (1):5–21.

Mikulincer, Mario, Victor Florian & Gilad Hirschberger (2003): 'The Existential Function of Close Relationships: Introducing Death into the Science of Love'. *Personality and Social Psychology Review*, 7 (1): 20–40.

Mikulincer, Mario, Omri Gillath & Phillip Shaver (2002): 'Activation of the Attachment System in Adulthood: Threat-Related Primes Increase the Accessibility of Mental Representations of Attachment Figures'. *Journal of Personality and Social Psychology*, 83:881–895.

Motyl, Matt, Joshua Hart, Tom Pyszczynski, David Weise, Molly Maxfield & Angelika Siedel (2011): 'Subtle Priming of Shared Human Experiences Eliminates Threat-Induced Negativity toward Arabs, Immigrants and Peace-Making'. *Journal of Experimental Social Psychology*, 47 (6):1179–1184.

Nagar, Mayaan & Sharon Rabinovitz (2015): 'Smoke Your Troubles Away: Exploring the Effects of Death Cognitions on Cannabis Craving and Consumption'. *Journal of Psychoactive Drugs*, 47 (2):91–99.

Pyszczynski, Tom & Pelin Kesebir (2011): 'Anxiety Buffer Disruption Theory: A Terror Management Account of Posttraumatic Stress Disorder'. *Anxiety, Stress & Coping: An International Journal*, 24 (1):3–26.

Pyszczynski, Tom, Adbolhossein Abdollahi, Sheldon Solomon, Jeff Greenberg, Florette Cohen & David Weise (2006): 'Mortality Salience, Martyrdom and Military Might: The Great Satan versus the Axis of Evil'. *Personality and Social Psychology Bulletin*, 32 (4):525–537.

Pyszczynski, Tom, Jeff Greenberg & Sheldon Solomon (1999): 'A Dual-Process Mode of Defense against Conscious and Unconscious Death-Related Thoughts: An Extension of Terror Management Theory'. *Psychological Review*, 106 (4): 835–845.

Pyszczynski, Tom, Jeff Greenberg, Sheldon Solomon & Molly Maxfield (2006): 'On the Unique Psychological Import of the Human Awareness of Mortality: Themes and Variations'. *Psychological Inquiry*, 17 (4):328–356.

Pyszczynski, Tom, Matt Motyl, Kenneth Vail, Gilad Hirschberger, Jamie Arndt & Pelin Kesebir (2012): 'Drawing Attention to Global Climate Change Decreases Support for War'. *Peace and Conflict: Journal of Peace Psychology*, 18 (4):354–368.

Pyszczynski, Tom, Zachary Rothschild & Adbolhossein Abdollahi (2008): 'Terrorism, Violence and Hope for Peace: A Terror Management Perspective'. *Current Direction in Psychological Science*, 17 (5):318–322.

Pyszczynski, Tom, Sheldon Solomon & Jeff Greenberg (2003): *In the Wake of 9/11: The Psychology of Terror*. Washington, DC: American Psychological Association.

Rosenblatt, Abram, Jeff Greenberg, Sheldon Solomon, Tom Pyszczynski & Deborah Lyon (1989): 'Evidence for Terror Management Theory I: The Effects of Mortality Salience on Reactions to Those Who Violate or Uphold Cultural Values'. *Journal of Personality and Social Psychology*, 57 (4):681–690.

Routledge, Clay, Jamie Arndt & Jamie Goldenberg (2004): 'A Time to Tan: Proximal and Distal Effects of Mortality Salience on Sun Exposure Intentions'. *Personality and Social Psychology Bulletin*, 30 (10):1347–1358.

Schimel, Jeff, Joseph Hayes, Todd Williams & Jesse Jahrig (2007): 'Is Death Really the Worm at the Core? Converging Evidence That Worldview Threat Increases Death-Thought Accessibility'. *Journal of Personality and Social Psychology*, 92 (5):789–803.

Soenke, Melissa, Jeff Greenberg & Uri Lifshin (in press): 'Are You Smarter Than a Cetacean? Death Reminders and Concerns about Human Intelligence'. *Society & Animals*.

Solomon, Sheldon, Jeff Greenberg & Tom Pyszczynski (2015): *The Worm at the Core: The Role of Death in Life.* New York: Random House.

Taubman-Ben-Ari, Orit, Victor Florian & Mario Mikulincer (1999): 'The Impact of Mortality Salience on Reckless Driving: A Test of Terror Management Mechanisms'. *Journal of Personality and Social Psychology*, 76 (1):35–45.

Vail, Kenneth, Jacob Juhl, Jamie Arndt, Matthew Vess, Clay Routledge & Bastiaan T. Rutjens (2012): 'When Death Is Good for Life: Considering the Positive Trajectories of Terror Management'. *Personality and Social Psychology Review*, 16 (4):303–329.

Van Tongeren, Daryl, Jeffery Green, Don Davis, Everett Worthington & Chelsea Reid (2013): 'Till Death Do Us Part: Terror Management and Forgiveness in Close Relationships'. *Personal Relationships*, 20 (4):755–768.

Vess, Matthew & Jamie Arndt (2008): 'The Nature of Death and the Death of Nature: The Impact of Mortality Salience on Environmental Concern'. *Journal of Research in Personality*, 42:1376–1380.

Vess, Matthew, Jamie Arndt, Cathy Cox, Clay Routledge & Jamie Goldenberg (2009): 'Exploring the Existential Function of Religion: The Effect of Religious Fundamentalism and Mortality Salience on Faith-Based Medical Refusals'. *Journal of Personality and Social Psychology*, 97 (2):334–350.

Wisman, Arnaud & Jamie Goldenberg (2005): 'From the Grave to the Cradle: Evidence That Mortality Salience Engenders a Desire for Offspring'. *Journal of Personality and Social Psychology*, 89 (1):46–61.

Yaakobi, Erez (2015): 'Desire to Work as a Death Anxiety Buffer Mechanism'. *Experimental Psychology*, 62:110–122.

Yaakobi, Erez, Mario Mikulincer & Phillip Shaver (2014): 'Parenthood as a Terror Management Mechanism: The Moderating Role of Attachment Orientations'. *Personality and Social Psychology Bulletin*, 40 (6):762–774.

Zestcott, Colin, Uri Lifshin, Peter Helm & Jeff Greenberg (2016): 'He Dies He Scores: The Effects of Reminders of Death on Athletic Performance in Basketball'. *Journal of Sport and Exercise Psychology*, 38(5), 470–480.

Zhou, Xinyeu, Jing Liu, Chenchao Chen & Zonghuo Yu (2008): 'Do Children Transcend Death? An Examination of the Terror Management Function of Offspring'. *Scandinavian Journal of Psychology*, 49 (5):413–418.

Zhou, Xinyue, Qijia Lei, Scott Marley & Jinsong Chen (2009): 'Existential Function of Babies: Babies as a Buffer of Death-Related Anxiety'. *Asian Journal of Social Psychology*, 12 (1):40–46.

5   The immortalisation of celebrities

David Giles

Introduction

What is so attractive about the idea of being famous? Leaving aside the obvious material benefits that tend to accompany worldly fame, the condition of celebrity brings with it a level of responsibility that can drive an individual to suicide, as in the case of Nirvana singer Kurt Cobain. Celebrities have a responsibility to their various audiences, to their families and friends, to the governance of the self, to moral and ideological public standards, that at times seems overwhelming. Being famous without being rich would seem a highly challenging occupation, a social role not to be lightly undertaken. Yet history teems with examples of people who seem content with posthumous glory. Fame for fame alone seems reward enough.

In my book *Illusions of Immortality* (Giles 2000), I suggested that the psychological roots of fame lie in the 'illusion' that is produced by the cultural replication of images, names and other phenomena pertaining to the celebrated individual. This is an illusion of immortality: its compulsion arises from the biological imperative to reproduce. Through media, celebrities replicate themselves to a bewildering degree. Thousands of images – still and moving – circulate. Words are spoken and written by and about the celebrity and reproduced in dizzying quantities. Dying tomorrow, they have left a trace in the world that can persist for centuries. Of course, in the digital age, we can all do this to some extent; hence the concept of 'microcelebrity' now popular in media and communication studies (Senft 2008). But this is simply the contemporary manifestation of a centuries-long tradition:

> The 'ethereal' immortality, immortality-through-other-people's-memory, remains astonishingly steady in its form over centuries … The novelty … is the promise … of merging a one-off experience of instant … immortality with the hope for its eternal duration: the (transient) state of 'being a celebrity' is an exercise (I repeat: yet untested) in such merger.
>
> (Zygmunt Bauman in interview with Michael Hviid Jacobsen in Jacobsen 2011:390)

If, then, the possibility of symbolic immortality is one of the fundamental driving forces behind individuals' desire for fame, celebrity may well be regarded as a *strategy* for achieving that goal (Bauman 1992). Through writing, visual representation on coins, banknotes, statues and portraits, and naming of public places and buildings, celebrated individuals throughout history have long been granted posterity for future generations. The invention of recording techniques, from the camera and the phonograph through to digitalisation, and their circulation through increasingly ubiquitous communication media, has brought about even more ways of preserving the public memory of specific individuals, with or without the recognition of statutory bodies.

In this chapter I am going to discuss the techniques and technologies that have evolved through history for bestowing immortality on individuals, and examine these in the light of the ever more crowded world of contemporary celebrity. It is important at this stage to say a little about the concept of celebrity, since it is a far from unambiguous term. I believe it is essential to differentiate fame from celebrity by treating the former as a social process and the latter as a cultural phenomenon (Giles 2000). One can become famous in a small community, such as a school, but it takes a mass medium to bring about the conditions necessary for celebrity. Even then, some find uncomfortable the label 'celebrity' applied to historically famous individuals such as writers and artists, and even to many famous individuals in contemporary society whose fame appears 'merited', or whose social standing (such as world leaders) guarantees them fame without needing the machinery of publicity associated with reality TV stars and other Barnum-like PR creations.

I think it is fundamentally misguided to try to distinguish some elevated stratum of famous individuals from a vulgar body of publicity-hungry attention-seekers. While Alice Marwick and danah boyd (2011) might describe celebrity as a series of practices, it must be conceded that the media have the last word on the matter. Practise celebrity all you like, but only the media can make it happen, and they can make it happen to anyone, regardless of the amount of practice they put in. An award-winning scientist, author, musician or academic can be treated as a celebrity in what Chris Rojek (2012:12) has called the 'washing machine' of contemporary culture. Celebrity, ultimately, is defined by its representation in the 'discursive regime' of media (Turner 2004).

But we are still not quite finished with definitions, because yet another constraint sees celebrity as an essentially modern phenomenon, defined by certain kinds of media – notably the film camera (Schickel 1985). The Hollywood framework for understanding celebrity has dominated much of the academic literature in the field of celebrity studies, but it is increasingly challenged by alternative models: James Bennett (2011) has outlined the very different conditions under which television produced its own celebrity system, while researchers of digital culture have to find ways of explaining how the 'micro-celebrities' of online technologies like YouTube are now emerging as bona fide celebrities through building massive followings on multiple platforms.

Meanwhile, historians of literary and musical culture have examined how the practices and representations of nineteenth-century media constituted celebrity for the likes of Byron and Rossini (Mole 2007, 2012).

Ultimately, if we think of media in Marshall McLuhan's (1964) terms as 'extensions of man [*sic*]', there is no need to specify some arbitrary cut-off point for the birth of celebrity culture. We can see celebrity as emerging gradually over time thanks to the evolution of ever-sophisticated and ubiquitous technologies. The thread that links PewDiePie, Marilyn Monroe, Mary Pickford and Byron can therefore be stretched as far as back as any medium that has the capability of representing and then replicating the trace of an individual.

Before examining the technologies of immortality in more detail, I would like to present two exclusionary criteria. The first is that, as Zygmunt Bauman (1992) has pointed out, immortality is not concerned with death and dying: it is about wishing death away. Therefore, tombstones, shrines, anniversaries and similar objects and practices explicitly linked to the passing of an individual are not elements of the strategy for immortality. Second, the practice of quasi-religious 'worship' of celebrities documented by Erika Doss (1999) and others is excluded because it similarly involves an acknowledgement that the person no longer exists. There are much better ways of keeping Elvis alive than making a 'pilgrimage' to Graceland on the anniversary of his death.

Biologically, of course, posterity is granted by the survival of an individual's genes in the form of descendants. But our offspring are only ever partial replications, and whatever unseen forces drive us to procreate, the production of children does not seem to deter individuals from continuing to seek fame, or to slow down its maintenance once established. Childless or not, the desire to remain alive in some form is a powerful force through history. In this next section, I am going to examine some of the ways that we have devised for cheating death.

Technologies of immortality

Visual representation

The art of sculpture constituted the earliest way of preserving the visual image of an individual. Leo Braudy, in his classic work on the history of fame (Braudy 1997:32), nominates Alexander the Great as the 'first famous person', not least because of the images celebrating his deeds: in addition to various writings, he was one of the first individuals to be depicted on coins, and the bronze statue by Lysippos, depicting Alexander with tousled hair and parted lips, came to serve as a much-mimicked template for portraiture right through to Hollywood. It certainly inspired the proliferation of visual images of famous Romans in the centuries that followed.

While in the Western world, the depiction of individuals largely died out following the collapse of Rome, the Moche civilisation of Ancient Peru developed its own tradition of honouring specific people by modelling them in the form of ceramic vessels. These portraits achieved sufficient accuracy not only that the individuals (mostly high-status males) would be recognisable but also that they captured aspects of their personality (Donnan 2004). Not only were leaders and warriors modelled, but also people famous for other reasons, such as wearing an exceptionally long beard (Benson 2004). In either case the motive for portraying individuals seems to have stemmed from the desire to honour their lives and preserve their memory for future generations.

Portraiture in the form of painting did not fully emerge in the West until the sixteenth century, when it became acceptable for artists to glorify secular subjects: as Leo Braudy (1997:267) puts it, 'faces were appearing everywhere'. While at first it was largely monarchs who were honoured in this way, the fashion for portraiture then spread to anyone with sufficient money to commission an artist. As in Ancient Peru, physiognomic accuracy became increasingly important as portraits were believed to represent the 'inner life' of the subject as much as the outward appearance (Woodall 1997). In preserving more than merely the physical self, realistic images were seen to immortalise personal identity in an era increasingly concerned with the glory of the public individual.

If the goal of portraiture is to make the individual seem alive in body and spirit, oil, bronze or marble are not the best materials for absolute verisimilitude. The Romans knew that the way to capture the exact details of the face was to place a wax cast over its features, but it was not until the eighteenth century, when wax was principally used to reproduce anatomical features for medical purposes, that Marie Tussaud developed her method for lifelike portrayal of famous figures. Her permanent exhibition in London, complete with models of Voltaire, Franklin and the pre-revolutionary French royals at the dinner table, has since expanded into a global industry. Branches of Madame Tussauds[1] can now be found everywhere from Tokyo to Las Vegas, each depicting a blend of local and global, historical and contemporary figures that is continually updated according to visitors' requests.

The illusion of mortality intrinsic to Tussauds wax models is encapsulated in the Merlin Entertainment Group's publicity for the attraction. 'Who do you want to meet?' the visitor is asked on arriving at the homepage of www.madametussauds.com. Early visitors were simply grateful for the opportunity to vent their spleen at unpopular politicians, but today our familiarity with photographic representation means that we are more discerning. Nevertheless, wax still has the potential to create an impression of life: there is a long tradition of celebrities posing as their wax figures and confusing the public (Arnold Schwarzenegger and One Direction are some of the most recent stars to have startled Tussauds visitors in this manner).

In a parallel development to the intimacy of social media, as well as the increased individualism of the age, the waxworks have gradually emerged from the tableaux that characterised the original museum, to be placed singly in positions that enable the public, as the marketing goes, to 'rub shoulders with our stars'. Literally, in some cases: the London branch keeps a spare

Amy Winehouse figure in the storeroom so that her trademark tattoos, worn away from constant handling, can be retouched (Barkham 2011). Taking a selfie with your favourite celebrity is now an intrinsic feature of the Tussauds experience.

The playful juxtaposition of celebrities and their wax doppelgängers is a clear reminder that death is not a necessary precursor for immortalisation. This stands in contrast to the death mask, which, whatever its creators might have believed at the time, does not immortalise its subject. It is worth noting that Marie Tussaud's original death masks were used, not to celebrate the lives of Louis XVI and Robespierre, but, mounted on pikes, to threaten the counter-revolutionaries at the height of the Reign of Terror with a reminder of the potential fate that lay in store for them.

Impersonation

Statues and waxworks immortalise their subjects by capturing their likeness in a single snapshot. The illusion of animation, however, requires more than a frozen moment. One way of preserving the living, breathing subject is to reincarnate him or her as a performance, so that the moves, the looks and the voice take up residence in another human body. Impersonators have been employed since the early days of Hollywood for commercial gain, and in popular music, 'tribute acts' have become a quick way of absorbing the glory from successful artists. Some celebrities, notably Elvis Presley and Marilyn Monroe, and increasingly Michael Jackson, have become so frequently rep-resented that the activity has become an industry in itself: there are regular US conventions solely devoted to Elvis impersonation, and it is estimated that there are 3,000 professional Elvis impersonators in the United States alone (Aho 2005). With Elvis remaining such a visible presence in contempo-rary culture, it is perhaps not surprising that many conspiracy theorists have claimed he is not really dead.

Like visual representation, impersonation does not begin with the death of the subject. Charlie Chaplin was immortalised at the first peak of his fame, in the 1910s, at a time when movie houses across the United States were clam-ouring for more screentime from the star. Billy West, later to become famous in his own right, began his career as a Chaplin impersonator to satisfy box office demand, and fake Chaplins sprang up throughout the film industry, even in as unlikely places as China and Japan (Sloan 2015). The impersona-tors soon began to attract fans of their own, some admirers claiming that they were better than the original: at one point, a Billy West fan accused Chaplin of trying too hard to imitate his imitator. There is a long-standing claim that Chaplin once entered, and failed to win, a Chaplin lookalike contest: the same claim has been made by (and on behalf of) other highly impersonated celebri-ties (Mejia 2015).[2]

To lose your own lookalike competition might seem to be failure on an absurd scale, but it speaks volumes about the art of impersonation.

Arguably the most popular subjects for imitation are those stars whose essence can be boiled down to a set of visual signifiers. The 'little tramp' hat, cane, moustache and waddle can easily transform any performer into Chaplin. In this way the basic iconography is established, and the impersonators then take their cues from other impersonators as much as the individual themselves (Ferris 2011). It is perhaps for this reason that Elvis 'interpreters' include lesbian drag kings, evangelists and skydivers, as well as representatives of many different ethnic groups and nationalities from Norway to Japan (Cowan 2010). 'Only a few key elements are needed to establish the required connection to Elvis', writes Marko Aho (2005:250): 'sideburns, jumpsuit, sunglasses – that's it.' Cultural commentators have often been baffled by the preference for Elvis impersonators to model his late, bloated, Vegas image rather than the far cooler figure cut during the 1950s, but the former collection of signifiers is more replicable, enabling a vast range of people to 'play Elvis', including an increasing number of females (Brittan 2006).

But the imitation game is not, ultimately, what immortalises figures like Elvis and Chaplin. Latter-day Las Vegas promoters do not shell out upwards of $200 for a ten-minute lookalike contest: Elvis imitators earn their crust because people want *to see Elvis*. He inhabits his interpreters to the point where they *become* Elvis, at least for a willing audience. This, like other visual forms of immortalisation, has nothing to do with death: the Dolly Parton impersonator interviewed by Kerry Ferris (2011) is addressed as 'Dolly' by all the members of the nightclub where she performs, even when out of costume. In this sense she becomes a conduit for the star. Whether or not the impersonator experiences a loss of self in the process, for everyone around her she has effectively become a proxy. As far as the star herself is concerned, the immortalisation process begins the moment she has been granted life in another human shell.

Recording

Up to now I have been discussing mainly the process of immortalising other people, but in the last 150 years technology has given us the option of directly immortalising ourselves, thereby seizing control over the whole process. Although much the same argument could be made for the written word (some, such as Elizabeth Eisenstein 1968, argued that celebrity began with the printing press), the physical trace left by the voice – whether on vinyl, magnetic tape or digital files – creates a sense of presence that engenders a feeling that the artist is somehow in the room with us when we listen to a recording. Phonography, argued Douglas Kahn (1999:9), 'wrenched the voice from the throat and out of time', presenting the listener with part of the singer's body, rather like the lipstick on a star's cigarette butt coveted by an ardent fan.

Once again, the issue of whether the recorded artist is dead or alive is irrelevant. Once they have left behind that semi-physical trace on record, they have effectively become immortal. Indeed, the early popularity of the phonograph lay predominantly in its ability to bring back the dead, although the mortal condition of the vocalist is largely a matter of audience interpretation, as fans of both Elvis and US rapper Tupac Shakur have cited recordings as evidence that the supposedly dead star is still alive (Sterne 2005).

Once again, a contrast should be drawn between the practices of immortalisation and those technologies that commemorate the dead individual. Among the latter are 'posthumous duets', whereby the voice of a living artist (either recorded or live) is laid over the recorded voice of a dead one to create the illusion of the two individuals performing side by side (Brunt 2015). This technique has been used to reunite legendary stars with their offspring (e.g. Nat King Cole and daughter Natalie) or to create unlikely collaborations (Roy Orbison with Westlife). These latter hybrids in particular have been the subject of much criticism on the grounds that they are inauthentic and even unethical, though, as Joli Jensen (2005) points out, even living artists have little control over their media representation. One exception to this rule might be soul singer James Brown, who, in later years, used samples of his early recordings to try to rejuvenate his flagging career (Jones 2009).

An alternative argument is that, once immortalised on record (audibly or visually), the star themselves *may as well be dead*. As John Frow (1997:205–206) has put it: '[the] absence of the recorded star, their presence as recording, is the reason why the worship of stars is a cult of the dead'. Once a recording achieves worldwide fame, it represents the artist to such an extent that their actual bodily self becomes almost secondary to its floating double. As a result, popular artists become haunted by their early successes: since these no longer represent the contemporary self, they find themselves trapped in a timewarp, fans interacting with a former (and possibly imperfect) version. Of course, the only way to combat this is to continually produce new recordings. It is notable that very few stars from the era of recorded music have ever wholly withdrawn from the recording process, no matter how low their profile has sunk during their lifetime.

Naming practices

One of the highest civic honours is to have a street or public building named after you. Of all immortalisation strategies this is perhaps the most effective, since it breaks the dependency of the individual on the immediate context of their fame and allows them to permeate other fields of human activity. Sir Alex Ferguson has a bronze statue immediately outside Old Trafford, Manchester United's football stadium, and a stand within the ground named after him, but it may be Sir Alex Ferguson Way that is his most enduring legacy. However, the naming of public places is entirely in the hands of statutory authorities and is subject, more than any of the technologies listed so far, to the ideologies and whims of legitimating bodies (not to mention the fluctuating fortunes of the famous).

Few could argue with naming streets after civil rights hero Martin Luther King: there are 900 of them in the United States. But other figures have provoked debate or outright embarrassment to the authorities that immortalised them. When the British celebrity presenter and charity fundraiser Jimmy Savile died in 2011, it was not altogether surprising that Scarborough Council should honour a local hero by naming a clifftop path after him. Mere weeks after unveiling the road sign on Savile's View, however, a criminal investigation had opened into hundreds of sexual abuse claims against him, and public pressure forced its prompt removal. Soon after, having initially held out in the hope of the accusations coming to nothing, a conference centre in Leeds had to spend £50,000 renaming Savile Hall.

As with the other technologies of immortalisation, having a street or building named after you does not require your death. Indeed, the most reliable way of ensuring your immortality is to achieve such a position of authority while alive that you can instigate the naming process yourself. Tyrannical dictatorship is a perfect opportunity, and it is no surprise that despotic leaders have wasted little time in immortalising themselves wherever possible, naming streets, airports and even entire cities after themselves – especially in recently conquered territories. Dozens of cities, urban districts and streets in the former Soviet Union were renamed after Josef Stalin in the 1920s and 1930s, and still others in Soviet-controlled Eastern Europe in the post-war period. The process of renaming German streets and squares after Adolf Hitler in the mid-1930s took even less time. If you can't authorise it yourself, then buy it: a Birmingham mosque bore the name of Saddam Hussein for 15 years to honour the Iraqi leader's £2 million financial donation that enabled it to be built in the first place (BBC 2003).

This is not a long-term strategy, however: as soon as the dictator dies, or loses power, the process of renaming gets under way all over again. Almost everywhere named after Stalin was famously 'deStalinised' in the early 1960s. The East German town of Stalinstadt, created in the early 1950s around a giant steel works, only bore his name for a mere eight years before being conveniently merged with neighbouring Schönfließ to form Eisenhüttenstadt in 1961. Two of the few places to survive deStalinisation were, oddly, streets in the south-east of England. Stalin Close in Colchester and Stalin Avenue in Chatham were both named by post-war planners to celebrate the Allied war leaders' success, with Roosevelt and Churchill honoured nearby. Residents of the Colchester cul-de-sac voted 'overwhelmingly' against a name change suggested by the local newspaper (Brading 2009), while the people of Chatham regard their street as an inescapable 'part of history' (*Kent Online* 2008).

The one exception to the immortalisation of place names is the 'blue plaque' tradition currently practised by English Heritage, a charitable institution that manages hundreds of historic buildings and sites in Britain. Since 1866, the characteristic plaques have been attached to London buildings to celebrate former residents – but only if those individuals have been dead for 20 years and are deemed sufficiently 'eminent' (Brierley 2000).

Reasons for immortalisation

The rush to eradicate the memory of undesirable individuals such as Savile and Stalin only serves to underline the brittle nature of reputation and the limits to unbridled self-promotion. Death relinquishes all control over the manipulation of the public persona, with only the interest of the bereaved friends and relatives to sustain the immortalisation process. At any stage, however, the motives for immortalising an individual will depend on the significance of that individual for the goals and values of others. This is where celebrity can be reduced simply to its usefulness as a promotional tool.

P. David Marshall (1997) has written of the 'cipher' status of celebrity, whereby the individuals themselves are essentially interchangeable. A good example of this can be seen in Mihai Coman's (2011) study of a Michael Jackson concert that took place in Bucharest in 1992, a few years after the downfall of the Nicolae Ceauşescu regime. Jackson's visit was framed by the Romanian press as a quasi-religious event, with crowds following him as he was driven from the airport to visit an orphanage and then on to the National Stadium as if on a pilgrimage. The concert itself was presented as a mystical experience: one reporter claimed that '100,000 people lived … moments of happiness and ecstasy that many had not thought they would ever experience' (Coman 2011:283).

Coman argues that Jackson's visit was an opportunity for the Romanian media to satisfy 'a desperate quest for a "prophetic" voice announcing the promised future' (Coman 2011:286), thereby filling a 'semantic void' with religious significance. With the collapse of communism, the decision to visit Bucharest made by a global American superstar represented the country's entrance into a new, more hopeful era. When Jackson returned to Romania four years later, despite exciting the same fervour among audiences, there was nothing like the same degree of mystical and religious imagery in the press coverage. His saintliness was no longer necessary.

In the remainder of this section I will discuss a number of different sets of motives for immortalising figures, dead and alive, whether to satisfy nationalistic, economic or sentimental purposes.

Ideological or nationalistic purposes

In the Sepik river culture of New Guinea, houses are protected by ancestral figures that represent important figures from the clan's history, often dating from many previous generations. Legends abound of these totemic wooden figures 'coming to life' and defending the clan when attacked by warriors from rival clans. One such celebrated figure, Minjemtimi, is currently housed in the Metropolitan Museum of Art in New York. Minjemtimi was said to have come to life during a battle but, despite putting up a good fight, was stolen by the rival clan and preserved in a men's ceremonial house until 'collected' by anthropologists. Since then he has served a similar function in an American museum, although it is not recorded how vigorously he resisted this most recent transfer (Kjellgren 2014).

Much like Minjemtimi, celebrities and other ancestral figures in recent history are kept alive – at least symbolically – so that they may continue to serve a role in promoting, and possibly defending, the nation. In a famous TV football commentary, Norwegian broadcaster Bjørge Lillelien celebrated a 1981 victory by his compatriots against England by reeling off a list of historical figures from Lord Nelson to boxer Henry Cooper, 'Lady Diana' and prime minister 'Maggie Thatcher'. At that moment, the defeated nation was represented not by 11 hapless footballers but by a roll-call of famous individuals.

James Caughey (1985) has argued that the role that celebrities occupy in contemporary society reflects that of gods and spirits (and ancestral figures) in earlier societies. We keep alive such figures because they provide important reference points for society, either as a 'primary basis' for socialisation (mention a famous celebrity to a stranger at a bus stop and you may strike up a conversation), or as important cultural knowledge. As Caughey notes, US psychiatrists may estimate a patient's sanity by asking them to list the last four presidents. Whether or not this is a good method for judging mental health status, it reveals the importance of public figures for cultural assimilation.

Today, Johann Sebastian Bach is normally thought of as a towering presence in music history: the godfather of Western classical music, the source from which springs some of the greatest achievements in the history of Western art. Bach is immortal in the sense that he speaks to us through his music in so many different places: the radio, the Web, the concert hall. Every day his music is broadcast to our homes. Compendiums of Western music carry his portrait and glorify his work. Tourists visit his (alleged) birthplace in Eisenach, the church in which he was baptised and sundry other locations connected to his life.

In the decades following Bach's death, however, his music became rather unfashionable, largely ignored apart from a few keyboard pieces that were used for technical exercises. Even his influence on subsequent composers, such as Mozart and Beethoven, has been exaggerated (Boyd 2000). It was not until he was championed some years later by composers discovering his work that he re-entered the repertoire at all. Most notable was a performance of the St Matthew Passion conducted by a young Felix Mendelssohn in 1829, described by Peter Mercer-Taylor (2004) as 'an event of epoch-making significance in the revitalisation of Bach's reputation'. The concert had a profound impact on writers such as Goethe as well as other contemporary composers, who gradually began to instal Bach as a major figure in music history: by 1900 over 200 books had been written about him, an exceptional figure for the period.

But Bach's revival was not just a matter of serendipity. As Malcolm Boyd (2000:242) says, it was 'a focal point for a re-awakening of German national pride'. German society needed heroes after the humiliation of the Napoleonic wars, and the religious content of the Passion and other choral works tapped into a contemporary surge in Protestantism. Bach had become *useful.* Furthermore, what the Leipzig audience got was not pure unadulterated Bach but Romanticised Bach: Mendelssohn actually rewrote large parts of the oratorio, scaling it down considerably for staging purposes and adapting vocal parts to suit available soloists, giving it a contemporary flavour quite distinct from its Baroque roots (Ashley 2005). Similar revitalisation has been described by Joli Jensen (2005) in relation to Patsy Cline and other posthumously celebrated popular artists. In each case the original is updated to suit the values of contemporary society.

Which figures are immortalised and which ones forgotten is essentially a moral issue. Kurt Cobain lives on for fans of rock music in the form of his recordings, Nirvana tribute bands, videos and a small memorial park in his birthplace of Aberdeen, Washington State. He could have had a nearby bridge renamed in his honour, Young Street Bridge, named after Alexander Young, a local pioneer. Cobain apparently dossed underneath it when at a low ebb. But the city council voted unanimously against it on the grounds that it would encourage suicide – presumably by diving off it, although Cobain's own life was taken with a shotgun in his home. 'We don't need to strip another part of our history away', said a local museum director by way of explanation (Michaels 2011).

Time will no doubt tell whether Aberdeen wishes to keep alive a legendary rock star or a nineteenth-century settler. Like Bach in the late 1700s, maybe Cobain is awaiting a rediscovery by subsequent generations at some point when his memory will be useful to Washington State. Heinrich Heine, nineteenth-century German poet, had to wait over a century before his native city, Düsseldorf, was able to resurrect him by giving his name to the local university. After his death in 1856, memorials were suppressed, largely due to anti-Semitism: one statue, the Lorelei Fountain, finally ended up in the Bronx;[3] another in a park in Toulon, southern France. But after the Second World War, Germans were finally able to honour a new generation of heroes: Heine's time had come.

Economic purposes

Celebrities and other public figures are immortalised because they are financially profitable. Business magazine *Forbes* has been publishing an annual list of the top-earning dead celebrities for several years now. Since his death in 2009, Michael Jackson has been hard to topple from the number one slot, raking in annual nine-figure-sum profits. Only for a year was he dethroned from this position, by actress Elizabeth Taylor, who stands fifth in the 2015 list. You may wonder which films Taylor is profiting from at the box office: in fact, her posthumous income derives from a range of perfumes (notably 'White Diamonds'), which continues to out-sell rival celebrity fragrances.

Endorsing a product is another way that living celebrities can impose their name and image upon cultural products and further the process of self-replication. It helps to be discreet about which products you choose to be associated with, of course: as Neil Alperstein (1991) found in a study of celebrity endorsement, inappropriate products can alienate fans who detect commercial opportunism. The endorsement of dead celebrities is, of course, even easier to procure: in 2015 the fourth top-earner was Bob Marley – not just from the proceeds of recordings, but because his name is attached to a drinks company (Marley Beverages) and an eco-friendly hi-fi company (House of Marley). There is no better example of how societies exploit their ancestral figures to meet contemporary economic requirements. As Dave Thompson (2001:159) wrote over a decade ago, Marley's radical, anti-capitalist legacy has been converted stealthily into 'smiling benevolence, a shining sun, a waving palm tree … the machine has utterly emasculated [him]'.

It is precisely for this reason that celebrities become economically more viable once they have died. Nowhere is this clearer than in the tourism industry, where significant locations in a star's history, largely anonymous during their lifetime, become visitor attractions with entrance fees and merchandise stores within years of their death. Freddie Mercury fans can travel to the Stone City in Zanzibar to visit his childhood home, eat in Mercury's restaurant and buy Mercury-related souvenirs, or they can visit the studio in Montreux which has been turned into a Queen museum (with a renowned statue of Mercury nearby). Fans of Omar Sharif can visit his holiday home in Las Palmas. But there are no tourist trails for living film legends such as Robert De Niro or Brigitte Bardot. The one exception to this rule may be US presidents: Bill Clinton's childhood home in Arkansas is already open for business.

Sentimental reasons

Of course, the most appealing aspect of immortality is to preserve the life of a loved one. Ultimately the early enthusiasts of the phonograph saw this as the primary function of recording technology (Sterne 2005): likewise the early video cameras were largely promoted for making home movies, to capture 'memories'. The erection of a statue or monument is seen as recognition of an individual life, and like the disembodied voice, the image represents the person in perpetuity. When a statue was unveiled of the singer Amy Winehouse in Camden, North London, it was regarded by sculptor and family as the continuation of a part of her unique being: designed to resemble her precisely, the sculpture was described by her father Mitch as 'like stopping her in a beautiful moment in time' (BBC 2014). Artist Scott Eaton claimed that the statue was intended to capture her 'attitude and strength, but also give subtle hints of insecurity … the hand on the hip, the grabbing of her skirt, the turned-in foot – these are all small elements that contribute to the personality of the piece'.

The Winehouse statue was claimed to be unusual because the local council agreed to waive its formal ruling that a figure had to be dead for 20 years before a statue could be erected (typically in the United Kingdom, the timespan is anything between 10 and 20 years). Presumably this rule is intended to prevent short-term celebrities from being honoured, since Westminster council allowed statues of Nelson Mandela and Ronald Reagan to appear within 10 years of their deaths. Likewise, permission is rarely refused for club requests for local footballing heroes to be put on a plinth in front of grounds throughout Britain while the players are still in perfect condition (Thierry Henry, Dennis Bergkamp and Tony Adams all adorn the surroundings of Arsenal's Emirates stadium).

One of the stranger examples of a statue erected out of sentimental reasons was the decision of Fulham Football Club's then owner Mohammed Al-Fayed to honour his friend Michael Jackson alongside the club's hero Johnny Haynes. Fulham fans objected immediately to the proposal, claiming that Jackson was 'controversial' and had 'no links with Fulham Football Club' beyond once attending a match as the owner's guest (Ronay 2011). Echoing the Winehouse parents' sentiments, Al-Fayed clearly saw the statue as embodying Jackson himself, saying 'I hope that Fulham fans will appreciate seeing the finest performer in the world in and among them'. Even Jackson fans objected, though this was more to do with the Fulham fans' reaction than the statue itself (although others have questioned its aesthetic qualities). Less than three years later, it was removed to the National Football Museum.

Even more unusual, although not entirely unconnected with its touristic potential, is the appearance of footballer David Beckham as a golden altar statue in the style of a *garuda* (guardian demon) at Wat Pariwas Buddhist temple in Bangkok. The intention of the sculptor, Beckham fan Thongruang Haemhod, is clear: he aimed 'to keep the memory of the football star alive for the next thousand years' (BBC 2000).

Celebrity, immortality and social media

With modern media technology, the opportunities for symbolic immortality have exploded to the point where social media potentially immortalises us all. However, the simple reproduction of imagery is not, by itself, sufficient for all users of social networks, as is clear from the efforts many users make to accumulate as many followers as possible, thus generating ever more reproduction. The advent of social media simply raises the bar: connecting to large numbers of people outside one's immediate social network seems to be as insatiable a desire as ever. As Michael C. Kearl (2010:59–60) has written, 'an immortalist *zeitgeist* now permeates American civic and popular cultures', particularly in digital culture, where 'one's images, behaviours, words, beliefs, and accomplishments exist indefinitely in this new electronic world'.

As through history, we have striven to eliminate the line between mortal and immortal by preserving individuals' visual appearance, by impersonating their bodies and recycling their names, so in the digital era the practice of 'microcelebrity' allows us to establish our own immortality by cultivating our own small patch of cyberspace. Unlike recorded voices, these allotments can be regularly tended and maintained so that they represent the most recent version of the self, so after death we are survived by a permanent trace that shows us as we would best like to be remembered. Whatever happens to those digital allotments in the future, we can rest assured that human ingenuity will always throw up some new way of representing and reproducing, and thereby immortalising, the individual.

Conclusion

In this chapter I have tried to extend the thesis advanced in my 2000 work, *Illusions of Immortality*, that the psychological core of fame and celebrity is the 'illusion' that one has replicated oneself through being represented, potentially massively and multiply, in contemporary media. This illusion transcends any material benefits accruing to the famous, so that in some cases individuals can crave posthumous fame by leaving a body of work to be 'discovered' by future generations. Although the desire to fame drives sometimes extreme behaviours, ultimately celebrity is a condition that is bestowed on individuals through media representation. While we can expend much effort striving for celebrity, we can never guarantee its success.

Much of the chapter discusses technologies for achieving this symbolic immortality, from ancient representations in manufactured objects to modern-day digital culture. Immortality can be bestowed on an individual the moment part of their person – a recognisable representation of their face, a name on a street or building, or a recording of their voice – is released into material culture through some form of communication medium. Alternatively the person may be housed in another human body, in the form of impersonation. Either way, the experience for the honoured individual is that of replication.

Throughout the chapter I have tried to separate the practice of bestowing immortality from the posthumous celebration of a life. Death is not by any means a precondition for immortalisation, even if many of its most explicit artefacts (statues, for example) are only brought into existence after death. Indeed, the immortalisation of celebrities is best understood as something that happens to the living, because, while we might finally settle for being 'discovered' by future generations, it will always remain the second choice.

Notes

1 The possessive apostrophe was dropped, followed by the honorific 'Madame', once the museum was bought by Merlin Entertainments.
2 The Chaplin story has been difficult to verify, some arguing it is an urban myth stemming from 1920s gossip columns. The same kind of story circulates, unsurprisingly, about Elvis. But Dolly Parton has confessed on camera to her own experience of the phenomenon (see: http://abcnews.go.com/Entertainment/dolly-parton-gay-rumors-losing-drag-queen-alike/story?id=17812138).
3 The fate of the Lorelei Fountain underlines emphatically the symbolic power of statuary: for various reasons, including racism and moral piety, it was bumped from pillar to post, being initially rejected by his home town of Düsseldorf, then

transported to New York, where it was repeatedly vandalised after being erected in the Bronx district. After years of neglect it was finally restored and moved a few blocks away in 1999 (Gray 2007).

References

Aho, Marko (2005): 'A Career in Music: From Obscurity to Immortality', in Steve Jones & Joli Jensen (eds): *Afterlife and Afterimage: Understanding Posthumous Fame*. Farnham: Ashgate Publishing, pp. 237–252.

Alperstein, Neil (1991): 'Imaginary Social Relationships with Celebrities Appearing in Television Commercials'. *Journal of Broadcasting and Electronic Media*, 35 (1):43–58.

Ashley, Tim (2005): 'The Butcher of Bach'. *Guardian*, 28 January. Available online at: www.theguardian.com/music/2005/jan/28/classicalmusicandopera.jsbach.

Barkham, Patrick (2011): 'What Makes Madame Tussauds' Wax Work?'. *Guardian*, 26 February. Available online at: www.theguardian.com/culture/2011/feb/26/madame-tussauds-why-so-popular.

Bauman, Zygmunt (1992): *Mortality, Immortality and Other Life Strategies*. Cambridge: Polity Press.

BBC (2000): 'Beckham Meets Buddha'. BBC, 16 May. Available online at: http://news.bbc.co.uk/1/hi/world/asia-pacific/742997.stm.

BBC (2003): 'City Mosque Abandons Saddam's Name'. BBC, 12 August. Available online at: http://news.bbc.co.uk/1/hi/england/west_midlands/3145109.stm.

BBC (2014): 'Life-Size Amy Winehouse Statue Unveiled in North London'. BBC, 14 September. Available online at: www.bbc.co.uk/news/uk-england-london-29190616.

Bennett, James (2011): *Television Personalities: Stardom and the Small Screen*. Abingdon: Routledge.

Benson, Elizabeth (2004): 'Varieties of Precolumbian Portraiture', in Dru Dowdy (ed.): *Retratos: 2,000 Years of Latin American Portraits*. New Haven, CT: Yale University Press, pp. 46–55.

Boyd, Malcolm (2000): *Bach*. New York: Oxford University Press.

Brading, Wendy (2009): 'Colchester: Stalin Should Stay!' *Essex County Standard*, 22 March. Available online at: www.gazette-news.co.uk/news/4216206.display.

Braudy, Leo (1997): *The Frenzy of Renown: Fame and Its History*. New York: Vintage Books.

Brierley, Natalie (2000): 'Immortal Discs: Blue Plaques'. *New Statesman*, 12 June.

Brittan, Francesca (2006): 'Women Who Do Elvis: Authenticity, Masculinity and Masquerade'. *Popular Music Studies*, 18 (0):167–190.

Brunt, Shelley (2015): 'Performing Beyond the Grave: The Posthumous Duet', in Catherine Strong & Barbara Lebrun (eds): *Death and the Rock Star*. Farnham: Ashgate Publishing, pp. 165–176.

Caughey, James (1985): *Imaginary Social Worlds: A Cultural Approach*. Lincoln: University of Nebraska Press.

Coman, Mihai (2011): 'Michael Jackson's 1992 Concert in Bucharest: Transforming a Star into a Saint'. *Celebrity Studies*, 2 (3):277–291.

Cowan, Sharon (2010): 'The Elvis We Deserve: The Social Regulation of Sex/Gender and Sexuality through Cultural Representations of "the King"'. *Law, Culture and the Humanities*, 6 (2):221–244.

Donnan, Christopher (2004): 'Moche Portraits: Masterpieces from Ancient Peru', in Dru Dowdy (ed.): *Retratos: 2,000 Years of Latin American Portraits*. New Haven, CT: Yale University Press, pp. 56–73.

Doss, Erika (1999): *Elvis Culture: Fans, Faith and Image*. Lawrence: University Press of Kansas.

Eisenstein, Elizabeth (1968): 'Some Conjectures about the Impact of Printing on Western Society and Thought: A Preliminary Report'. *Journal of Modern History*, 40 (1):1–57.

Ferris, Kerry (2011): 'Building Characters: The Work of Celebrity Impersonators'. *Journal of Popular Culture*, 44 (6):1191–1208.

Frow, John (1997): 'Is Elvis a God? Cult, Culture, Questions of Method'. *International Journal of Cultural Studies*, 1 (2):197–210.

Giles, David (2000): *Illusions of Immortality: A Psychology of Fame and Celebrity*. Basingstoke: Macmillan.

Gray, Christopher (2007): 'Sturm und Drang over a Memorial to Heinrich Heine'. *New York Times*, 27 May. Available online at: www.nytimes.com/2007/05/27/realestate/27scap.html?_r=0.

Jacobsen, Michael Hviid (2011): 'Sociology, Mortality and Solidarity: An Interview with Zygmunt Bauman on Death, Dying and Immortality'. *Mortality*, 16 (4):380–393.

Jensen, Joli (2005): 'On Fandom, Celebrity and Mediation: Posthumous Possibilities', in Joli Jensen & Steve Jones (eds): *Afterlife as Afterimage: Understanding Posthumous Fame*. New York: Peter Lang, pp. xv–xxiii.

Jones, Steve (2009): 'James Brown, Sample Culture and the Permanent Distance of Glory'. *Fibreculture Journal*, 15. Available online at: http://fifteen.fibreculturejournal.org/fcj-103-james-brown-sample-culture-and-the-permanent-distance-of-glory.

Kahn, Douglas (1999): *Noise, Water, Meat: A History of Sound in the Arts*. Cambridge, MA: MIT Press.

Kearl, Michael C. (2010): 'The Proliferation of Postselves in American Civic and Popular Cultures'. *Mortality*, 15 (1):47–64.

Kent Online (2008): 'Dictator Stalin Still Honoured on Medway Street'. *Kent Online*, 18 September. Available online at: www.kentonline.co.uk/kent/news/dictator-stalin-still-honoured-o-a44077.

Kjellgren, Eric (2014): *How to Read Oceanic Art*. New York: Metropolitan Museum of Art.

McLuhan, Marshall (1964): *Understanding Media: The Extensions of Man*. New York: McGraw-Hill.

Marshall, P. David (1997): *Celebrity and Power: Fame in Contemporary Culture*. Minneapolis: University of Minnesota Press.

Marwick, Alice & danah boyd (2011): 'To See and Be Seen: Celebrity Practice on Twitter'. *Convergence*, 17 (2):139–158.

Mejia, Paula (2015): 'Five Strange Facts about Charlie Chaplin'. *Newsweek*, 16 April. Available online at: www.newsweek.com/five-strange-facts-charlie-chaplin-322850.

Mercer-Taylor, Peter (2004): 'Mendelssohn and the Institution(s) of German Art Music', in Peter Mercer-Taylor (ed.): *The Cambridge Companion to Mendelssohn*. Cambridge: Cambridge University Press, pp. 9–25.

Michaels, Sean (2011): 'Nirvana Singer's Hometown Says No to Kurt Cobain Bridge'. *Guardian*, 29 July. Available online at: www.theguardian.com/music/2011/jul/29/nirvana-singer-kurt-cobain-bridge.

Mole, Tom (2007): *Byron's Romantic Celebrity: Industrial Culture and the Hermeneutic of Intimacy*. Basingstoke: Palgrave/Macmillan.

Mole, Tom (ed.) (2012): *Romanticism and Celebrity Culture, 1750–1850*. Cambridge: Cambridge University Press.

Rojek, Chris (2012): *Fame Attack: The Inflation of Celebrity and Its Consequences*. London: Bloomsbury.

Ronay, Barney (2011): 'Fulham Fans Cry Foul over "Bizarre" Michael Jackson Statue'. *Guardian*, 1 April. Available online at: www.theguardian.com/football/2011/apr/01/fulham-michael-jackson-statue-fans.

Schickel, Richard (1985): *Intimate Strangers: The Culture of Celebrity in America*. Chicago: Ivan R. Dee.

Senft, Terri (2008): *Camgirls: Celebrity and Community in the Age of Social Networks*. New York: Peter Lang.

Sloan, Will (2015): 'The Only and Original: How Billy West Nearly Out-Chaplined Chaplin'. *Partisan*, 22 July. Available online at: www.partisanmagazine.com/blog/2015/6/5/the-only-and-original.

Sterne, Jonathan (2005): 'Dead Rock Stars 1900', in Steve Jones & Joli Jensen (eds): *Afterlife and Afterimage: Understanding Posthumous Fame*. Farnham: Ashgate Publishing, pp. 253–268.

Thompson, Dave (2001): *Reggae and Caribbean Music: The Listening Companion*. San Francisco, CA: Backbeat.

Turner, Graeme (2004): *Understanding Celebrity*. London: Sage Publications.

Woodall, Joanna (1997): 'Introduction: Facing the Subject', in Joanna Woodall (ed.): *Portraiture: Facing the Subject*. Manchester: Manchester University Press, pp. 1–25.

6 The contemporary imaginary of work

Symbolic immortality within the postmodern corporate discourse

Adriana Teodorescu

Introduction: work, meaning and immortality in contemporary Western society

Work represents a fundamental human experience whose understanding and socio-cultural practice is performed more and more from the point of view of its ability to provide personal meaning to people (Baumeister 1991:116; Dik *et al.* 2013). Western contemporary society pays unprecedented attention to work. Beyond its obvious practical, individual and social necessity – namely, ensuring material support for the existence of the individual and his role in the settlement of the market economy – nowadays, work tends to be imbued with immense positive meaning. Work is regarded as the social environment where the postmodern individual (henceforth 'he/him') can manifest and further develop human and technical abilities and innate talents, and where he can build valuable social relations. Work legitimates individuals as persons who are important to themselves (an increase in self-respect) and to others (a confirmation of a socially superior status). The discourses that praise the virtue of work intertwine with the criticism (Hodgkinson 2007; Klontz 2013; Safi 2014; Sennett 1998) that points out that work begins to be over-evaluated in terms of its ability to give life meaning and from this place negative effects are derived, such as workaholism.

The current importance of work in contemporary social practices, but especially in the contemporary social imaginary, is illustrated by an ample study from 2005, which underlines the fact that *busyness* – a strong avatar of work – became 'the new badge of honour' (Gershuny 2005). The same study highlighted the fact that current society does not necessarily devote as much time to work as it used to, but – a major change compared to other historical periods – longing for work overtakes longing for leisure. The importance of work in the contemporary imaginary can be explained through the fact that in a world where robust, metaphysical truths are destroyed, the individual is continuously menaced by insignificance, so that 'maintaining meaning and identity became ever more complex' (Strenger 2011:15).

Because work is a matter more and more tied to the human search for meaning, death influences contemporary socio-cultural construction of work to a high degree. Getting work closer to one's death might seem, at first glance, a bizarre aspect. However, the absence of labelling death within certain socio-cultural dimensions does not presuppose that death is less present than in the areas where it is considered to play a significant part.[1] On the contrary, as Zygmunt Bauman notes, the impact of death is many times greater in the areas where nothing seems to make it so:

> The impact of death is at its most powerful (and creative) when death does not appear under its own name; in areas and times which are not explicitly dedicated to it; precisely where we manage to live as if death was not or did not matter, when we do not remember about mortality and are not put off or vexed by the thoughts of the ultimate futility of life.
>
> (Bauman 1992:7)

By searching for a life meaning in and through work, postmodern society tries to quench its anxiety in the face of death: 'Death is hard to keep in mind when there is work to be done: it seems not so much taboo as unlikely' (De Botton 2010:324). Because of this, the contemporary imaginary of work abounds in elements whose cultural logic can be defined as being anti-thanatic. To better circumscribe the concept, anti-thanatic logic is the cultural logic that can acknowledge the unavoidable human reality of death, while contrarily lacking the ability to elaborate proper strategies for understanding life according to this idea. Driven by what is deemed to be an abnormal fear that emanates from the reckoning of death, anti-thanatic logic actively engages in a (virtually) perpetual fight against this enemy. It seeks to withstand death by any means, while at the same time maintaining a peaceful outward appearance. Efforts to counteract death must always be veiled. The semiotics corresponding to anti-thanatic logic is characterised by a fracture between a signifier that seems to totally forget the signified within which death and mortality can no longer be ignored. This entails the manifestation of a permanent concern for annulling those aspects that might awaken the consciousness of human mortality. Thus, this cultural logic resorts to non-literal, symbolic immortality (Lifton & Olson 1974; Lifton 1979) as a strategy for constructing the elements that form the contemporary imaginary of work.

In what follows, I want to illustrate that one of the fundamental vectors constructing the contemporary imaginary of work is the pursuit of symbolic immortality. This is achieved by overusing some essential features of postmodernity: *narcissism*, the imperative of *breaking the limits* and *infantilisation* – traits commonly united by an anti-thanatic orientation. I will refer especially to the postmodern corporate imaginary, because work in transnational corporations has specific features, which makes it unique in the general employment landscape.[2]

Through symbolic immortality this study takes into account both the meaning given by Robert Jay Lifton and the explanations Bauman offers regarding the way in which symbolic immortality functions in postmodern times. In line with Lifton's theory, symbolic immortality is a cultural reality generated by the universal human will to nurture a feeling of continuity and transcendence in the face of death, a feeling reached through symbolic means. Lifton gives privilege to the positive meaning associated with symbolic immortality, showing that, when symbolic immortality is inhibited, people experience profound psychological difficulty (Lifton 1968). On the other hand, from a more critical perspective, Bauman defines the relationship of contemporary society with immortality in terms of deconstruction. Immortality is broken into a set of smaller or greater immortalities, all within reach. From this point of view, immortality does not refer so much to an imaginary projection of the self after death – an after-death immortality, for example through family, art, nature or work – but rather to immortality as the postponement of death, a temporary victory against it (a before-death immortality): 'Each moment, or no moment, is immortal. Immortality is here – but not here to stay. Immortality is as transient and evanescent as the rest of things' (Bauman 1992:164). In both complementary senses, symbolic immortality is a social-cultural strategy meant to activate defensive mechanisms against death and to support the idea that life is meaningful.

The corporate work culture and the social features of symbolic immortality through work

As a form of economic organisation typical to capitalism, the corporation appears in the late nineteenth century and is settled by the early twentieth. Anthony Giddens (2009:799–800) notes that one of the most important features of modern-day post-Fordist corporations is the paternal attention given to employees. There are two major structures in today's corporations: human resource management, understood as the internal management of relations with employees; and the necessity to make people aware of the *corporate culture* – namely, a set of values specific to that company, occasionally leading to ideology-driven thinking (Thompson & Findlay 1999) – which is implemented through various strategies and practices. Human resource management postulates that there is no serious conflict between the employees and their employer (Giddens 2009:894–898) and privileges the work seen as a 'calling' (Baumeister 1991:125–126), while, without being left aside, other meanings associated with work, the job and career, tend to be slightly neglected. The logic behind this is relatively clear: to be able to compete with other companies, the corporation must function in a unitary and homogeneous manner, and must eliminate any internal difference of opinion. Corporate culture is aimed at increasing the trust and loyalty of its employees (Brown 2009:19). For this to happen, there needs to be a nurturing of those mechanisms that stimulate the growth of group cohesion. Cohesion is achieved through a series of rituals such as: fun activities, celebrating various events, community service, etc. Nowadays, corporations are preoccupied not only with constructing and continuously reinforcing employees' motivation – a strategy of giving meaning to work (Sievers 1994) – but also with entertaining a friendly relationship with the public and valuing its opinions. Issues such as corporate ethics and social responsibility are more and more widely discussed (Nash 2009).

Among the most important features of corporate work, we need to mention the use of an extremely persuasive discourse that seeks to deliver a positive image of the company, especially towards current and potential employees,[3] as well as to the general public. This type of discourse can be noticed on company official pages and blogs, Facebook pages or other online networks and social communities. In the making of this type of discourse, we can easily detect techniques that seek to underline the relationship between work and meaning (work gives meaning to life) and to place this relationship within the symbolic immortality imaginary. What should be mentioned is the fact that the imaginary of symbolic immortality through work is determined not only by the plurality of corporate discourses in the internal world of the company, or in public, but also by the corporate social practices and the way in which the company is organised.[4] Moreover, the reverse relationship is also true: corporate practices and discourses contribute to the way in which the postmodern imaginary of work is shaped.[5] It is extremely important for this twofold factor to be understood, since the construction of corporate discourse does not need to be consciously performed by symbolic references to immortality. On the other hand, this does not exclude the manipulative aspect of these discourses, in the sense that, consciously or not, they do exploit the wish of the postmodern individual to transcend death by resorting to cultural substitutes for immortality. Actually, as has been observed, work itself, through its very nature, beyond any particular feature, forces society to adopt a manipulative behaviour:

> Society needs to get people to do a large number of dull things that they don't particularly want to do. Work requires exertion and sacrifice, and somehow society has to induce people to make these exertions and sacrifices.
>
> (Baumeister 1991:118)

> It is quite astonishing that our contemporary organization theories and, more specifically, the increasing concern for organizational and corporate culture seem to mainly ignore the issue of immortality. This is even more surprising as our contemporary institutional and societal practice is full, not to say plastered, with our attempts to install immortality.
>
> (Sievers 1994:99)

The fact that, on one hand, symbolic immortality through work tends to be more and more important in the contemporary collective imaginary and, on the other, tends to be used more and more intensely, consciously or not, by transnational companies as a strategy to increase work appeal and attractiveness, is due to its direct connection with some fundamental cultural traits of postmodernity. In comparison with other symbolic immortality structures (through nature, through children, through art), which have a certain degree of independence from history, immortality through work is deeply rooted in the epoch that makes it possible. There are three important strands in post-modern society that essentially contribute to the cultural motivation of symbolic immortality through work. I will discuss them by focusing on the way in which they materialise in the contemporary imaginary of work and on their anti-thanatic potential, therefore on their ability to trigger the fiction of immortality. These strands are interrelated, as they are determined by the same postmodern cultural energies that nurture each other. The first strand is linked to the identification of a place for existential meaning; the second strand is linked to the dynamics of the place in which the existential meaning resides; while the third strand focuses on nature and on the qualitative functioning of existential meaning.

Narcissism: towards a new place for meaning

At first glance, narcissism is nothing but the radical expression of adamant individualism promoted by Western, hyper-consumerist society. However, as noted by many researchers, culturally speaking, narcissism might be defined as the pathological reflection of the individual into himself, as a result of the loosening of relationships with the world, set against the backdrop of a general mistrust in the ability of social structures to ensure order (Lasch 1991) and in the ability of reality to provide meaning (Baudrillard 1977; Debray 2008). A by-product of postmodernity, narcissism can be understood in the way that Christopher Lasch first saw it, as a set of 'survival strategies' destined to counteract the anxiety that haunts the postmodern subject because of his inability to anchor himself in the contemporary world.[6] This is a world whose relativity hides (Javeau 2007:146) the exhaustion of social and political solutions that become incapable of preserving two things in the collective imaginary: the past, which is important in the definition of human identity, and the future, as a dimension of hope for the better and of trust in posterity:

> Having no hope of improving their lives in any of the ways that matter, people have convinced themselves that what matters is psychic self-improvement ... To live for the moment is the prevailing passion – to live for yourself, not for your predecessors or posterity.
>
> (Lasch 1991:4–5)

The present becomes the only temporal dimension that matters – the dimension in which the unrooted postmodern subject projects his life. This is performed fairly easily, because postmodern society endows the present with show-like characteristics (Lipovetsky 1992). Moreover, the existential intensity of the present is diminished to increase its attractiveness and to avoid, with the help of image proliferation (Gauthier 1998), the encounter with non-representable death (Baudrillard 1977; Debray 2008; Le Breton 2004:1027).

As a survival strategy, determined by the weakening of ties to the world, narcissism raises the problem of identifying a place for the existential meaning of the postmodern individual. However, the present is too extensive, too vast to be able to pinpoint a specific place for meaning. There has to be more – which, in this case, is less.

The superficiality of the contemporary world is the background that stimulates, by means of compensation, and coaxes the postmodern individual to engage in the search for an authentic self, which is largely synonymous with identifying an existential meaning. This quest for authenticity has nothing in common with the quest intensely debated by existential philosophy and anthropology, according to which the ultimate authenticity of an individual is closely tied to the facing of one's own mortality as an essential condition of human nature (Heidegger 1962; Sartre 1943). On the other hand, the authenticity concept was criticised as well, the majority showing it to be a cultural construct, and that making authenticity equivalent to the acceptance of death is abusive (Adorno 1973; Ellis 2001:162). What is certain is that postmodern authenticity is not defined with death being its starting point, but is based rather on an immortality understood as deconstruction, as a projection of how immortality is felt in the present (Bauman 1992). It is interesting to notice that the hyper-consumerist ideological shadow of postmodern authenticity is happiness (Lipovetsky 2006), which can be understood as a temporary abolition of death anxiety.

The postmodern individual is truly searching for an authentic self – one to which he feels fully entitled – without yielding his maximal psychological comfort. Therefore, he has to search for sufficient strength to make a stand in the face of the reality of the external world. He is encouraged to ensure that his psyche will not suffer as a result of this process. Of course, what is at stake here is the therapeutic psychology intensely criticised by researchers (Foley 2011; Lasch 1991; Lilienfeld *et al.* 2010; Lipovetsky 2006), precisely because placating the individual with 'everything will be all right' and 'you just have to want it' is based on concealing helplessness and individual death – both of which occur naturally – a concealment meant to increase an individual's trust in his own powers. This determines an adhesion to a paradoxical self: an ideal self (a self that has to be reached) and, at the same time, a self that already exists (alluded to by 'be yourself' references). Moreover, this dual, twofold self is captured by a dialectical thinking rich in Nietzschean and existentialist echoes, which are prevalent in self-help books and positive thinking discourse found on the Internet, such as 'become what you are'. It is interesting to notice that what is left aside by this type of phrasing is death itself. Death is abstracted from the natural process of transformation (any life ends in death), a transformation that ends in and through the present time.

A proper place for the existential meaning of the narcissistic individual, combining the need for authenticity with psychological comfort, might be family. Until recently, family was seen as having the role of contributing to the psychological well-being of the individual. In contemporary Western society, the triumphant discourse on individual happiness within the family and on its ability to ensure enhanced psychological comfort fades in terms of their persuasive impact (Bruckner 2010; Klinenberg 2013). This occurs despite the fact that many studies continue to confirm Durkheim's idea according to which, the more an individual is involved in family relations, the more he/she is protected from death (Vaillant 2012). However, strictly from the perspective of *fulfilling the self* – the ultimate postmodern value and another name given to postmodern authenticity – these discourses enter the category of obsolete social discourses, to which there is a certain nostalgia attached, inspiring numerous movies and heart-wrenching books. The problem is that, beyond their intrinsic quality, the social discourses of fulfilment through family life are prone, in their vast majority, to suffer from the stigmata of a lack of seriousness: for current-day society, family is not a means of finding meaning, but, at best, the domestic support for it.

The postmodern individual does not find the proper environment to carry on his *conquest of self* within the family, since the family is earmarked for death. Because those who make up the family cannot be co-narcissistic individuals for a long time – sources of pleasure without problematic, ontological depths. In fact, they reveal themselves to be, sooner or later, true *beings-towards-death* (Heidegger 1962). It is not even necessary that they die to induce the postmodern individual to confront the reality of death. Elements such as disease, misunderstanding, abandonment or existential fragility are generally sufficient.

However, the triumphant discourses on the happiness of the individual through work abound within mass as well as within organisational culture. Work, especially the work carried out in transnational corporations, corresponds to the aspirations of narcissistic fulfilment of the self, in a far superior manner than the family could hope to achieve, its great advantage being that, on a social imaginary level, it functions according to principles similar to those regarding the symbolic embodiment of the self. If the self must become involved in an alert race towards perfection (Foley 2011), then postmodern work needs to be plastic, as it entails a continuous transformation, mobility (from one project to the other, from one location to the other), a continuous present that tames the perspective of an unknown future, and which thus contains the promise of discovering the true, so desired self:

> Because we want you to thrive at Oracle, we work to enhance your quality of life, help you invest in your future.
>
> (Oracle 2016)

> No need to predict the future, you can create it.
>
> (BMW 2016)

> Daimler as an employer. Shape your future. Change the world ... We can offer you the best possible chance to forge a successful future. And not just professionally, but personally too.
>
> (Daimler 2016)

GE offers you a fantastic work environment and unmatched opportunities to build a successful future.

(General Electrics 2016)

Work entails the confrontation with and overcoming of one's own limits, with the help of the specialists in human resources and of many, ever-growing development training opportunities marketed by the majority of public relations specialists hired by companies: 'We invest time, resources and energy to support each IQuest member take full control of their talent' (IQuest Group 2016). However, that which remains is still work (as opposed to family life) – despite the emphasis laid on the team – as an individual activity (the salary and the bonuses are attributed to one individual and one only). The narcissistic self also remains individual, being forced to rely only upon himself. Therefore, work has all the advantages to be a privileged place for the meaning of the postmodern individual.

The purpose of work is to offer not only the means through which the self introspects by means of its narcissistic mirrors, projecting itself at the centre of its idealised narratives about the future, but also to supply a symbolic aid in creating a place for meaning outside of the individual. No matter how focused on himself he is, the postmodern individual needs to position his existential meaning outside of himself, otherwise the risk of implosion and, consequently, of existential annulment becomes extremely great. Actually, things seem clearer if we consider that work is the main trigger and maintainer of the economy paradigm. Economy becomes an instrument in evaluating social and cultural elements, which leads to an overlapping of economy with Western culture. Carlo Strenger talks about this almost inevitable, economic measurement of reality in critical terms: 'the mindless dogma that what really matters must be measurable in economic terms' (Strenger 2011:2). Strangely enough, in the contemporary imaginary of work, economy is devoid of the negative connotations that surround the idea of instability and arbitrariness. Thus, the positive meaning, which characterises the postmodern myth of work that sets one free (from poverty, from boredom, repetitiveness and ultimately death) and brings happiness, is gladly maintained (Warr & Clapperton 2010).

Given these aspects, we can better understand that the narcissistic comfort that the postmodern individual finds in work resides in stabilising his existential meaning in a place from which death is banished. Even admitting that death might linger within the self, the postmodern individual creates for himself the illusion that, in contrast to his self, his existential meaning is not enslaved by death, because this meaning is achieved not only *through* work, but also *in* the work itself:

We not only offer you a job, we also give you something to identify with: more than 80 percent of all Bosch associates are proud to be part of the company.

(Bosch 2016)

Together we can make a difference – We accomplish extraordinary things every day. Our teams support various causes ... Here, you'll make a difference.

(J. P. Morgan 2016)

Or, as Alain De Botton puts it, there can be no death as long as there is work to be done:

Work does not by its nature permit us to do anything other than take it too seriously. It must destroy our sense of perspective, and we should be grateful to it for precisely that reason, for allowing us to mingle ourselves promiscuously with events, for letting us wear thoughts of our own death and the destruction of our enterprises with beautiful lightness, as mere intellectual propositions.

(De Botton 2010:324)

Breaking the limits: an expanding place for meaning

Breaking all limits is one of the postmodern fundamentals. The contemporary epoch highlights and exults man's need to outrun himself, to become better and more performant at what he does. The ancestor of limit-breaking is the project. Among the founding philosophers of the project, Jean-Paul Sartre (1943, 1946) is a prominent figure. Sartre views the being as inherently ontologically organised as a project (*being-for-itself*), but believes that man must acknowledge his project-like nature, assuming an anti-essentialist perspective according to which the individual is thrown into the world, a pure reflex of arbitrariness. Men embody their essence as they advance through life, needing to become their own project precisely because there is no meaning that precedes their birth. For Sartre, assuming the self as a project is a way of defying the absurdity of death, which, as the French philosopher argues (in full Heidegger-like apostasy), is not even an integral part of the being (Sartre 1943:584).

There are two major, correlated resemblances between Sartre's project and the expanded postmodern self: first, the fact that both are means of deconstructing the future through the pretence of structurally subordinating it to the present, and then the fact that both of them run from death. However, the fundamental difference lies in the fact that, if the Sartre-like soul runs, through the project, from an absurd death it is aware of, the postmodern self runs from death because of fear. Unconsciously, the postmodern being knows that death is part of his structural ontology, but does not possess the means to confront it. From here derive the differences between the Sartre project and the postmodern project of breaking limits. Sartre's project is not based on progressive principles: *being-for-itself* is simply meant, via its ontological nature, to aim for the future. And, despite the fact that he refuses a meeting with death, he does not delude himself that his (true) fulfilment will ever happen. Breaking the limits is perceived by postmodernity in a positive, vertical light: the self conquers itself not only from a purely ontological perspective, as with the Sartre model, but also pragmatically, quantitatively and qualitatively. In this respect, the project of breaking the limits – ode to the power of the individual – is more of a romantic, rather than an existentialist one.

From the point of view of the social imaginary of work, the cultural imperative of breaking the limits – together with its variants or sub-structures: surpassing the self, excellence, potential, performance, success at any cost – is also tied to the place where the postmodern individual projects his meaning on a mental basis. In addition, breaking the limits indicates that it is not enough for the postmodern subject to find an anchoring-place for meaning, but, in agreement with generic postmodern logic, this place must continuously evolve, must continuously expand:

> Work Hard. Have Fun. Make History. Go beyond what's expected and reinvent normal.
>
> (Amazon 2016)

> We set ourselves goals we know we can't reach yet, because we know that by stretching to meet them we can get further than we expected.
>
> (Google 2016)

> [W]e'll support and encourage you to push your boundaries, explore new opportunities and meet new people ... We can help you get where you want to go.
>
> (J. P. Morgan 2016)

> Our mission is to go beyond the client expectations by bringing together technology, talent, innovation, and the highest quality standards.
>
> (Luxoft 2016)

Breaking the limits refers not only to what the postmodern subject is and can become, but also, to a great extent, in agreement with capitalist logic, to what he does and can do (Safi 2014). In both respects, breaking the limits is authorised because it is based on the idea that a person's *potential* greatly surpasses what the individual currently is and does. The potential is directly tied to the narcissistic structure of postmodern individuals who are constantly told that they are entitled to obtain things, to be better, to go further, etc. (Baudry 1991; Javeau 2007; Lasch 1991; Naish 2009:130). The strong belief in individual potential has been haunting postmodern society to exhaustion and holds a special spot in the collective imaginary of work. Work-related discourses praise the idea that every individual must attain maximum potential. These discourses also stress that work (or a particular company) is the ideal place where potential can be fully reached. Without being an exclusive feature of the work imaginary, *potential* is one of the prominent myths it propagates (De Botton 2010; Sievers 1994), as it can be found in internal and external PR discourses, and hence why many companies massively invest in programmes meant to enhance the professional abilities of their employees (Foley 2011:35):

> ExxonMobil is a dynamic, exciting place to work. We hire exceptional people, and every one of them is empowered to think independently, take initiative and be innovative.
>
> (ExxonMobil 2016)

> Everything starts with passion at BMW. It turns a profession into a vocation. It drives us to keep reinventing mobility and bringing innovative ideas onto the roads.
>
> (BMW 2016)

> Joining us at one of our international locations means taking on new challenges and gives you access to a professional universe like no other in the world.
>
> (BNP Parisbas 2016)

> You are young, talented and looking for a career in which you play a meaningful part in millions of lives. If this is you, you might be up for a change of a life time.
>
> (ING 2016)

The myth of potential develops as a result of the deconstruction of immortality, so that the symbolic immortality it promises consists of a life that becomes better not only quantitatively, but also qualitatively. The things that are not yet experienced are more important than what the individual has already experienced, so that the postmodern individual constantly brings the future into the present, instead of plunging in and making real advancement towards the future:

> It became the enduring project of our modern cultures of redemption – cultures committed above all to science and progress – to create societies in which people can realize their potential, in which 'growth' and 'productivity' and 'opportunity' are the watchwords … Once the promise of immortality, of being chosen, was displaced by the promise of more life – the promise, as we say, of getting more out of life – the unlived life became a haunting presence in a life legitimated by nothing more than the desire to live it.
>
> (Phillips 2013:xiv–xv)

The symbolic immortality promised by the myth of potential refers not only to the present (immortality through deconstruction), but also to a post-mortem immortality. This is due to the fact that the myth of potential is symbolically constructed by contamination with the myth of artist. Work functions in a very similar way to immortality through art (Baumeister 1991:126): work promises to fulfil the artistic experiences of the worker, engendering a feeling of immortality through the sensation of time suspension and artistic catharsis while, on the other hand, giving the sensation that he will be acknowledged, through his accomplishments, even after his death. Sociologists have shown that the artist myth is more and more frequently encountered in the way individuals view their work, even in the case of categories such as engineers, which, until recently, were considered incompatible with this model (Baumeister 1991:126, Béra & Lamy 2003). Work offers the postmodern employee the possibility to discover an existential meaning in a similar way that art, in the past, would offer itself to those determined to serve it. Innovation, creativity, originality – words used extensively by the postmodern discourses related to work become true contemporary rhetorical hallmarks, if not stereotypes. These are qualities that postmodern employees can and must have, and which enable them to perform all work activities in a climate of intensified life:

> What do we expect from you: Creative and fresh thinking in your work and your life, regardless of your role.
>
> (Coca-Cola 2016)

> This job is not a simple task and we make sure that our people have the possibility to create innovative solutions … We are respected engineers of the imagination.
>
> (Luxoft 2016)

Even more so, these also promise that the work of the postmodern subject will not be left unknown after he is gone, that the results of his work will be treated similarly to art products, answering not only to the practical necessities of the public/society, but also to artistic necessities (Sievers 1994:114). Many companies, through their discourses, exploit the impulse towards a post-mortem immortality, towards survival beyond any personal life boundaries:

> Do you think the future starts today? So do we. In the spirit of our company founder Robert Bosch, we have actively shaped the future for more than 125 years by developing innovative solutions for future generations.
>
> (Bosch 2016)

> GE is a company of ideas. A place where ideas are nurtured and grow into beautiful things that make the world work better.
>
> (General Electrics 2016)

Numerous postmodern and work experts criticise *breaking the limits*, as a survival strategy and as a trigger for the immortality chimera. The main objections include:

1   Entitlement is an illusion: not everybody has the right to succeed, professional and personal success are correlated with an individual's professional and personal abilities, so that those who succeed in a field represent the exception, rather than the rule (De Botton 2010:279). Failure is absolutely inevitable throughout human life, but it has still become a taboo (Foley 2011:87; Sennett 1998).[7]

2   The over-emphasis on creativity, innovation and originality at any cost highlights the accent on youth and change (Sennett 1998), and therefore on a deformed vision of the world, promoted by the atrophy of rational to the detriment of positive thinking, a magical thinking centred on pure will. The mere idea of wanting something strongly enough seems sufficient in the postmodern imaginary. The quality of work permanently assessed in terms of innovation, change and cure for 'the fear of aging and death' (Lasch 1991:45) has a perverted side effect. When it incorporates a normal monotony, fleeting as it may be, the postmodern subject will perceive the quality of his work as destabilising on a psychological level. Practically, these objections have commonality in the abandonment and fictionalisation of reality that conceals avatars of death.

An interesting interpretation that can account for the pitfalls of the anti-thanatic orientation of the cultural imperative of breaking the limits can be found in the work of French sociologist Patrick Baudry (1991). He shows that contemporary, consumerist society develops and promotes a discourse and practical register he calls *suicidal*. This behaviour is recognisable in corporate culture, in the appraisal given to some qualities such as excellence and performance in work or to the free consent to participate in collective activities that entail life-threatening risks (e.g. team-building exercises involving risk). According to Baudry, *breaking the limits*, positively highlighted by many sectors of postmodern society, offers the illusion of suspending death through the contemptuous gesture of choosing death. Actually, in a symbolically geographic pattern, we can consider that when man exits or surpasses himself, there is no other place to go than death.

Burkard Sievers (1994:59–136), in his book on the symbolic process of mortality and immortality within recent corporations, describes work within a company as being a collusive quarrel about taking part in immortality. Immortality, Sievers believes, is wanted by everybody, but can only be gained by some – usually management and leaders (see also Vandevelde 1996:123).[8] It may be that Sievers's Neo-Marxist approach is not the most appropriate in the context of transnational corporations where power-sharing is blurred and it no longer automatically generates master–slave relations.

From the point of view of visibility, the authority of managers dilutes itself (De Botton 2010; Foley 2011; Lasch 1991:183–186). Traditional authority would not be an elegant solution for those who, just like true artists, break their limits continuously. This is one of the conclusions that result from the file report by the French publication *Philosophie Magazine* (2010). It argues that the dissolution of this authority, correlated to encouraging postmodern individuals to take responsibility for the projects they are engaged in, triggers a specific kind of alienation through the work of each individual. It explains how the tendency of the postmodern individual to expect everything from the workplace and from the performed work is praised, emulated by managers and sustained by cunning organisational policies. The comfortable conditions that are made available, the fast pace of promotion, together with the discourses that stress the need for continuous career development, all lead to alienation through excessive commitment. In this case, the individual is determined to exhibit responsible behaviour by making responsible behaviour a self-triggered reality, and by turning obligation into commitment (another term heavily used in the postmodern discourse of work):

> Employees are entrusted with more responsibility and more opportunity than most comparable companies. Since we have a high hiring bar, once you are in, we bet on you. We allow you to influence change and help us grow.
>
> (Amazon 2016)

> ING stimulates a performance culture, in which employees make their own decisions.
>
> (ING 2016)

Practically, the corporate employee tends to internalise the manager figure and the external supervision attached to it, effectively becoming their own employee. The struggle for immortality within the company, discussed by Sievers, is interiorised, the social aspects of struggle giving way to the psychological aspects.[9] Far from being a struggle between two separate instances, immortality becomes a struggle with the self. The more the self is moulded to agree with the progressive principles of hyper-capitalism, the more it becomes closer to gaining immortality.

The (new) infantilisation: re-enchanting meaning

Infantilisation can be noticed at various levels of contemporary social life, ranging from the Western fascination with television, advertising, fantasy movies and the entertainment industry in general, to postponing the decisions that involve long-term responsibility (choosing a career, marriage, having children). The latter is also known as Peter Pan syndrome, the term being coined by Dan Kiley in 1983, referring also to the obsession with work specific to some of the subjects afflicted by this syndrome. Another indicator of social infantilisation is, according to a considerable number of researchers, the contemporary obsession with children, to whom attention has been given to a degree unprecedented in Western history (Ariès 1965; Douglas & Michaels 2004; Jong 2010; Warner 2006). Infantilisation also includes the team-buildings and the fun activities that define the vast majority of trans-national corporations. A reaction to the age of liberation (Foley 2011:37–38), the *infantilisation* of the postmodern individual is a fairly well-documented fact, which continues to attract numerous critics, chiefly because it implies a very serious denial of human finiteness by perpetuating the desire for a state of eternal youth (Elias 1985/2001). The major consequences of this denial are a lack of responsibility towards others (Lipovetsky 1992) and the diminishment of all defence mechanisms in the face of social manipulation.

Infantilisation may hide a search for a meaning obscured by stern hyper-capitalism, but actually it stems from the need to re-enchant the meanings of a life menaced by pragmatism and death, to reinvest them with mystery and passion, to make them able to contribute to the happiness of the individual (the hedonist imperative of the current epoch). Infantilisation does not entail a return to childhood, but the creation of a childhood surrogate, an idealised childhood – a dangerous one – which eliminates loss. In fact, this sham childhood established through the cultural process of infantilisation is a construction that incorporates a subtle yet resolute stance against death and especially against dying. For example, Steven B., Product Support Helpdesk Specialist at Garmin, describes his career as playing with toys and proudly states that he never has to grow up. As Kiley said, the infantilised individual refuses to grow up and is caught 'between the man he didn't want to become and the boy he could no longer be' (Kiley 1983:23).

From the perspective of the contemporary collective work imaginary, infantilisation focuses on the qualitative functioning of existential meaning. If narcissism indicates work as a possible location for meaning, and surpassing boundaries shows that this place must continuously expand to keep meaning attractive and to diminish the fear of death for the postmodern individual, then *infantilisation* shows that work must redefine itself by borrowing aspects regarding the magic of childhood. Thus, happiness, which, for the current epoch, becomes a true obsession in relation to work (De Botton 2010:106), is an essential feature of this magic.

One of the most visible signs of workplace infantilisation is the team-building and fun activities that define the vast majority of transnational corporations. Corporate webpages abound not only in discourses that emphasise their ability to create an enjoyable, fun work and extra-work atmosphere, but also in proofs that sustain this idea, including pictures or videos of team-building and other fun activities, along with employee testimonials. Such proofs reveal that, far from being accidental, excellence and discourses exalting the extraordinary traits of the model employee run alongside having fun, as if functioning as the new value gauge for postmodern corporations and also as a central feature of the contemporary work imaginary. In their *301 Ways to Have Fun at Work*, David Hemsath and Leslie Yerkes (1997) observed that having fun is indeed a recent corporate value, a powerful resource that should be implemented as an organisational strategy meant to facilitate employee searches for creativity and innovation, while preventing both stress and absenteeism:

> We're all in it together, which is why we think it's important to have a good time and bond within the team while producing excellence for our customers every time.
>
> (IQuest Group 2016)

> Our offices and cafes are designed to encourage interactions … and to spark conversation about work as well as play.
>
> (Google 2016)

Ten years after the publication of Hemsath and Yerkes' book, journalist Matt Labash (2008) conducted a field investigation spotlighting the idea that fun is 'the new core value on the loose' within the contemporary corporate environment. The point being, Labash notices, precisely that: because fun is now a fully fledged corporate value, it functions in a prescriptive way, so that the infantilisation of the workplace is defined by a 'coercive' fun. As the Labash analysis goes on to show, to have fun is, or at least carries a high risk of becoming, mandatory. Taking this into account, the oppressive nature of corporate infantilisation becomes visible. Nestled within the magic and happiness of this second, surrogate childhood lurks the spectre of a necessary obedience.

Infantilism in the workplace can be understood in Sievers' terms, from a Neo-Marxist perspective, as a relatively conscious strategy developed by management in order to impose power on employees and to exclude them from the secular immortality offered, on a symbolical level, by multi-national companies. Although Sievers' explanations of infantilisation could be helpful in our understanding of the contemporary corporate situation, overall, the cultural paradigm of childhood, which supports Sievers' approach on work, is not postmodern in nature, but rather modernist. It is an approach based on the subordinate relationship between parent and child that does not perfectly describe the relationship between the postmodern company and its employees:

> The infantilization of the worker means that he is not responsible for his work. It is an expression of the fundamental splitting in our work enterprises according to which those at the top are seen by themselves and by others as adults and those at the bottom are seen as children.
>
> (Sievers 1994:74)

Years before Sievers, Christopher Lasch tried to describe the unexpected, yet powerful correlation between the different models of child-rearing and the way in which companies are organised. He explained that business and organisational sociology cultures tend to go hand in hand with postmodern parenting theories, arguing for empowerment of the child and for a diminishment in restrictions imposed by the authoritarian figure of the parent. This does not mean that the power structures disappear, but that what Lasch (1991:218–236) calls *paternalism without father* is triggered. It is a valuable idea for understanding the contemporary corporate infantilisation.

Expanding upon Lasch, Michael Foley (2011:162) discusses benign paternalism and the *Big Baby*, whose needs and whims must be fully satisfied (Foley 2011:39). He also tackles *new infantilism*, which entails the pursuit of personal satisfaction no matter what. It is an infantilism that companies exploit to their benefit, because, by giving the postmodern individual the fun he needs, companies manage to significantly increase his loyalty to the workplace to the detriment of his personal life (Foley 2011:102–105) – the increase in the importance of work colleagues vs a decrease in the importance of family – and also to the detriment of trust in his ability to solve work problems on his own. As far as personal life is concerned, John Naish (2009:118–122) notes that the fact that postmodern work makes the management of family ties more difficult has become taboo. This happens because life inside the company is more simplified through fun and focusing on the problems of the company, rather than on the more complex problems (including death and dying) of the individual himself.

Indeed, work relations with colleagues are, in fact, rather infant–infant type relations, built on a psycho-cultural regression to childhood. Work becomes a game (Hall 2015) for which the postmodern individual needs partners, needs a team. And since there are more and more aggressive tendencies to invade the individual's personal space, through practices such as team-building or nights out or various facilities offered by more and more corporations, work is designed to be no longer just a game, but a perpetual adventure:

> The corporations have become self-contained worlds with their own shops, cafes, bars, restaurants, gyms, hairdressers, massage rooms and medical facilities. The workplace is a new village, a community offering not merely employment and status but all essential services, a rich varied social life and fun, fun, fun, fun.
>
> (Foley 2011:162–163)

It has been shown that any group offers the possibility of personal self-transcendence, functioning at a relatively comfortable low level compared to other forms of transcendence (Baron & Branscombe 2011). By identifying with the group, the postmodern individual can unburden himself from his very own *self* and from his mortality as well. The process is even easier in the case of the corporate group, which is placed, within the imaginary of postmodern work, under a utopian horizon: a superior human organisation that has nothing to do with inter-personal conflicts and which succeeds to ethically and fairly manage its tasks. The team is an important operational and ideological unit of the corporate environment, imbued with unprecedented positive value. In his chapter dedicated to the examination of the main characteristics of the contemporary workplace, Robert Rowland Smith (2010:47) observes that the postmodern work team is configured in a similar way to the perfect sports team – noticeable also in the language used to describe it and in the propensity for organising team-building events as sport competitions. This 'sportive' configuration – privileged version of the game – is intended to contribute to making the team sacrosanct without negatively affecting the narcissism of the individuals. Indeed, the employees remain players – the childlike essence is evident – endowed with special talents, yet conceding their incompleteness, their dependence upon others. When seen against the background of team rhetoric, the vertical imperative of exceeding personal limits appears to be only a small piece of a much larger puzzle: the limits that need to be left behind relate not only to personal and professional skills, but also to an ontological interpersonal dimension. While instilling the need to abandon the comfortable, familiar self, this interpersonal dimension sustains the bizarre transformation of the self into what it (already) is: one cannot fall when he is surrounded and even compounded by others. The narcissism of the postmodern employee is not only preserved, but also reinforced: the Others are perfect mirrors of the self.

The team or the work group utopia is based on death denial in several ways. First, the fact that, with the great help of the rhetoric of fun, otherness is seen exclusively through a positive lens – an otherness placed in the full cultural paradigm of rendering the *Other* as positive (Deloro 2009; Lesourd 2007; Vattimo 2002) – entails a process of denying human evil:

> The Other has become a commercial slogan: love one another, the Other 'is good for you' ... but this is not true. The more we pacify our relations, the less the Other exists. We have become *human, too human!* We thus see the Other break in abstract and terrifying manners, which make the world a place of horror and transforms subjectivity into a battlefield.
>
> (Deloro 2009:14)

> Teamwork, though, takes us into that domain of demeaning superficiality which besets the modern workplace. Indeed, teamwork exits the realm of tragedy to enact human relations as a farce.
>
> (Sennett 1998)

If there is such a thing as evil in the corporate imaginary of work, it originates from within the individual and not from the Other, although it can be discarded, being the result of a lack of (corporate) education, not of an ontological deficit or of a normal social context. Without ontological depth, the Other does not bring sadness or misery, does not corrode the narcissistic nature of the postmodern individual, either by being better and thus engendering hatred, or by being worse and thereby breeding contempt. No death drive could arise from the confrontation with this immature, child-like Other. Possible conflicts between employees – which are not considered to have a serious cause (just as among children) – can be solved through the golden path of communication, one of the universal healers of the corporate work imaginary.

Liaison abilities are a 'must' and for this reason become the focus of training courses. Communication also goes through a massive process of positivisation that condemns and banishes difference. Nowadays, communication almost exclusively transforms itself into something commonplace, into necessary agreement and into the need to send a clear message:

> Great ideas sometimes come from singular inspiration, but more often they're a result of collaborative effort ... To spark engagement and team building, we sponsor on-site events, such as seminars and cookouts, as well as opportunities to serve our community through philanthropic organizations and services.
>
> (Garmin 2016)

> A spirit of collaboration – you thrive when you work with a diverse range of people.
>
> (Coca-Cola 2016)

In Aristotelian terminology, a pragmatic logos prevails over a semantic logos. David le Breton (1990) considers that *transparency imagery* is a modern-day hallmark when it comes to the way in which we tackle the body. This imagery gets activated also in the case of communication and relationships. Transparency imagery might be explained, the French researcher claims, through society's need to oppose death and deny dying. By taking control of the body through images, by making it totally visible, society creates the illusion that it could master its own death. Being a means of simplifying the world and of offering an optimistic interpretation of reality – accessible, stable, meaningful – the corporate transparency ideal, in terms of communication, is just another reflex of infantilism.

A further clue for the process of infantilisation occurring in contemporary corporations is the growing preference for younger employees. The hidden logic seems, in fact, to be 'the younger, the better'. In 1998, Richard Sennett observed in his book that this age discrimination is a worrisome phenomenon that can be explained by the corporate necessity to control its employees in an unflashy, cunning manner. Traits such as flexibility and innovation render the middle-aged employee not so well suited for corporate work, especially when work is performed within technological companies where the pace of change is more intense than in other fields. Nevertheless, underneath these practical reasons lies a certain social inability to integrate the biggest variable, the greatest project of all: the human life – encompassing not only old age and death, but also other values that come with experience such as commitment, stability or critical thinking. In a nutshell, the re-enchantment of meaning that the infantilisation of work offers is strictly dependent on the ability of work to ban, through discourses and practices, the shadow of death from within inter-human relations and to provide a glamorous image of the inter-personal relationships.

Conclusions

The present chapter has striven to disclose the presence of symbolic immortality within the contemporary imaginary of work, especially in relation to recent corporate discourses, and to analyse the ways in which the fact that immortality can function as a survival strategy is used to contribute when socially constructing the idea that work is a valuable source of existential meaning. Special attention was given to the three features of postmodernity that participate to a great extent in articulating the current vision of corporate work: narcissism, the imperative of breaking the limits and the cultural process of infantilisation. The study pointed out that all of these features are characterised by an insidious rejection of human mortality, manifesting what was defined as an anti-thanatic orientation. As the chapter has emphasised, symbolic immortality through work often goes hand in hand not only with the need to endow work with meaning, but also, importantly, with equating this meaning to the purpose of life as a whole.

Up to a point, it may not be unethical for corporations to take advantage of the human need for meaning and transcendence. The problem lies not in the mere existence of symbolic immortality through work, but in the fact that, thus structured – having a collective and even stereotyped configuration – it tends to exclude other forms of symbolic immortality and, most of all, the personal and creative aspects of symbolic immortality in general. Symbolic immortality has as a direct beneficiary the company itself, rather than its employees. Also, the corporate shaping of symbolic immortality tends to block the communication channels for discontent or frustration, which are so human. In fact, the mechanisms via which infantilisation occurs in companies, the retention of the employee in a narcissistic psycho-cultural state and constant stimulation of the individual's growing desire to break limits, all have many disadvantages at the level where the postmodern employee configures his life.

Work might be closer to death than to immortality. This happens especially when it is practised excessively. Medical and sociological studies insist on aspects such as the exhaustion of the contemporary employee through over-time work, the significant increase in stress levels and the risk for cardiovascular diseases, the decrease in libido and increase in depression. Moreover, the quality of the existential meaning that the employee can discover in work might be affected by the fact that work in current corporations triggers a 'corrosion of character' (Sennett 1998) and questions the identity of the employee who is forced to negotiate between work and personal life. Many of the explicit and implicit requirements of corporate culture – visiting the company offices and the customers, abnegation, spending after-hours time with the team – conflict with a series of personal and family values such as responsibility and loyalty to family. Work–life balance remains more of a promise than a solution.

Indeed, it is quite astonishing to notice that while the contemporary corporate imaginary of work is built around the idea that working gives full meaning to life and constitutes a successful solution to death anxiety by triggering the fiction of either surviving corporeal death or by engendering a sense of permanence, the reality can be quite different. It is an aspect that was explored some decades ago by Richard Sennett (1998), who examined the difficulties of postmodern employees to compose a coherent, meaningful narrative of their lives. Sennett underscored how even if monotonous and routinised, traditional work had a great advantage: the power to create meaning and to protect the individual from stress, depression and anxiety. The problem with postmodern work is that exactly the very values for which it is praised – such as the above-discussed flexibility, excellence, originality, breaking the limits and taking risks – become difficult to manage from a personal point of view. Engineered to continuous transformation, postmodern work shatters life into fragments that can hardly be said to produce a narrative – a consistent feeling that life has or had meaning. Today, Sennett's observations are more than ever of interest for both a sociology of work and for a proper understanding of the negative side effects of symbolic immortality – of the gap between how it is designed at a social level and how it is perceived and lived from an individual perspective.

It is obvious that the work imaginary cannot fully determine the way in which the individual understands how to equate the meaning of work with the meaning of his personal, entire life, nor the way in which he allows himself to be engaged in the fiction of a corporate immortality capable of postponing death or even ensuring his post-mortem continuity, through the major achievements that will outlive him. Nevertheless, the influence of the work imaginary (the imaginary in general) on human life cannot be denied. There should be a growth in vigilance when it comes to poignant discourses and practices concerning ethical values and life meanings of the individual, especially when these appeal to death and immortality as survival strategies. Because neither of them are good in themselves.

Notes

1 Actually, it would be impossible to find a socio-cultural dimension that is not in any way connected to death if we think that human culture, as a whole, is generated by death (Heidegger 1962) and that the same culture functions as a means of counteracting death (Kastenbaum 2007).
2 Although the word *corporate* has a wider and quite controversial meaning (Lind 2014), this chapter will consider corporations to stand only for transnational companies.
3 The employees considered here are those from the middle class.

4 In what concerns the corporate practices, it should be noted that companies are not limited to symbolic immortality, but also aim towards absolute immortality. This is the case with IT companies when, to the contemporary imaginary of work, the contemporary imaginary of science and technology is also added. Technological progress is seen as the universal key to every human problem, death included (*Philosophie Magazine* 2014).
5 For these practices to be discussed from the perspective of direct observation, it is necessary to perform fieldwork that was not possible up to now. Therefore, this study acknowledges the partial nature of its methodology and of its obtained results. The approach this chapter uses will be theoretical, but there will be examples of corporate discourse.
6 Narcissism can be understood also as a trigger that questions the values and the humanistic dimension of contemporary society.
7 A good example is the start-up, which has been extremely fashionable in recent years. A very small portion of these manage to succeed over time.
8 Symbolic immortality seems to be more easily obtained by company leaders rather than the simple employees; the company itself, in the event of the leader's death, contributes to the preservation of their memory, like in the case of former CEO and co-founder of Apple, Steve Jobs (Bell & Taylor 2016).
9 This interpretation explains the apparent conflict between responsibility and desire, a synonym of the conflict between critical thinking and magical thinking, a conflict hosted (also) by the contemporary work imaginary.

References

Adorno, Theodor W. (1973): *The Jargon of Authenticity*. Evanston, IL: Northwestern University Press.
Ariès, Philippe (1965): *Centuries of Childhood: A Social History of Family Life*. New York: Random House.
Baron, Robert A. & Nyla R. Branscombe (2011): *Social Psychology*. Boston: Pearson Education.
Baudrillard, Jean (1977): *L'échange symbolique et la mort*. Paris: Gallimard.
Baudry, Patrick (1991): *Le corps extreme: Approche sociologique des conduits à risque*. Paris: L'Harmattan.
Bauman, Zygmunt (1992): *Mortality, Immortality and Other Life Strategies*. Cambridge: Polity Press.
Baumeister, Roy F. (1991): *Meanings of Life*. New York: Guilford Press.
Bell, Emma & Scott Taylor (2016): 'Vernacular Mourning and Corporate Memorialization in Framing the Death of Steve Jobs'. *Organization*, 23 (1):114–132.
Béra, Matthieu & Yvon Lamy (2003): *Sociologie de la culture*. Paris: Armand Colin.
Brown, Megan (2009): *The Cultural Work of Corporations*. London: Palgrave Macmillan.
Bruckner, Pascal (2010): *Le mariage d'amour a-t-il échoué?* Paris: Grasset.
De Botton, Alain (2010): *The Pleasures and Sorrows of Work*. London: Penguin Books.
Debray, Régis (2008): *Vie et mort de l'image: Une histoire du regard en Occident*. Paris: Gallimard.
Deloro, Cyrille (2009): *L'autre: Petit traité de narcissisme intelligent*. Paris: Larousse.
Dik, Bryan J., Zinta S. Byrne & Michael F. Steger (eds) (2013): *Purpose and Meaning in the Workplace*. Washington DC: American Psychological Association Press.
Douglas, Susan J. & Meredith W. Michaels (2004): *The Mommy Myth: The Idealization of Motherhood and How It Has Undermined Women*. New York: Free Press.

Elias, Norbert (1985/2001): *The Loneliness of the Dying*. London: Continuum.

Ellis, Christopher (2001): 'Static and Genetic Phenomenology of Death'. *Contretemps*, 2 (5):157–163.

Foley, Michael (2011): *The Age of Absurdity: Why Modern Life Makes It Hard to Be Happy*. London: Simon & Schuster.

Gauthier, Alain (1998): *Du visible au visual: Anthropologie du regard*. Paris: Presses Universitaires de France.

Gershuny, Jonathan (2005): 'Busyness as the Badge of Honour for the New Superordinate Working Class'. *Working Papers of the Institute for Social and Economic Research*, paper 2005–9. Colchester: University of Essex.

Giddens, Anthony (2009): *Sociology*. Cambridge: Polity Press.

Hall, Alena (2015): 'The Key to Happiness at Work That Has Nothing to Do with Your Actual Job'. *The Huffington Post*, 2 April.

Heidegger, Martin (1962): *Being and Time*. Oxford: Blackwell Publishing.

Hemsath, Dave & Leslie Yerkes (1997): *301 Ways to Have Fun at Work*. San Francisco, CA: Berret-Koehler Publishers.

Hodgkinson, Tom (2007): *How to Be Idle: A Loafer's Manifesto*. New York: Harper.

Javeau, Claude (2007): *Les paradoxes de la postmodernité*. Paris: Presses Universitaires de France.

Jong, Erica (2010): 'Mother Madness'. *Wall Street Journal*, 6 November.

Kastenbaum, Robert (2007): *Death, Society and Human Experience*. New York: Pearson Education.

Kiley, Dan (1983): *The Peter Pan Syndrome: Men Who Have Never Grown up*. New York: Dodd Mead.

Klinenberg, Eric (2013): *Going Solo: The Extraordinary Arise and Surprising Appeal of Living Alone*. London: Penguin Books.

Klontz, Brad (2013): 'Are You a Workaholic. Do You Work over 50 Hours a Week?'. *Psychology Today*, 18 July.

Labash, Matt (2008): 'Are We Having Fun Yet? The Infantilization of Corporate America'. *Weekly Standard*, March–April.

Lasch, Christopher (1991): *The Culture of Narcissism: American Life in an Age of Diminishing Expectations*. New York: W. W. Norton & Company.

Le Breton, David (1990): *Anthropologie du corps et modernité*. Paris: Presses Universitaires de France.

Le Breton, David (2004): 'Le macabre en spectacle: Leçons d'anatomie', in Frédéric Lenoir & Jean-Philippe de Tonnac (eds): *La mort et l'immortalité: Encyclopédie des savoirs et de croyances*. Paris: Bayard.

Lesourd, Serge (2007): 'La mélancolisation du sujet postmoderne ou la disparition de l'Autre'. *Cliniques méditerranéennes*, 75 (1):13–26.

Lifton, Robert Jay (1968): *Death in Life: Survivors of Hiroshima*. New York: Random House.

Lifton, Robert Jay (1979): *The Broken Connection: On Death and the Continuity of Life*. New York: Simon & Schuster.

Lifton, Robert Jay & Eric Olson (1974): *Living and Dying*. London: Wildwood House.

Lilienfeld, Scott O., Steven Jay Lynn, John Ruscio & Barry L. Beyerstein (2010): *50 Great Myths of Popular Psychology: Shattering Widespread Misconceptions about Human Behavior*. Oxford: Wiley-Blackwell.

Lind, Michael (2014): 'The "Corporatist" Confusion: Why a Prominent Political Term Needs to Be Retired'. *Salon*, 5 January.

Lipovetsky, Gilles (1992): *Le crépuscule du devoir*. Paris: Gallimard.

Lipovetsky, Gilles (2006): *Le bonheur paradoxal: Essai sur la société d'hyperconsommation*. Paris: Gallimard.

Naish, John (2009): *Enough: Breaking Free from the World of Excess*. London: Hodder.

Nash, Laura (2009): *Ethics without Sermon*. Boston: Harvard Business Press.

Phillips, Adam (2013): *Missing out: In Praise of the Unlived Life*. London: Penguin Books.

Philosophie Magazine (2010): 'Le travail nuit-il à la santé?' [Dossier]. *Philosophie Magazine*, 39, May.

Philosophie Magazine (2014): 'Liberté. Inégalité. Immortalité: Le monde que vous prépare la Silicon Valley' [Dossier]. *Philosophie Magazine*, 83, October.

Safi, Omid (2014): 'The Disease of Being Busy'. *On Being*, 6 November.

Sartre, Jean-Paul (1943): *L'être et le néant: Essai d'ontologie phénoménologique*. Paris: Gallimard.

Sartre, Jean-Paul (1946): *L'Existentialisme est un humanisme*. Paris: Gallimard.

Sennett, Richard (1998): *The Corrosion of Character: The Personal Consequences of Work in the New Capitalism*. New York: W. W. Norton & Company.

Sievers, Burkard (1994): *Work, Death and Life Itself: Essays on Management and Organization*. Berlin: Walter de Gruyter.

Smith, Robert Rowland (2010): *Breakfast with Socrates: An Extraordinary (Philosophical) Journey Through Your Ordinary Day*. New York: Free Press.

Strenger, Carlo (2011): *The Fear of Insignificance: Searching for Meaning in the Twenty-First Century*. London: Palgrave Macmillan.

Thompson, Paul & Patricia Findlay (1999): 'Changing the People: Social Engineering in the Contemporary Workplace', in Larry Ray & Andrew Sayer (eds): *Culture and Economy after the Cultural Turn*. London: Sage Publications.

Vaillant, George E. (2012): *Triumphs of Experience: The Men of the Harvard Grant Study*. Cambridge, MA: Belknap Press.

Vandevelde, Toon (1996): 'Participation, Immortality and the Gift Economy: An Introduction to the Work of Burkard Sievers'. *Ethical Perspectives*, 3:123.

Vattimo, Gianni (2002): *After Christianity*. New York: Columbia University Press.

Warner, Judith (2006): *Perfect Madness: Motherhood in the Age of Anxiety*. New York: Riverhead Trade.

Warr, Peter & Guy Clapperton (2010): *The Joy of Work? Jobs, Happiness and You*. New York: Routledge.

7 The neuronal identity
Strategies of immortality in contemporary Western culture

Gianfranco Pecchinenda

Introduction

As we know, every society passes on to its members a certain image of man, an idea of himself and his identity, together with a vision of the sense of existence and a culture of immortality. Until the end of the twentieth century, the majority of psychologists and social scientists refused to admit that the roots of the psyche were in the biological brain. In the last three decades of the century, after some fundamental discoveries about how the brain works, there emerged a new, particular category of man: the *Neuronal man*.

The psyche, wrote French neurologist Jean-Pierre Changeux (2013), 'has an anatomy and a biology'. The gelatinous mass of the brain is made up of tens of billions of nerve cells, neurons, which are linked by vast numbers of connections, the synapses. These neurons carry electrical impulses and chemical substances, neurotransmitters. Each neuron has an individuality, but participates in operations that mobilize other neurons in other brain areas. Each area has a different function that new technologies – scanner, electronic microscope, positron camera – have identified and even enabled us to observe their operation. Knowing the wiring and how the elements fit together were the first steps.

After proving that 'identity' can be reduced to physico-chemical properties, it is possible to apply new knowledge to specific behaviours that explains how the brain works when its owner feels pain, experiences ecstasy, analyses a problem, speaks, acts, thinks. We are in the heart of the machine. And it can be exciting. But be wary of describing the same event with the language of the neurobiologist or that of the social sciences; be wary of reducing man to a set of mechanisms, or of reducing the human brain to a computer; be wary of evacuating all metaphysics and beliefs of immortality and reducing them to scientific knowledge.

The aim of this chapter is to analyse and discuss the most recent contributions to these issues in the social sciences. I start by briefly analysing the relationship between the process of the social construction of reality and human mortality (e.g. Schütz 1972). The specific condition of the human being – the only species conscious of its finitude – is the subject on which I focus in the first part of the chapter, in order to explain the sociological importance of what I define as the 'culture of immortality'. In the following paragraphs, I propose a classification that, though general, is – in my opinion – a useful ideal-type model to explain different worldviews. So the *Natural Aristotelian man*, the *Cartesian man*, the *Structural man*, the *Communicating man*, the *Genoma man*, the *Neuronal man* are *figures* that represent how men are related to death in different socio-historical configurations. In this way, I believe, it is possible to understand the broader transformation of the image of man and the world that has occurred gradually in the course of human development. Finally I consider, in short, what the social impact of the changes has been on immortality.

Images of man and different strategies of immortality

First it should be noted that society – any society, in any era – is a collective enterprise whose main goal is to conceal the finite nature of life. Whatever image of man emerges from time to time – according to the different socio-historical configurations – it always demonstrates this fundamental *dik-tat*: instil doubts about man's mortality. It is fair to say – as indeed I did elsewhere (Pecchinenda 2014) – that societies have produced, throughout history, many different strategies of immortality: these matrices of meaning, shared by whole epochs, are useful to define 'mimetic systems'. They have a very hard task to accomplish: the struggle with anguish caused by an irrefutable awareness. In fact, the human being is the only animal that knows that death comes inexorably to end the physical life. You can even assert, without fear of contradiction, that the ultimate legitimacy of every culture rests on it being a *culture of immortality*. Analysing the various and very ingenious ways by which men, historically, have created whole universes of meaning to transfigure their inescapable condition of finitude is of high importance for the sociological discipline. It can indeed be argued that the phenomenon of 'death' – understood in terms specified here – is the crucial variable for the analysis of collective behaviour. The more a theoretical approach of this kind seeks to identify the presence of death in institutions, practices and rituals that, prima facie, would attribute the fulfilment of social functions radically alien to it, the more it can be useful. The success of such cultural devices is measurable in some way. Understanding how a society can stand the display of the *Absurd* – feeling that death leads inexorably to it – represents a strong indicator of the broader transformations of human habitus: as the many forms of everyday life are placed away from such intrusions, most human beings will enjoy a relative degree of 'ontological security' (Giddens 1999) and vice versa.

Clearly, depending on the different ages and social groups, even very different strategies have been implemented to protect the order painstakingly built by humans: chaos – the overwhelming metaphor for death – has been kept under control, for millennia, from polymorphic immortality mythologies based, precisely, on the belief of a life after death. They have produced a very heterogeneous patchwork of rituals, cults and narratives based on the conviction that there is a continuous link between the mundane world and the transcendent world (e.g. Bauman 1995). Such complex symbolic forms of 'self-deception', on the other hand, guarantee the perpetuation of the species as those materials: to underestimate the importance of collective imagery means to culpably ignore an essential component of human life. The institutions governing the different forms of organization of human life systematically legitimized cultures based on this sort of self-deception. This, in fact, responds to an inescapable anthropological necessity. The unconscious desire of immortality is embodied in different social forms that can be placed on a continuum whose poles range from a magical-religious-type model to a rational-scientific one. In the first case, human life is fully embedded in a sacred universe governed by immutable principles established by tradition (e.g. Berger 1973).

This state of affairs convinces humans of the illusory nature of the End: in this regime of *assigned immortality*, compliance with the *nomos* established in *illo tempore* (Eliade 1975) by the community means gaining nothing other than the overcoming of death itself. At the other end of the continuum are worldviews based on rational explanations. In this type of culture the being-in-world meanings are intensified by indefinitely postponing the moment of death. Again, though, men have a nearly fideistic attitude, basing their hopes on the powerful ideology of progress. Indefinitely postponing – at least on the level of imagery – the threat of death coincides, in the last instance, with a more technically sophisticated desire of eternity: in this case we define this cultural device as *acquired immortality*. In the first case we are dealing with a social scenario in which the means of salvation are typically derived from a sacred cosmos, where the universe of meaning thus belongs to a magical-religious model; in the latter case, scientific achievements are absolute protagonists, especially by means of medicine, modern Western society's proudest achievement in its progressive conception of the world. In any case, it remains to be pointed out that – as some strategies are more effective than others – none of this guarantees an unshakable shield against the disintegrating forces of death. For the modern man, the welcoming embrace of the *routine* remains the last bastion to oppose the anomic threat posed by the long shadow of death: the steady pace of daily life reassures human beings through the repetition of small gestures that are not systematically open to question. So, predictable existential landscapes that are not constantly subject to the grip of doubt are embedded in nearly the entire life of human beings. What phenomenology calls 'marginal situations' are just the various strategies of a struggle for immortality. Against them, these strategies try out their solidity and plausibility – or, in other words, their degree of legitimacy (Berger & Luckmann 1991, 2010). The mythology of immortality typical of the modern age – that is to say, that based on the ideology of the indefinite progress of medical science – has caused remarkable psychological consequences, which reopen at 'blame' scenarios that seemed overcome by the transition from traditional societies to subsequent ones (Pecchinenda 2007). Being healthy, in the modern cosmology based on efficiency, becomes a duty that, if breached, can turn into punishment to be expiated, even with a 'well-deserved death'. In this regard, the immense technical knowledge and expertise made available by the majestic achievements of science does not accept failure (e.g. Beck & Beck-Gernsheim 2002): according to this symbolic universe, disease and death, when glimpsed in the world, can and must be driven away; to fail to do so means not having fought hard enough, means surrendering to an enemy against which, shamefully, you have not made the maximum effort (e.g. Sontag 1989). All in all here – although we are only in the initial stage of the process – a renewed system of 'moralization of physical evil' comes to light, similar, in some respects, to that existing in pre-modern communities (Camorrino 2015:116–139).

As noted above, every society passes on to its members a certain image of man, an idea of himself and his identity, together with a vision of the sense of existence and a culture of immortality. The hypothesis is that, since the mid-1980s, the transformation that takes place causes the birth of the so-called *Neuronal man.*[1] Proceeding step by step, it is possible to propose a chronology of six images of mankind, which have emerged in the course of our history:

1   The *Natural Aristotelian man.*
2   The *Cartesian man.*
3   The *Structural man.*
4   The *Communicating man.*
5   The *Genoma man.*
6   The *Neuronal man.*

In the following paragraphs I will deal with these images one by one and then relate them to each other.

The Natural Aristotelian man

The first anthropological type, whose heritage comes directly from ancient Greece, is the *Aristotelian man* (Wolff 2010). It is perhaps useful to recall the characteristics of the relationship between man and the world at this stage. As stated by the great scholar Jean-Pierre Vernant, human beings during this time were 'spontaneously cosmic' (Vernant 1994:44). The worldview of the ancient Greek was therefore based on a complex representation of the self and of the universe. It is evident, according to Vernant, that he was aware of the fact that the human being was somehow different from other humans and non-humans in the world and in the supra-world, but the knowledge of this property

> does not cut man off from the world; it does not lead him to posit against the universe as a whole – a domain of reality irreducible to any other and

whose very existence places it at the fringe, with man and his thought constituting an entirely separate world.

(Vernant 1994:44)

Anyway, in this perspective, any human being is considered a *rational animal*, the interpretive archetype is derived directly from the natural sciences and the human being, firmly situated in the centre of the universe, represents the basis for comparison with any other living being (the human being is an integral part of nature, but differentiates itself from every other living being by being rational) (e.g. Brague 2005). It is an image of the human being that, as we know, refusing the Platonic idea of dualism, rejects the idea that the soul can be divided from the body.

A biological and naturalistic point of view was counterposed to Plato's ethic and epistemological point of view. While Plato's theory, which in the modern age was to coincide with René Descartes's, tried to identify an entity (the soul, or the mind) existing in every living being, the Aristotelian one referred to some abilities or functions. In Aristotle's works, the *soul* was a term that indicated the carrying out of functions that an organ-equipped body is suitable to perform, and not an entity located inside a living body. From Aristotle's point of view, the soul is the entirety of the body's organic functions, and those can exist only if the object performing them is present. Only from an abstract point of view can we separate the soul from the body. So, the Aristotelian theory is not compatible with a dualist theory, because the soul is not detached from the body's functions.

Still, in spite of Aristotle's break, Western thinking proceeded along Plato's path, because its dualistic conception was compatible with the biblical tradition. The religious beliefs regarding immortality, combined with the Platonic theory, sharpened the dualism between body and soul, therefore laying ground for the philosophical thinking of the Middle Ages and, later, Descartes's theory. However, it should be remembered, the Cartesian view is not entirely comparable to the Platonic one. We cannot find anything that looks like the 'modern self' during this era, since all the features that modernity will recognize as particular to the individual are still not present. Things like uniqueness, interiority or ownership of individual rights – in short, what distinguishes the modern self – are not yet developed (Vernant 1994:48).

Finally, departing from here we find the theories of mediation or reductionism. The former considered the soul and the body as two entities different on a quality level, but interconnected; the latter supposed that spiritual categories are needed to explain what has not yet been explained by biological science. If it is true that in the post-Renaissance era Plato's authority was undermined, it is also true that the model proposed by the great Greek philosopher continues to influence modern imagery. It seems that Plato's conceptual universe works like an unavoidable matrix of meaning. Plato must be considered, ultimately, as the one who conceived of a model of reality consisting of intelligible archetypes, the nature of which is substantially mathematical (Pecchinenda 2014:22–26).

The Cartesian man

In the seventeenth century, a new cosmology postulated that the mechanism of the universe operated by itself, following the immutable laws of mathematical nature: free from the ties imposed by supernatural aid, the philosopher had access to the status of out-of-the-world thinker (e.g. Husserl 2008; Prigogine & Stengers 1999). The anthropological type corresponding to this renewed cosmology is that of the classic *Cartesian man*. Beginning in the seventeenth century, a new idea of the human being emerged in philosophy and science, replacing the 'rational animal' derived from Aristotle's work. It was a new human being for a new science. There was a new philosophical method (Descartes's, which no longer followed Aristotelian logic) (e.g. Koyré 1996); also, there were the necessities of a new conceptual paradigm, modern mechanics, instead of the ancient zoology or cosmology (e.g. Horkheimer & Adorno 1966; Shapin 2003). Therefore, an anti-naturalistic and dualist idea of the human being was affirmed (*res cogitans* and *res extensa*).

This dualist distinction was to preoccupy the whole philosophical thinking of the Middle Ages. The liability of physicality in itself would prevail; physicality would be recognized as the opponent, the obstacle and the wretched companion of the soul, to which were ascribed the weaknesses, the downfalls and all the most humiliating defeats of mankind (e.g. Le Goff 2008).

This detached and intellectual anthropological concept was supported by many religious tendencies, monasticism above all (e.g. Le Goff 2000; Mumford 2011), which saw in the flesh the weakness of mankind. The ethics of religion recommended desisting from the urges of flesh and to chagrin himself in the body and in all the senses, the 'windows of soul from which the solicitations of sin come in'. The body had to be restrained; it had to avoid the possibility of reacting. Later, humanists, Platonists, Aristotelians, mages and philosophers of the Renaissance would consider that mankind sat between nature and the supernatural (e.g. Rossi 1989, 2006; Yates 2006, 2010). Human beings would no longer be nature's provisional guest, the soul would no longer be the body's provisional guest: mankind would be a natural being. However, humans are the only natural beings with culture, arts, language, history; that is to say, thought and knowledge. So it is natural but also original, therefore irreducible to any other being.

We can consider this conception as antithetical to the scientific conception of the world. Modern science, overtaking magic and animism, sure enough would produce a vision of nature as inanimate, made up of bodies that move according to entirely mechanical laws (e.g. Kuhn 2008). This was to mark deeply the body–mind dilemma, only to deliver it to us in the shape in which we still argue about it. Biological and physical sciences started to use the machine model to explain the world and living beings. And, in this respect, scholars 'may be monistic or dualistic; they may credit the "mind" with qualities of "matter" or "matter" with qualities of the "mind", all these propositions try to account for the whole in terms of its parts' (Elias 1956:248). We have to underscore that it was impossible that this complex and articulated process would not affect different and essential fields of human culture: the concept of mankind governing and dominating the natural environment; the concept of mankind freeing itself from any divinity; the concept of mankind that can begin to plan 're-creating' creatures in his likeness, which would eventually reach an extraordinary expression in the science fiction depictions of the Frankenstein figure (e.g. Lecercle 2002).

The Structural man

As Michael Foucault (2009) pointedly supposed in *The Order of Things*, before the end of the eighteenth century 'man did not exist'; that is, human beings had not yet acquired the theoretical foundations of a scientifically knowledgeable entity.

Between the late eighteenth century and the early nineteenth, however, the theoretical foundations of the human being significantly changed: the human being was no longer regarded as the 'king of knowledge', the one who occupies the centre of the scene,[2] obtaining instead an ambiguous spot. The human being became the 'object' of a specific field of knowledge and, at the same time, the 'subject' who knows: unlike the *Cartesian man*, the *Structural man* would no longer be a subject detached from nature who (because of its peculiar and unmatched traits) is fit to scientifically know nature itself; instead, it would become an object among others that is itself scientifically knowable.

Beginning in this epoch, and during the twentieth century, new sciences developed – human and social sciences, indeed – whose essential challenge was to make the human being a legitimate *object* for scientific knowledge, but at the same time to keep it in the situation of the subject who knows. The human being, as conceived of by human and social sciences, is a subjective performer in particular situations, perceiving meaning, bearing intentions, free in its choices – sometimes systematically rational (as in the *homo economicus*) – as well as, on the other hand, being a passive carrier of social and historical events, a product of an individual (psychoanalytical) or social history, or an interchangeable member of a community that ascribes to him or her a proper role and proper beliefs (a particular sociology). It is as the cause (of global effects) or as the effect (of global causes), or both cause and effect of an interaction process (according to some methodological currents shared by many social sciences).

Therefore, to determine which anthropological typology appears behind approaches that are so different and, sometimes, contradictory is seemingly difficult without resorting to a specific emerging model. Effectively, there was a time, during the twentieth century, when a series of different disciplines, autonomously from one another, resorted to the same model of human being, grouped together in the same 'scientific paradigm'. It was during this period that the cross-concept of *structure* was affirmed, that is, the idea that objects (and individuals) do not exist in and of themselves, or in their singularity, but that it is possible to consider them only according to the differences between them and others (objects and individuals), and according to the connections that tie them.

In studying structures (in languages, in rules of kinship, in social relationships, in the unconscious, etc.), the human and social sciences gave themselves an invariable, formal and strictly determined object (as if it were a mathematical object), which did not rely on local variations, individual points of view or on the actors' conscience.

During the twentieth century, many researchers, in an independent and probably unaware way, proposed the fundamental traits of this 'structural' model of the human being. Karl Marx for history, Émile Durkheim for sociology, Sigmund Freud for psychology and Ferdinand de Saussure for linguistics proposed a *paradigm* that many social scientists successively endorsed, therefore characterizing an historical phase when anthropology acquired three distinguishing traits that differentiated this structural model from the other two previous models:

1   Unlike the *Aristotelian man* and *Cartesian man*, the *Structural man* does not have any essence;
2   Unlike the *Artistotelian man*, the *Structural man* is not a neutral being;
3   Unlike the *Cartesian man*, the *Structural man* is not capable of independently determining its thoughts and its will.

The most characteristic among those traits, the one that would have major consequences for representations of the human being in this phase, is the loss of singularity and autonomy.

The human and social sciences therefore did not study the human being in general, although, time after time, they studied – in accordance with the specific method and the specific science – a highly determined part of humanity: social facts (sociology), cultures (ethnology or cultural anthropology), the evolution of societies (history), conscious functions (psychology), unconscious functions (psychoanalysis), language (linguistics). In conclusion, for the first time, the human being was to lose its wholeness to become subject to a new look; a look pointed towards a man who is a subject-subjugated, that is, anti-natural, dualistic and not-essentialist man (Wolff 2010).

The Communicating man

Among the main causes of the cosmological and anthropological transformation that took place between the nineteenth and twentieth centuries and grew in importance from the end of the Second World War, there is certainly the large significance acquired by the development of communication technologies (e.g. Kern 2007). Philosopher of communication theory Marshall McLuhan (1976) already suggested an interpretation of man as a being defined by his technological prosthesis properties.

More specifically, McLuhan should be considered a pioneer of the idea of the *Neuronal man*, given his original idea on the basis of which human thought would be shaped not by its contents but especially by forms suggested by technological prosthesis in which the human being is immersed, and his other idea that media directly influence our bodies and our senses. According to some researchers, this phenomenon should have led to the appearance of a real mythology. In a study of some years ago, Philippe Breton (1996) attempted to find the roots of this mythology among the work of earlier researchers in cybernetics. The French researcher started with the premise that informatics and communicational features had become the frame-value of our age, although today's situation is not very new. After all, to communicate, and to develop procedures with this aim in mind, are anthropological constants and like a framework of practices strongly connected to historical backgrounds. It may seem obvious to say so, but communication and its techniques are fundamental aspects of mankind, and despite the primitivity of prehistoric man, there is no doubt he spent a great part of his energies in order not only to communicate, but even to 'meditate' on communication.

The theory according to which the very foundation of mankind developed from such 'reflection' is by no means without basis, however speculative it may seem. According to this point of view, humans are communicating beings, partially structured by a sort of impulse to show himself, to 'get himself out' that motivates him. Precisely by such intensification of this anthropological constant the contemporary social system has been structured, always increasing human opportunities and so going beyond one's bodily limits.

The basis of modernity simulates this early system, perfected thanks to high technology. For a turn in the evolution of communications technology, the era of two world wars was crucial. The origins and the achievement of the new 'information and communication society' would establish the reaction of modernity and the redefinition of itself. Born into the troubles of a long world war and the start of a tragic decay in social relationships, the universal resort to communication is therefore linked to certain historical occurrences, giving it social sense and range. According to Breton, the birth and diffusion of cybernetic thinking, joined with the traumas caused by the two world wars, makes urgent the need for redemption, caused by the loss of reference points: 'Everything is called into question.' It is from this perspective that media development emerges as a priority. Alongside the ideological crisis is, at the same time, the need for a value working as a leading agent of change in a society totally based on communicative transparency: in this way, it was thought – argues Breton – no dark plan would have been possible, least of all historical tragedies like Nazism and the Holocaust. Communication, transparent and immanently satisfying social needs, begins to be an obsession that constitutes a perfect response to twentieth-century crisis.

The novelty of this communication paradigm is accompanied by a new way to make science, a new definition of human being, the introduction of some concepts that fed new theories to the science of communication. This new conception of originality does not inhabit just the centrality conferred to notions of *Information* and *Communication*, but in considering information exchanges and relations that are entirely constitutive of natural and artificial events. Breton maintains that *Homo Communicans*' features, traits and 'character' are inscribed in the disciplinary model of cybernetics, since cybernetics is the 'science of men and machineries unified controls'. By means of communication, he writes, 'every entity is the sum of information that can exchange in networks in which it can enter'. It is here that we find the idea that 'in new society everything is communication', establishing the basis of an argument that can be defined as *utopian*.

The assault on the functional classic scientific method concerns all conceptions that postulate whichever phenomenon of the inner being, stating that everything can be explained in terms of relations, then implying that everything is situated outside our interiority. Every phenomenon, or every being, can be metaphorically likened to an onion, as if it were a set of overlapping appearances without an internal nucleus, because the whole which is inside is put outside; from this fact also arises the new conception of *Homo Communicans*, a being which is at this point deprived of his interiority, immersed in relations and information exchanges with his counterparts and within his social structure. This can also be explained as an achievement of media, of a bond with TV and computer: a new vision of reality, prefigured by Cybernetics; a real redefinition of the human being and his relations with reality.

The Genoma man

Yet, in the last decades – that is, the era of the widespread success of the myth of information (Pecchinenda 2009) – a deterministic view of the body based on the centrality of the biological factor at the expense of the social variable seems to become prominent. This view, which is in some respects very reductionist, is a direct consequence of the popularity obtained by a new image of man: what I have called *Genoma man*. In some respects it is a contemporary fulfilment of some features that were already part of *Man-Machine* – the typical image of modern man that I have analysed elsewhere (Pecchinenda 2008:92–102). In contemporary society, great importance is attached to the fascinating constellation of genetics. Yet, the vision of the human body as an organism whose parts are modifiable or exchangeable with those of other bodies, or even with artificial organs, is not far from that conceptualized by the *Homme-Machine* theorists (especially by Offroy Julien de La Mettrie (1709–1751)). The very important discoveries made in the field of genetic research also showed how subtle the boundaries are between the animal kingdom and the human one: if humankind shares more than 90 per cent of its gene pool with the higher primates, a certain continuity in the 'Great Chain of Being' again seems guaranteed. The *Genoma man* is the product of what we might call a *biologizing utopia*, an unprecedented narrative model capable of reforming the modern cosmology and replacing – albeit in a gradual process that is still in progress – the myth of the machine with that of information. *The cyborg*, even if in different terminological versions – artificial man, creature, robot – finds its origins in the field of mythology. Rather, among all the myths created by man, that of the automaton – even though it is among the oldest – is probably the narrative model that has succeeded, to great effect, in regenerating itself over the centuries, to the extent that we can state that every epoch has seen an updated version of the myth of the artificial being impose itself on the collective imagery. In fact, it is a fascination that has perpetuated itself in its basic structural themes, even while undergoing notable and sometimes significant transformations. In this case, for example, it is neither absurd nor ingenuous to speak of a determinism of the body. *Genoma man* appears to us, in this sense, as a sort of realization of the *man-machine*, with whom he shares in the collective imagery a series of important elements.

We shall see in what sense this is the case: above all, in both cases, the determining factor in the constitution of man is clearly outlined by biology and no longer by society; in both cases the possibility of rendering man more self-sufficient is an object followed stringently. More than ever, man feels that he is the master of his own destiny and of his own body, seeing that he is capable of foreseeing and controlling his own destiny, which was once subject to the will of God or the caprice of Nature (as, for example, in the determination of sex and of other genetic characteristics). From the ethical standpoint – as La Mettrie upholds, among other things – everything can be evaluated either positively or negatively. With regard to the reductionist aspects connected with the new emerging paradigm, here, too, it is possible to find a certain continuity of La Mettrie's idea. If the actual valorization of the body and of physical well-being – and of the various components connected to them – is considered to be a positive movement, from another standpoint critical observations may be made on the sometimes profane use of the human organism. That which, for centuries, was considered to be the sacred container of the most precious and admirable characteristic of the human being – his soul – has been violated, banalized, manipulated and commercialized. The new form of valorization of the mechanical body has acquired a price in the new paradigm. Organs can be bought and sold. As in La Mettrie's works, the human body is considered by modern science to be a machine with spare parts to be inserted. So, as in the past, the soul and the spirit were educated and improved, in the actual imagery the perfection of the body has acquired value (Pecchinenda 2007).

The Neuronal man

Before considering the image of the *Neuronal man*, as it now appears to be emerging, it is useful, first of all, to take a step back in order to better understand the historical and social conditions that allowed it to appear. A new representation of the anthropological imagery begins to emerge, indeed, in the late nineteenth and early twentieth century. According to a certain view, man – 'thrown' in the world – is no longer supported by transcendence, by a guiding or ruling force located within the self, or even by historical or biological heritage. He is the being who is called upon to invent himself, without the benefit of a normative ideal assigned once and for all. His relations with the community, in this context, can be considered only from the point of view of a *choice*. Entering the social life becomes an infinitely hard mission to accomplish, and rejecting the social world and its conventions is not represented as a dramatic gesture, but as a kind of basic right for everyone (Pecchinenda 2014).[3] He seems to be part of an *inaccessible community*. However, in many other cases, he is committed to a party, a group, a cause, a way of life. These ties have been neither given nor defined previously; in fact, the individual is neither constant nor loyal, like when he was committed to old or new form of idealism, but is simply *available*. Sometimes the community he wants to join obstinately refuses him, sometimes it imprisons him, sometimes it persecutes him, but never is it able to assimilate him, to integrate him, so the truth of separation, be it an exclusion or a point of departure, remains always primordial. Like Narcissus, the individual finds true happiness contemplating his own face and satisfying his own drives. Having lost the desire to look around, he contemplates, he listens, he acts without thinking, led by his drives, which he does not want and cannot control. It seems the freedom to constantly shape himself remains intact, but as the range of awareness and action is greatly reduced, and since the impetus of the drives, which are beyond consciousness, is always stronger, this freedom is, indeed, barely perceptible. It is an overall metamorphosis, related to a highly significant series of technological and cultural transformations, which will lead to the emergence of a new interpretative paradigm of man and of his place in the cosmos.

The essential trait that shaped, during the nineteenth century, the relationship with death and immortality, a relationship born as a consequence of the so-called *Structural man* – and which in turn shaped the previous anthropological images – is the emergence of some very unusual features in human history:

- Since the end of the nineteenth century death has no longer been seen as a *transition* from one side to another but as a *boundary* situation (as Jaspers said, death is converted into the 'boundary-situation'), so men are increasingly less interested in what lies beyond or behind this boundary, and begin to be more interested in knowing the boundary in itself; that is, death.
- Death (and immortality) is not related to a double man (body and soul) but to a man living in existential unity (to some extent there is something of the *Aristotelian man*).
- Hence the problem of immortality, or of personal and individual perpetuation, becomes an existential phenomenon related to a hermeneutic dimension, to an interpretation of life itself.

Leaving aside the issues related to the link between the meaning of life (existentialism) and the rational perception of the inevitability of death, with all its ambivalence (issues analysed in detail by existentialist philosophy), we come to the *Neuronal man* and to the image of the contemporary man and immortality. This new paradigm is not born in the realm of human and social sciences, but by virtue of the *coalition* between an unprecedented arrangement of new and developing sciences: neuroscience (related to the study of brain images and to the new technologies of molecular biology that allow observation of the brain in action),[4] evolutionary biology, primatology, ethology, palaeoanthropology and other new, related fields of research. The development of these subjects has brought the emergence of a new naturalist paradigm, the *cognitivist* one, that can also be extended to various human and social sciences; and on the other hand the appearance of some new human and social sciences, born as a result of this naturalist turn, such as socio-biology and evolutionary psychology.

The characteristic of such interdisciplinary research, grouped around this new cognitive core, is the sharing of the same methodological position (the naturalist explanation), of the same metaphysical presupposition (materialistic monism) and – most importantly – the same image of man, considered a living being like everyone else, the result of evolution and adaptation to the environment. The methodological postulate of all cognitive science is to consider the processes that lead to knowledge (perception, memory, learning, imagination, language, reasoning, planning actions, etc.), and more generally the mental processes (thoughts, consciousness, emotions, etc.), as natural phenomena. The cognitive paradigm is gradually replacing the structuralist paradigm, both in the study of man and his image. Today these two competing paradigms, however – as noted by the French philosopher Francis Wolff (2010:126–127) – have some important things in common, such as interdisciplinarity and a unifying philosophy. But the most significant factor, in my opinion, is that they are both considered scientific paradigms, in the sense given to that concept by Thomas S. Kuhn (1978). That is, they represent a scientific theory that establishes itself as a model for all the other sciences, thanks to its *exemplary model*. In the case of structuralism, it is the so-called theory of 'relevant features' that is found at the origin of phonology: a theory according to which the phonetic system of any language can be described by the simple contribution of a few tens of phonemes definable as a series of discrete sections. To think is to talk, and speech is, first of all, the articulation of phonemes. This theory formed the core of all linguistics, and later of cultural anthropology and all the other social sciences, which derived from it the methodological assumption that human phenomena depend on internal structures of dependence, unconscious and detached from individuals. In the case of cognitive science, the exemplary model is undoubtedly the application of the calculation theory for the functioning of mental processes, which is its foundational moment: as we noted about the emergence of so-called *homo communicans* (which is nothing if not a variation on *Neuronal man*), thought comes to be regarded as a common 'treatment of information' and can therefore be described in terms of a calculation that, in turn, can be considered as a series of logical operations performed on abstract symbols (Pecchinenda 2003).

The situation when computational theory meets neuroscience, which in turn strive to map the brain, must be placed at the origins of the generalization and expansion of this new paradigm: the theory, initially applied only to certain intellectual operations, and which later will serve as a model for the description of all other mental processes (cognitive psychology), gradually incorporates anthropology, sociology, economics and religion too. From this exemplary model, cognitive science will derive its own methodological postulate: mental phenomena are a particular kind of natural phenomena. Going back to some topics already discussed in the previous pages, it is also necessary to not underestimate the fact that, as noted by Roland Gori (2013:31ff.), such models of mathematical formalization of mental processes, developed by cognitivism and the cybernetic models linked with them, find themselves ever more often prodigiously interconnected with brain sciences when it is understood that the principles of mathematical logic can give an account of its operation. From this point, connectionism, by extending ordinary cognitivism, begins to consider the whole brain as a deductive machine able to encode, an information processor and memorizer in forms identical to those of the symbolization of logic. This scientific view of how the brain works proceeds in harmony with the dream of the Turing programming language to find and fabricate a formal language suitable to describe reality and to promote that part to take the part of the whole, to the point that neuroscience researchers consider their heuristic models to be real. Cognitive sciences are a writing of the world and not the world itself. One should not confuse the map with the territory. Now, faced with certain things, we are no longer in the presence of heuristic construction, but in the presence of the same reality that these sciences are trying to study: the spirit would be the natural computer that could experience itself through an isomorphic machine. Hence the conception of the brain as the sole and authentic subject of behaviour. Sense, history, social, psychological and political meanings tend to disappear entirely from the scene. Their values are reduced by message syntax, which is real information at the expense of sense. Technological advances have combined computer science and its extensions, cognitive science, neuroscience and, more recently, neuroeconomics. The concept of information – as we said previously – resembling more and more that of knowledge, is proving to be extremely powerful in the biological sciences, in particular in genetics. Code presents itself as the carrier of genetic information that produces the proteins necessary to the message of life. A genetic education programme is regarded as the true generator of the whole living system, as well as of its regularity and its anomalies. All this can only lead, inevitably, to the success of this new anthropological figure of a human being, which we defined as *Neuronal man* (e.g. Churchland 2012; Edelman 2005; Le Doux 2012).[5]

Conclusion: the social impact of changes in immortality

It is clear that the different anthropological profiles outlined in this chapter show, in their turn, social worlds with very different characteristics. Of course this chapter was not intended to exhaust such a vast and complex subject. But it is possible – in my opinion – to find in these general categories tools to enable us to better understand the different ways in which men of different ages perceived the world around them and their own identity.

As we have seen, the *Natural Aristotelian man* looked at himself as a rational entity, but not yet divorced from the cosmic scenario that embraced him. The Greek social landscape – although giving way to the affirmation of a rational man – not yet transformed by technical activity, did not allow a split to be introduced between the human being and the world. So man – even if perceived as a rational animal – remained an organism among organisms.

The identity transformation, of which the *Cartesian man* becomes the absolute protagonist, reveals a broader social change. The mechanistic universe stands out as the image of the emerging modern society. The first successes of the economic system, commerce and industry, are the symbolic engine for the affirmation of this new anthropological type, whose dualistic identity is made up of a body and a *cogito* that act in a world subject to the mathematical domain of the laws of nature.

In the nineteenth century there is a further transformation. The birth of the social sciences changes the image of man. *Structural man* is not only the person who knows the world – the classical view of the natural sciences – but also the object of knowledge. The concept of structure imposes itself transversely in the academic disciplines, creating a new image of man whose thoughts and whose actions are no longer seen as expressions of an isolated subject but, on the contrary, as the product of tensions that largely transcend the man himself. The man's identity is then analysed only by studying the social structure in which he is an actor among others. A radical change of perspective – from the subject to the structure – is therefore realized in this period.

In the second half of the twentieth century, as a result of the tragic spectacle of the Second World War, comes a new anthropological type. Closely linked to the growing expansion of new communication technologies and discoveries of cybernetics, the *Communicating man* emerges. A new, transparent identity, completely extrovert in relationships made possible by new media, appears to be a plausible answer to the crisis: a world where people know everything about everyone would not allow any *lager*.

With *Genoma man*, the perspective changes again. Attention is focused on the biological factor and no longer on the social one. The extraordinary promises made by genetics – whose success is a result of the great discoveries that have marked the initial phase of this field of research – promote a *biologizing utopia*. The myth of information is the peculiar imagery within which this new image of man comes to light. Somehow, *Genoma man* is an advanced version of the *homme-machine* proposed by La Mettrie – an *homme-machine* immersed in a universe dominated by the myth of information.

Neuronal man is an image of man that has emerged gradually over the last few decades. As we have seen, not only neuroscience has contributed to the success of this new anthropological type (internal to a cognitive paradigm). For example, increasingly sophisticated technologies applied to molecular biology have made it possible, as never before, to map brain functions while these are activated. Indeed, we are facing a naturalist turn: if earlier *Structural man* defined the social nature of human beings, now *Neuronal man* defines the natural roots of human sociability. So the social sciences absorb this new anthropological image and *Neuronal man* becomes the model of their analyses. Cognitive sciences again consider – a bit like going on *Natural Aristotelian man* – the human being and all its manifestations and features to be, precisely, natural phenomena. The success of this type of explanation allowed the *Neuronal man* paradigm to become an 'exemplary model' for many other disciplines.

It is certain that this brief reconstruction cannot give a full account of the long socio-historical period considered in this chapter, just as it is certain that the *Neuronal man* is the last image of man in chronological order, but certainly not the last ever. Social, technological, economic, cultural and even religious transformations that will follow in the future will create a new image of the world and, with it, a new image of man. To understand what will take the place of the *Neuronal man*, we can only wait on the bank of the river.

Notes

1 A further phase of the process that I have defined as 'biologizing utopia' – a phenomenon that I will mention briefly below.
2 Emblematic, in this regard, is the reference to the work of the painter Diego Velazquez.
3 This is very often the cause of the distress of the central characters in twentieth-century novels. Leaving aside this intricate and vast debate, I prefer a more attractive and useful perspective for a work like this, so I consider it more fruitful to more deeply analyse these issues by studying some of the many novels, short stories or other artistic works that have stressed, more or less directly, these issues.
4 The human brain is, for this peculiar vision of man, a bioethical structure whose main purpose is to create the best conditions for the organism to survive. In simple terms, the brain, and the body in which it is integrated, must survive. This is the diktat. To complicate the issue, think about the 'mind', shaped by the union between the two: a kind of physical/conceptual medium – like, approximately, the pineal gland of René Descartes – between the entities considered. In any case, the fundamental purpose of the mind is to avoid the thought of the body's mortality and, very important for our analysis, to think of it as immortal. The point is that – according to my hypothesis – the more the strategies implemented by the different social consortia for 'self-deception' about their mortality are prepared adequately and in a sophisticated way, the more man is able to always shape more developed societies.
5 The relevance of such a figure is confirmed by the great interest aroused by scientific works and essays, also informative, that have been published on the subject.

References

Bauman, Zygmunt (1995): *Il teatro dell'immortalità: Mortalità, immortalità e altre strategie di vita.* Bologna: Il Mulino.

Beck, Ulrich & Elisabeth Beck-Gernsheim (2002): *Individualization: Institutionalized Individualism and Its Social and Political Consequences.* Thousand Oaks, CA: Sage Publications.

Berger, Peter L. (1973): *The Social Reality of Religion.* Harmondsworth: Penguin Books.

Berger, Peter L. & Thomas Luckmann (1991): *The Social Construction of Reality: A Treatise in the Sociology of Knowledge.* Harmondsworth: Penguin Books.

Berger, Peter L. & Thomas Luckmann (2010): *Lo smarrimento dell'uomo moderno.* Bologna: Il Mulino.

Brague, Rémi (2005): *La Saggezza del mondo: Storia dell'esperienza umana dell'Universo.* Soveria Mannelli: Rubbettino.

Breton, Philippe (1996): *L'utopia della comunicazione: Il mito del 'villaggio planetario'.* Turin: UTET.

Camorrino, Antonio (2015): *La natura è inattuale: Scienza, società e catastrofi nel XXI secolo.* S. M. C. V.: Ipermedium libri.

Cavicchia Scalamonti, Antonio (1984): *Il senso della morte: Contributi per una sociologia della morte.* Naples: Liguori.

Cavicchia Scalamonti, Antonio (1991): *Tempo e morte.* Naples: Liguori.

Cavicchia Scalamonti, Antonio (1993): *La camera verde: Il cinema e la morte.* Naples: Ipermedium libri.

Cavicchia Scalamonti, Antonio (1997): *La morte: Quattro variazioni sul tema.* Naples: Ipermedium libri.

Cavicchia Scalamonti, Antonio (2015): *L'illusione senza avvenire.* Naples: Ipermedium libri.

Cavicchia Scalamonti, Antonio & Gianfranco Pecchinenda (1992): *La memoria e I silenzi: Una città e il suo cimitero.* Naples: Colonnese.

Cavicchia Scalamonti, Antonio & Gianfranco Pecchinenda (1996): *La memoria consumata.* Naples: Ipermedium libri.

Changeux, Jean-Pierre (2013): *Il bello, il buono, il vero: Un nuovo approccio neuronale.* Milan: Raffaello Cortina.

Churchland, Patricia S. (2012): *Neurobiologia della morale.* Milan: Raffaello Cortina.

Damasio, Antonio R. (2000): *Emozione e coscienza.* Milan: Adelphi.

Edelman, Gerald M. (2005): *Più grande del cielo: Lo straordinario dono fenomenico della coscienza.* Turin: Einaudi.

Eliade, Mircea (1975): *Il mito dell'eterno ritorno.* Milan: Rusconi.

Elias, Norbert (1956): 'Problems of Involvement and Detachment'. *British Journal of Sociology,* 7 (3):226–252.

Foucault, Michel (2009): *Le parole e le cose.* Milan: Bur.

Gamba, Fiorenza (2016): *Mémoire et immortalité aux temps du numérique.* Paris: L'Harmattan.

Giddens, Anthony (1999): *Identità e società moderna.* Naples: Ipermedium.

Gori, Roland (2013): *La Dignité de penser.* Arles: Actes Sud.

Horkheimer, Max & Theodor W. Adorno (1966): *Dialettica dell'illuminismo.* Turin: Einaudi.

Husserl, Edmund (2008): *La crisi delle scienze europee e la fenomenologia trascendentale.* Milan: Il Saggiatore.

Kern, Stephen (2007): *Il tempo e lo spazio: La percezione del mondo tra Otto e Novecento.* Bologna: Il Mulino.

Koyré, Alexandre (1996): *Lezioni su Cartesio*. Milan: Tranchida.

Kuhn, Thomas S. (1978): *La struttura delle rivoluzioni scientifiche: Come mutano le idee della scienza*. Turin: Einaudi.

Kuhn, Thomas S. (2008): *La tensione essenziale e altri saggi*. Turin: Einaudi.

Lecercle, Jean-Jacques (2002): *Frankestein mito e filosofia*. S. M. C. V.: Ipermedium.

Le Doux, Joseph (2012): *Il Sé sinaptico*. Milan: Raffaello Cortina.

Le Goff, Jacques (2000): *Tempo della Chiesa e tempo del mercante: Saggi sul lavoro e la cultura nel Medioevo*. Turin: Einaudi.

Le Goff, Jacques (2008): *L'immaginario medievale*. Rome-Bari: Laterza.

McLuhan, Marshall (1976): *La galassia Gutenberg: Nascita dell'uomo tipografico*. Rome: Armando.

Mumford, Lewis (2011): *Il mito della macchina*. Milan: Il Saggiatore.

Pecchinenda, Gianfranco (2003): *Videogiochi e cultura della simulazione: La nascita dell'homo game*. Rome-Bari: Laterza.

Pecchinenda, Gianfranco (2007): 'The Genome and the Imaginary: Notes on the Sociology of Death and the Culture of Immortality'. *International Review of Sociology*, 17 (1):167–185.

Pecchinenda, Gianfranco (2008): *Homunculus: Sociologia dell'identità e autonarrazione*. Naples: Liguori.

Pecchinenda, Gianfranco (2009): *La narrazione della società: Appunti introduttivi alla sociologia dei processi culturali e comunicativi*. S. M. C. V.: Ipermedium.

Pecchinenda, Gianfranco (2014): *Il Sistema Mimetico: Contributi per una Sociologia dell'Assurdo*. S. M. C. V.: Ipermedium.

Prigogine, Ilya & Isabelle Stengers (1999): *La nuova alleanza: Metamorfosi della scienza*. Turin: Einaudi.

Rossi, Paolo (1989): *Introduzione a La Magia naturale nel Rinascimento: Testi di Agrippa, Cardano Fludd*. Turin: Utet.

Rossi, Paolo (2006): *Il tempo dei maghi: Rinascimento e modernità*. Milan: Raffaello Cortina.

Santoro, Alessandra (2016): *Il paradiso può attendere: Strategie dell'immortalità e società contemporanea*. Doctoral thesis, Università degli studi Federico II, Naples.

Schütz, Alfred (1972): *The Phenomenology of the Social World*. Evanston, IL: Northwestern University Press.

Shapin, Steven (2003): *La rivoluzione scientifica*. Turin: Einaudi.

Sontag, Susan (1989): *L'aids e le sue metafore*. Turin: Einaudi.

Vernant, Jean-Pierre (1994): 'Greek Man'. *Bulletin of the American Academy of Arts and Sciences*, 47 (8):44–50.

Wolff, Francis (2010): *Notre humanité: D'Aristote aux neurosciences*. Paris: Fayard.

Yates, Frances A. (2006): *Giordano Bruno e la cultura europea del Rinascimento*. Rome-Bari: Laterza.

Yates, Frances A. (2010): *Giordano Bruno e la tradizione ermetica*. Rome-Bari: Laterza.

8   Toward post-human

The dream of never-ending life

Nunzia Bonifati

Introduction

In *Isthmian*, the ancient Greek poet Pindar warned us: 'Seek not to become Zeus! / You have everything, if a share / Of these beautiful things comes to you. / Mortal ends befit mortal men'.[1] Nevertheless, one of the most whimsical trends in our millennium is to believe that one day we will achieve eternal youth and beauty, like the Greek gods, thanks to science and technological knowledge and tools. Realistically, it does not seem a good idea, especially if you consider we will end up with an epochal demographic crisis due to a scarcity of land and natural resources. Wars of conquest would break out, with many dead and injured, because biological immortality does not protect us from accidental death. Moreover, in order to live in peace, probably nobody should procreate any more.

This scenario is awful, but apparently humankind prefers to dream about immortality without consequences in order to alleviate their anguish about dealing with death. If being aware of one's own senescence and death is too painful to deal with, the creative alternative to immortality is a good lifeline. After all, as psychologists say, the ability to imagine ways out of a bad situation is an excellent tool to overcome the traumas of life (van der Kolk 2014).

The important fact is that nowadays the fast-paced development of science, technology and biotechnology allows humankind to hope for a potential overcoming of its own biological limits. However, what if the dream comes true, at least partially? Theoretically, it is possible to extend the human lifespan to over 120 years, and maybe achieving this is only a matter of time (Lytal 2015; Masoro & Austad 2006). Nevertheless, would humans be able to meet this epochal challenge? What would the implications be for human freedom and human values? Moreover, would the concept of humanity change for the better or for the worse? These are important questions, which we cannot answer yet. Presently we can only speculate on the possible consequences of extending the lifespan beyond its current limits and enhancing the human body and its capacities.

In this chapter I will try to answer such questions, keeping in mind that they require a multidisciplinary approach and a thoughtful analysis carried out by philosophers, sociologists, anthropologists, theologians, scientists, engineers, medical doctors and so on. Summing up, I will just frame the search for eternal life as an attempt to find a practical solution to the 'problem of death'. In the first section, I will briefly consider the ancient dream of eternal youth. In the second, I will mention post-human philosophy and discuss its being conditioned by the concepts of *hýbris* and the 'will to power'. In the third section, we shall see how recent developments in science and technology have created in the collective imaginary the illusion of really conquering immortality. In the fourth section, instead, I will talk about the different paths outlined by techno-scientific research on the way to enhancing human beings, while in the fifth section I will summarize some of the paradoxical consequences of these technological paths to human enhancement. Lastly, I will sum up the discussion and outline the risks of the obsessive research to overcome human biological limits. Indeed, my purpose is to show the extraordinary complexity and riskiness of the paths aiming to research into eternal youth.

From dream to reality

Let us start from the origin. The dream of eternal youth, physical potency and beauty is as old as history, and is rooted in most of the world's cultures. Since ancient times, human communities have believed in the existence of an ancestral place or source of happiness, such as a fountain of youth. There are references to blessed eras or places in the Greeks myths (the Golden Age), in the Bible (the Garden of Eden), in Indian and Chinese sacred texts, and also in the Sumerian, Egyptian and Mexican ancient traditions (Graf 1892/2002:34). The dream of earthly immortality has a very complex and articulated history and we cannot address it comprehensively in a few words. However, it is worth mentioning briefly, in order to better understand how today the ancient dream of never-ending life is going to take shape.

The first human communities attributed divine power to nature – the earth, the sun and the moon – and saw death as a mystery, maybe the result of sorcery. However, they did not think of immortality (Pettazzoni 1957). The idea of eternal life arose with polytheistic religions, as an exclusively divine attribute that is absolutely denied to humans. The ancient Greeks judged people who aspired to immortality and the powers of the gods to be suffering from a severe form of mind-blindness. The cause of disease was a serious fault called ὕβρις (*hýbris*) – 'hubris'. The ancient Greeks thus considered it wise and healthy to accept their own biological limits; in Apollo's temple at Delphi, the inscription γνῶθι σαυτόν (*gnôthi sautón*) – 'know yourself' – warned people of the risk of *hýbris*. Plato, in 'Socrates' apology', interpreted the famous Delphic aphorism *gnôthi sautón* as an admonition to suggest the practice of self-consciousness, the foundation of the Socratic awareness of 'not knowing'. Furthermore, the ancient Greeks knew very well they could not go back to the original 'Golden Age', a long-lost time of happiness when humans lived in peace and blessedness. The only immortal human attribute admitted was the soul. However, because they considered the soul – at least partially, as Aristotle said in 'On the Soul' – to be inseparable from the body, not all the philosophers agreed. Death for the ancient Greeks was synonymous with annihilation, but they accepted their faith, and the Romans, too, carried on the tradition. As the epicurean Lucretius wrote in *De Rerum Natura* (III 830): *Nil igitur mors est ad nos neque pertinet hilum / quandoquidem natura animi mortalis abetur.*[2] The same concept is found in Seneca's equally famous quotation in *Troades* (II v. 398–399): *Post mortem nihil est* ('After death nothingness').

Starting with the great monotheistic religions – Judaism, Christianity and Islam – the idea of an afterlife of eternal happiness and beatitude emerges, as God's compensation for a life lived in conformity with divine law. Christian and Muslim worshipers believed in an immortal afterlife, Jews in the *Olam Ha-Ba*, 'the World to Come'. Furthermore, God's realm offered hope in the final redemption, a promise of exceptional value and spiritual strength. The idea of earthly immortality was vain. After all, the Garden of Eden was part of the Genesis, and nobody had experienced either the source of immortality or the tree of life. Pursuing the vain idea of earthly immortality meant that believers would have committed the sins of pride and idolatry, and thus risked losing the Heavenly Realm.

Nevertheless, neither the warning of the Delphic oracle nor the promise of the Heavenly Realm were ever able to diminish the dream of eternal youth. This vision has continued, through the centuries, to stimulate the creativity of artists, writers and poets, who, from the Middle Ages onwards, have imagined conquering immortality by means of a covenant with the devil, the *daimones* able to seize the human soul (D'Agostino 2004; Rudwin 1931). Conversely, the dream also motivated the alchemists searching for the philosopher's stone or the elixir of life; and nowadays it continues to stimulate the creativity of scientists as well.

In the wake of the ancient dream of never-ending life, scientists today are studying how to overcome human biological limits as much as possible, and how to improve and strengthen the human body well beyond the goal to cure and prevent illness. Actually, this attempt to overcome human limits should not be seen as an intentional and organized attempt to pursue the dream. Rather it emerges as a trend, in the wake of the ideology of the progressive advancement of scientific knowledge, inherited from positivism and neo-positivism (Niiniluoto *et al.* 2004; Rossi 1988).

Toward post-human

Nowadays, the only ones with a real human enhancement program are the worldwide transhumanist movement (Hughes 2004). The transhumanists assess positively the process of the gradual transformation of the human being into an enhanced creature, physically and mentally superior. This school of thought takes the shape of a liberation movement from the biological limits of the human being, which is seen as a creature that has the moral duty to improve itself until perfection. In order to reach the goal, the transhumanists study, encourage and plan the process to transform the human being into a post-human, in an ethical and humanistic framework. The transhumanist utopia, with its messianic vision, helps to ease the anguish unleashed by the awareness of our own mortality and our physical and psychic fragility (Hughes 2012). The scientific community does not consider the transhumanist movement with approval, above all because its members declare themselves to have a vast metaphysical perspective on the development, direction, goals and values of conscience and life (More 1990–1996). Nevertheless, transhumanists are among the few to question systematically the potential ethical and social consequences of what they see as a species jump from human to post-human. For this reason, we should consider their argumentation seriously, while sharing neither their ideas nor their program.

Oddly, society seems to accept with pleasure the human enhancement proposal. However, many thinkers raise doubts about this trend, which they see as *hýbris* or as idolatry (see, e.g., Agar 2014; Baudrillard 2000; Fukuyama 2002; Longo 2003; Sandel 2009). After all, as the philosopher Emanuele Severino says, in our age the 'will to power' is showing its true face: the set of tools of the technically advanced societies become the ultimate purpose of those same societies (Severino 1988:38). From a different point of view, the sociologist Zygmunt Bauman underlines the novelty of a science that is becoming a sort of religion: 'With the Enlightenment came the enthronement of the new deity, that of the Nature, together with the legitimation of science as its only orthodox cult, and of scientist as its prophets and priests' (Bauman 1989:68).

The power to change nature

Human beings have always wanted to increase their power over Nature, with the assumption that this power would make them, among other things, able to defeat death and pain (Severino 2008). Death is in fact an irreversible event, and this is enough to make it unbearable in Western culture, which is conditioned by the will to transform things and Nature (see, for example, the 'will to decision and action' in Edmund Husserl, and the 'will to power and self-creation' in Friedrich Nietzsche). In order to control death, we use the technique that modern science has transformed into the most powerful tool to change the world (Severino 1988). In fact, by reading any handbook of genetics, nanoscience or robotics, we can see how much our power over the world has grown.

The great leap forward happened in 1997, when in the Scottish laboratory of the Roslin Institute, the scientist Ian Wilmut successfully cloned Dolly the sheep, using the nuclear transfer technique. At that moment, the world knew that scientists were able to intervene in the genome of a mammal in a conscious, organized and effective way. The impact of the news on public opinion was impressive. It seemed that there was no longer any limit to the power of science (Jensen 2014). Since Dolly, biotechnological techniques have improved so much that animal cloning now seems to be child's play, and it is becoming more and more common to hear about laboratory animals being genetically modified, like 'Oncomouse', the famous rodent genetically modified to get cancer, developed by Harvard University.

Life science and biotechnology are directly involved in the process of the physical and functional enhancement of human beings, and so they deserve a closer look in the post-human perspective. Biomedicine especially – the successful synthesis of biology and medical practice – gives us a glimpse of extraordinary perspectives in the prevention of aging, in the treatment of many diseases, and in aesthetical treatments. Thanks to biomedical science, maybe one day we will become more beautiful, healthier and longer-living. Meanwhile, bioengineers work together with scientists and medical doctors in the design and testing of new models to understand human physiology, biomaterials suited to transplant, artificial organs, and robotic prosthesis able to connect to the central nervous system, and much more (Bonifati 2012).

In particular, we see a rapid improvement in new diagnostic and surgical techniques, in gene therapy and regenerative medicine, giving us hope, for example, of finding a cure for cancer and diabetes. However, it is an illusion to believe that new therapies and techniques (biomedical, surgical, biotech and so on) will not be used to improve the body's appearance and enhance physical and mental performance. After all, the history of medicine and surgery proves it, and the best example is plastic surgery.

During its history, plastic surgery has always been used both to treat deformation or damage, and to restore or improve part of the body (Cosmacini 2003; Haiken 1997). Despite the risks to health, such as the potential development of infections or anesthesia and post-surgery complications, people have never eschewed aesthetical improvements. In the same way, as soon as the safety and therapeutic efficacy of a new treatment is proven, it could also be used for the purposes of enhancement, and people would accept the risks. It is hypocrisy to think that this will not happen, because to do so pretends to ignore the fact that every technical tool (from knife to robot) has always had an ambivalent use, for good or evil (Longo 2001). Furthermore, it is also dangerous, because it assumes that the evaluation of the lawfulness of such techniques is confined to the Authority and Bioethical committees, as if this problem did not actually concern the increasingly more competitive model of society we are building, and its consequences on humankind (Sandel 2009). It is evident in fact that we have taken a path that, at least at the moment, concerns only the individual and her/his own personal ambition of perfection, and not the human community as a whole. The issue is highly controversial. However, let us consider some of the most controversial paths outlined by techno-scientific research on the way to enhancing human beings, keeping in mind that all of these are convergent and intertwined.

Human enhancement technology paths

Human enhancement technologies are complex and articulated paths, straddling the human dreams of immortality and the need to survive the human condition of mortality. The goal is to enable the human being to overcome mental and physical fatigue, to improve physical appearance, to become more resistant to disease and to increase lifespan. This kind of enhancement is powered mainly by electronic and robotic devices, drugs, medical devices, regenerative medicine and gene therapy.

Wearable technologies

These electronic or robotic devices for augmented reality are in constant development. They are various in type and complexity. The simpler ones are wearable devices (bracelets, belts, accessories and clothing) to monitor, record and elaborate data related to vital signs (i.e., breathing, heart rate, blood pressure, body temperature), minerals (in sweat), calorie consumption, distance walked, altitude, external temperature, and so on. Usually athletes use these devices to monitor their performance during training. Sometimes, people who operate in dangerous environments, like construction workers, use them as well. Other wearable electronic or robotic devices that record physiological parameters (blood pressure, heartbeat, glycaemia, minerals and so on) are used by people who need to keep their health status under control. In addition, smart-watches and smart-glasses are promising wearable devices for augmented reality. There are also other very useful wearable devices currently under research and development, called 'tactile sensors technologies'. These devices make it possible to communicate tactile perceptions remotely, exactly as we currently do when sharing photos and videos with friends. A very promising tactile device, for example, works like this: a person (the transmitter) wears a special glove equipped with sensors. The transmitter touches an object and her/his tactile feeling is recorded, reduced to a strength signal and transmitted wirelessly and in real time to another person (the recipient). The recipient wears another glove, equipped with many small engines, that apply pressure on her/his hand, thus simulating the feeling perceived by the transmitter (Prattichizzo *et al.* 2010). This experimental technology is finding application in medicine and nursing, but when simplified, people will use it as an augmented reality device to share tactile sensations with friends.

Other promising wearable robotic technologies are exoskeletons, which increase physical power and reduce fatigue. They all came from US military research, especially from DARPA, the US defense agency committed to advanced research. On the other hand, the first to take an interest in civilian use have been the Japanese, who developed a robotic exoskeleton to facilitate movement for people who have difficulty walking (Bonifati 2010). Currently there are various robotic exoskeletons, used to help permanently paralyzed people to walk again. These robotic suits are requiring less and less space and are becoming easier to wear. Tomorrow they could become as comfortable and practical as a tracksuit and people could use them for practical purposes like doing heavy work or walking uphill without feeling fatigued.

Organs and tissues

A research field that offers interesting perspectives on health improvement and human enhancement is regenerative medicine and tissue engineering. This branch of medical science seeks to repair damaged tissues and organs by exploiting the potential capabilities of stem cells. These cells are well suited for this therapeutic scope because of their own surprising capabilities to repair and regenerate themselves in vitro, giving rise to all the cells of which a body is composed. Exploiting the capabilities of stem cells, it is possible to create 'spare parts' of organs and tissues. Currently the skin can be successfully cultivated, likewise other tissues, and there are promising results with corneas (Rama *et al.* 2010). In order to make these tissues grow, medical doctors remove a tiny flap of tissue from the patient's body, put it in a culture and wait for the tissue to grow to the expected dimensions. Finally, the tissue is used for transplant. However, skin and corneas are epithelial tissues, which are very simple to cultivate in vitro. For other, more complex kinds of tissues (connective, muscular and nervous), we await the results of the many clinical studies currently under way. By exploiting the incredible vitality of stem cells, maybe in a few decades we will be able to cultivate many different tissues. Should this be the case, medical doctors could transplant patients with their own cells, without the risk of rejection. Obviously, aesthetic surgery is very interested in this research field – though it is not without controversies (Khunger 2014) – and every day it reveals its latest successes to the public.

Studies on the spontaneous regenerative capacity of tissues are also interesting. The salamander, for example, has the capability to regrow large body parts whenever it is accidentally mutilated. A study (Heber-Katz *et al.* 2010) has revealed that the gene that regulates the regenerative process – also found in other amphibians and, for very marginal aspects, in humans – is the p21. When the gene is inactive, the severed limb fibroblasts regress to an embryonic stage of their development, to recall how to rebuild the different parts of the body. Then they start to recreate tissues exactly as they did before. Conversely, when the p21 gene is active, it inhibits the spontaneous regeneration process of tissues. In theory, it would be enough to turn off the p21 gene in order to stimulate the regeneration process when needed. Unfortunately, keeping the gene turned on is also very useful to prevent cancer, because it inhibits cell proliferation in the case of damaged DNA. Therefore, turning off gene p21 could be very dangerous. Anyway, researchers continue to study processes of spontaneous self-regeneration, looking for better tools for regenerative medicine (Bonifati 2012).

Drugs and hormones

Another well-trodden path to enhance physical and mental performance and strengthen the physical structure of the body is the use of chemical substances: pharmaceutical drugs, vaccines, hormones and supplements, smart drugs. But this type of enhancement can sometimes be dangerous for one's health, and so not always effective in extending the lifespan. For example, ephedrine, a chemical stimulant of the nervous system similar to amphetamine, is often used by students to increase concentration when studying and by athletes to improve physical performance (the World Anti-Doping Agency deems it a doping substance). Nevertheless, this substance, which today has very limited therapeutic indications (hypotension caused by drugs, narcolepsy), can cause serious damage to the nervous system and, ultimately, permanent changes to the body's physical structure. On the other hand, a popular substance that could be used for the purpose of improvement is growth hormone. Because some controversial studies show that this hormone could be safe and healthy, national or federal agencies for the evaluation of medical products may one day extend the hormone's therapeutic indications, for example, as an anti-aging or a slimming substance.[3] Furthermore, in the United States, pediatricians have spread the practice of prescribing the growth hormone to short children to make them grow taller. Considering the supposed healthy virtues of the growth hormone, this practice could become common, for example, in countries where the average height is low.

A hormone that could be used for the purpose of moral enhancement (Douglas 2008; Persson & Savulescu 2012a) is oxytocin – the hormone of motherhood. The supply of oxytocin would reduce aggressiveness, enhance empathy and confidence toward others and act as a hate attenuator. Therefore, it could be used to improve human behavior. Also antidepressant drugs, such as selective serotonin reuptake inhibitors (SSRI alter physiological processes in the brain, acting on neurotransmitter receptors) could be useful for the purpose of moral enhancement. According to its promoters, moral enhancement may be necessary because the vast development of technology has made humans potentially more dangerous, but there has not been a corresponding improvement in moral awareness (Persson & Savulescu 2012b). However, moral improvement creates many more problems than it would solve (DeGrazia 2013). For example: who should decide what kind of moral enhancement should be chosen? Which moral paradigm should be our source of inspiration? Are we sure that influential groups would not try to impose their moral model inspired only by their own advantage? And finally, wouldn't a single moral paradigm impoverish society, denying the possibility to confront people with different moral perspectives? (Balistreri 2015:119).

Implantable devices

We can define a cyborg as a healthy human being implanted with various prostheses and devices, in order to become more powerful. The scenario is tempting. However, this kind of path to enhancement carries potential risks for human health. Therefore, it makes no sense to follow it, at least not in order to increase human lifespan. Actually, technologies and advanced surgical techniques in theory would allow the implanting of different kinds of prostheses and electronic devices, like cameras, artificial cochlea, pacemakers, processors and so on. For example, it is possible to implant the so-called RFID (Radio Frequency Identification) in the arm of a transplanted person. These devices can be used to store crucial medical information about the person that can be extremely useful in emergency cases. For years, the public have been discussing the possibility of implanting RFID in children's arms to prevent kidnapping (Taylor 2015) or in the arms of Alzheimer's patients in order to locate them easily should they go missing. A further example is the implant of Deep Brain Stimulation (DBS) devices (Coenen *et al.* 2009:80–86). Today DBS are used with some success in facilitating the recovery of memory in Alzheimer's sufferers and in the treatment of motor symptoms in Parkinson's disease and other movement disorders. Also under way, not without controversy, is the extension of this therapeutic implant to neuropsychiatric conditions such as severe major depression or refractory obsessive-compulsive disorder (Alivisatos *et al.* 2012; Fried 2015).

The possibility cannot be excluded that in the future these brain stimulators could be used as enhancement tools. Nevertheless, the extension of the use of therapeutic implants to allow physical and psychic enhancement is dangerous for the health and ethically controversial. Risks to health are well known and listed by every ministry of health and by regulatory agencies in each country, and should persuade everyone not to follow this path (Bonifati & Longo 2012). From the ethical perspective, problems arising from the use of such devices concern mainly the potential violation of human dignity and privacy (EGE 2005). These wireless devices in fact contain sensitive information, and the implanted people could be controlled without their knowledge or subjected to forced control.

GM babies

The purpose of eugenics, in the context of human enhancement, is to improve humans by selecting the genetic traits seen as advantageous to increase health, longevity, beauty, physical and mental power and sensory capabilities, through promoting favorable genetic factors and preventing the transmission of unfavorable genetic factors (Coenen *et al.* 2009:71–79). Considering the boldness of its goal, it is clear that in the collective imagination this type of human enhancement appears to be the most critical since cloning times (see, e.g., Agar 2010; Baudrillard 2000; Jensen 2008, 2014; Sandel 2009). Nevertheless, the possibility of enhancing human beings using gene therapies is still a distant one.

Today, genome editing technologies are the most topical field of research, specifically CRISPR (Clustered Regularly Interspaced Short Palindromic Repeats), genome editing technologies that allow modification of the genome of gametes or embryos of human and non-human animals. The objective of these technologies is the treatment of genetic diseases in an embryonic state (or at a germinal level). However, scientists are currently very cautious, because these tools could cause health risks (Lanphier *et al.* 2015). Meanwhile, in January 2016 the United Kingdom's Human Fertilisation and Embryology Authority approved a license application to use genome editing in research at the Francis Crick Institute in London. It is the first European experimentation on human embryos, but it will be illegal for scientists to implant the modified embryos into a woman.

This UK study aims to provide an understanding of the earliest moments of human life, and, scientists reassure, it will not be used for creating genetically modified babies. However, the road is open. Not by chance, scientists are discussing genome editing in international symposia, evaluating the therapeutic perspectives, ethical constraints and possible consequences in regard to human evolution (Friedmann 2016). There are concerns that, when genome editing technologies improve, it will be difficult to confine their use exclusively to therapeutic purposes. The techniques will offer parents the opportunity to 'design' their own babies, choosing the gender, height, skin color, longevity and so on.

Beyond the genetic supermarket, genome editing opens a new perspective concerning human evolution. At the very first stage of development of life, prior to embryo formation, the improvements made to the 'bad genome' would be transmitted to the descendants. Gene therapy will hence be useful in the treatment of genetic diseases on a large scale. These diseases, being no longer transmittable to children, in the end would disappear. If this were the case, in a few generations we could succeed in an enterprise that has so far been the exclusive domain of Nature, with unpredictable consequences. For the first time we could become the masters of our own genetic destiny.

Other minor futuristic paths

The 'technological singularity' theorists (such as the futurist Ray Kurzweil) are convinced that we can reach a disembodied immortality through transferring the data of one's mind to a digital support, whereby linking all the 'Artificial minds' to one another creates a sort of single planetary and immortal mind (Kurzweil 2005). This offers a vision of a disembodied immortality made of bytes, digital memories, computers or robots that can keep the 'copy' of the mind of departed people, so that they can go on living. The goal is to 'transfer' or 'upload' a conscious mind from a human brain to a computer. Nevertheless, it is a controversial research field, because it tends to assimilate the computational capability of a computer to human intelligence. However, it is very simplistic to compare the brain to the computer and the computer to the brain (Bonifati & Longo 2012, ch. 4), the more so because, as neuroscientists say, we know very little about the human brain.

Another futuristic path is to try to extend longevity toward the 120 years imprinted in our genetic code without the side effects of aging. The researchers' goal is to prevent aging, seen as a disease, by reducing every inflammatory and oxidative process (Masoro & Austad 2006). To this end, scientists are studying the telomeres and the telomerase, the embryonic stem cells and the cells' regenerative capabilities. Other studies concern biologically immortal organisms, such as bacteria, jellyfish and, particularly, the tardigrades, which are able to change their genes to adapt from time to time to environmental adversity (Boothby *et al.* 2015). The goal is to discover the secret of their longevity and try to imitate them. However, they are very simple organisms, not comparable with the complexity of other animal species, like mammals. In addition, the numerous studies on the genetic characteristics of centennial people might shed light on the secret of longevity (Sebastiani *et al.* 2012). Furthermore, since there is a strong correlation between longevity and calorie-restrictive diets, scientists are studying the effects of such diets in humans (Ravussin *et al.* 2015) and in animals (Sinclair 2005).

Living as sick to die healthy

Meanwhile, in wealthy countries people live longer and in better health conditions (WHO 2014). According to the World Health Organization's (WHO) *World Health Statistics*, the increase in life expectancy mainly depends on family planning, low infant mortality, prevention and treatment of diseases, a healthy lifestyle, a healthy environment and so on. In short, it depends on the meticulous monitoring of human and environmental health. The greater the control, the greater the chance to live longer. The obsession with health monitoring paradoxically ends up considering the various development stages of life, with specific diseases requiring palliative care, psychological resilience and adequate strategies for survival (Conrad & Maturo 2009; Rovatti 2008). From pregnancy to old age, every stage of life is under diagnostic and pharmacological medical supervision. Pregnant women take folic acid to prevent birth defects; infants get vitamin D for the development of bones; students and adults undergo immune-stimulation to increase the immune system; the elderly take antioxidants and so on. In addition, the 'symptoms of life' connected to the different life stages are under medical scrutiny, and if necessary treated with appropriate therapies. It is enough to think of the excessive vivacity of children that is often associated with ADHD (Attention Deficit Hyperactivity Disorder), and in some cases treated pharmacologically with methylphenidate, a central nervous system stimulant.

The obsessive control of health status reduces human life to the expression of optimal parameters and optimal vital functions. It is a very narrow view. Since the cellular aging process ends with biological death, we tend to view life, especially old age, like a slow and progressive terminal illness. After all, the tendency to consider aging as a disease rather than a stage of human development also has a medical justification in the vision of health offered by WHO in 1946: 'Health is a state of complete physical, mental and social wellbeing and not merely the absence of disease or infirmity.'[4] Actually, it is very difficult to reconcile the symptoms of old age due to cellular degeneration with the WHO definition of health. How many elderly people without infirmity or illness enjoy 'a state of complete physical, mental, and social well-being'? Evidently, in 1946 we did not expect the significant increase in life expectancy that we see today in wealthy countries. However, there is something more to say.

Since the last century, the concept of well-being has been connected to the 'will' as a principle of rational action. To offer some examples, in the 1930s – in the midst of the Great Depression – the imperative of physical beauty (synonymous with well-being) emerges, which everyone has to achieve through will and perseverance (Vigarello 2004). Then, starting from the 1970s, in line with the WHO concept of health, we begin increasingly to control health in all its forms: beauty, posture, dexterity and physical strength, intellectual capacity and so on. Consequently, the idea of medicalization of life takes shape: each life stage begins to be kept under strict medical supervision (Illich 1975).

In the context of life medicalization, we can consider human enhancement technologies as a kind of palliative care of the terminal illness called 'life'. An extreme and rather bizarre example of survival strategy from the human mortal condition is the cryopreservation of gametes or embryos. Such a practice is not yet popular, but some young couples have already cryopreserved their gametes (or embryos) to ensure the generation of their offspring from young and healthy gametes even in their mature age (or even post-mortem). However, the result of this unconventional use of assisted reproductive technologies is to have children in old age, or to generate children who are orphans even before they are born. You could have the illusion of becoming the master of your own biological destiny, but a question arises: would the children agree?

Conclusion

Is it worth freeing humankind from its biological constraints? Along with death, we should also cancel the decrepitude of old age, that which mythology, art and literature have always linked to unhappy or unfortunate creatures. Like the despised and hated 'Struldbrug', depicted harshly in *Gulliver's Travels*. Or like Dr. Faust, the title character of the masterpiece by Wolfgang Goethe, who receives damnation, but in the end dies in bliss and goes to heaven. The madness of a never-ending life is clearly shown in Jorge Luis Borges's tale, 'The Immortal' (1947): 'to draw out the span of a man's life was to draw out the agony of his dying and multiply the number of his death' (Borges 2004:5).

Apparently, neither the teachings of ancient Greeks, nor the Latin *memento mori*, nor the promise of heaven, nor the awful scenario of an immortal life have been capable of changing the minds of those pursuing the project to overcome human limits. Transhumanists like James Hughes (2004, 2012) and Nick

Bostrom and Julian Savulescu (2009) assert that following a technological and scientific program, which includes human moral improvement, immortality would not create any side effects, and in the end everybody would share its benefits. However, the demographic issue remains unresolved. Moreover, history shows that technological and scientific progress has never made human beings more virtuous or ethically better. As far as moral enhancement goes, as suggested above, it brings forth more issues than solutions. However, transhumanists are not the only ones pursuing the program to improve the human species. According to political scientist Francis Fukuyama, human enhancement is implicit in the research agenda of contemporary biomedicine, and all of the 'new procedures and technologies emerging from research laboratories and hospitals ... can as easily be used to "enhance" the species as to ease or ameliorate illness' (Fukuyama 2009). Fukuyama believes that human enhancement is the most dangerous idea of the millennium, because it would endanger mainly the principle of equality, according to which 'all men are created equal' (US Declaration of Independence). In fact, not everyone would have access to the improvements, and there would be citizens who would perceive themselves as superior, claiming to have more rights over others.

American philosopher Michael Sandel declared his opposition to the human enhancement program, especially where eugenics is concerned, although, as with many other thinkers and scientists, he claims that enhancements aimed at therapeutic purposes are permissible and should not be hampered: 'The need for healing arises from the fact that the world is not perfect and complete but in constant need of human intervention and repair' (Sandel 2009:101). According to Sandel's moral perspective, it is immoral to try to use biotechnology to enhance humans in order to lift some people above the norm, because this is a sort of consumerist ethic, far from the values of medicine.

If bioengineering made the myth of the 'self-made man' come true, it would be difficult to view our talents as gifts for which we are indebted, rather than as achievements for which we are responsible. This would transform three key features of our moral landscape: humility, responsibility, and solidarity.

(Sandel 2009:86)

A slightly different perspective is found in the provocative, sarcastic and hopeless considerations of the French philosopher and sociologist Jean Baudrillard, according to whom the illusion of immortality is entirely uncritical: 'blindly we dream of overcoming death through immortality, when all the time immortality is the most horrific of all fates' (Baudrillard 2000:6).

The latest consideration concerns the unpredictable consequences of techno-scientific applications that would allow the overcoming of human biological limits. As suggested in his time by the father of cybernetics, Norbert Wiener (1950, 1964), we have over time accumulated a huge amount of technical and scientific knowledge and skills. However, the uncertainty connected to the use of such knowledge is more problematic now than in the past. The more the techniques improve, the more complicated and capable of getting out of our control the processes become. Therefore, the process of overcoming our biological limitations calls for caution, balance and a sense of responsibility.

This is especially important because, for more than half a century, science and technology have advanced *motu proprio* and very quickly, leaving behind meditation, which of course needs time to make the most of its possibilities. If this gap is not reduced, I think, it is likely that we will have many problems in steering techno-scientific and biotechnological applications. Reducing this gap then becomes the biggest cultural challenge of the 'knowledge society', even more than the research of biological immortality itself.

To close, in this chapter I have outlined the ancient dream of eternal youth and explored the post-human philosophy with its concepts of *hýbris*, 'will to power' and 'medicalization of life'. I have showed how the latest developments of science and technology have created, in the collective imaginary, the illusion of a potential conquest of immortality, and the different paths outlined by techno-scientific research on the way to enhancing the human being. In summary, just like the other thinkers and philosophers quoted in this chapter, I have attempted to show the significant complexity and risks of the paths taken by human enhancement technology and some of their paradoxical consequences. However, at the end of the journey my research raises more questions than answers. Nevertheless, there are some key points that clearly emerge from my work that I would like to underline. First, the fast-paced development of science and technology has created the illusion that it is possible to achieve the ancient dream of eternal youth. Second, it is probably not worth extending the human lifespan beyond its limits. Third, there is an ever-extending gap between techno-scientific improvement on the one hand and moral and cultural improvement on the other. Fourth, eugenics, with its own ethical dilemmas and risks, is one of the potential outcomes of the human enhancement program. And finally, following the human enhancement technology paths with a philosophical outlook is undoubtedly one of the most critical challenges of our near future.

Notes

1 Pindar, *Isthmian 5*, p. 49.
2 Lucretius: 'So death is nothing, and matters nothing to us once it is clear that the mind is mortal stuff', in *De Rerum Natura: The Poem on Nature*, p. 97.
3 For brief information and therapeutic indications about the growth hormone, see the website 'The Growth Hormone Research Society (GRS)' at: www.ghresearch-society.org/GRS%20hGH%20Indications.htm. For the controversial studies, see the following: Bartke (2008); Bartke *et al.* (2013); and *HGH Controversies* on Wikipedia, available at: https://en.wikipedia.org/wiki/HGH_controversies#cite_note-NYTPoison-5.
4 WHO (1946): Preamble to the Constitution of the World Health Organization as adopted by the International Health Conference, New York, 19–22 June, 1946; signed on 22 July 1946 by the representatives of 61 States (Official Records of the World Health Organization, no. 2, p. 100) and entered into force on 7 April 1948.

References

Agar, Nicholas (2010): *Humanity's End: Why We Should Reject Radical Enhancement*. Cambridge, MA: MIT Press.

Agar, Nicholas (2014): *Truly Human Enhancement: A Philosophical Defense of Limits*. Cambridge, MA: MIT Press.

Alivisatos, Paul et al. (2012): 'The Brain Activity Map Project and the Challenge of Functional Connectomics'. *Neuron*, 74 (6):970–974.

Balistreri, Maurizio (2015): 'La medicina e il dogma della normalità nel dibattito sul potenziamento morale'. *Lessico di etica pubblica*, 1:118–126.

Bartke, Andrzej (2008): 'Growth Hormone and Aging: A Challenging Controversy'. *Clinical Interventions in Aging*, 3 (4):659–665.

Bartke, Andrzej, Reyhan Westbrook, Liou Sun & Mariusz Ratajczak (2013): 'Links between Growth Hormone and Aging'. *Endokrynologia Polska*, 64 (1):46–52.

Baudrillard, Jean (2000): *The Vital Illusion* (edited by Julia Witwer). New York: Columbia University Press.

Bauman, Zygmunt (1989): *Modernity and the Holocaust*. Cambridge: Polity Press.

Bonifati, Nunzia (2010): *Et voilà I robot: Etica ed estetica delle macchine*. Milan: Springer-Verlag Italia.

Bonifati, Nunzia (2012): 'Tre livelli di ibridazione uomo-macchina', in Silvia Garagna et al. (eds): *Le sfide della biologia sintetica e la fine del naturale*. Pavia: Collegio Ghislieri, Ibis.

Bonifati, Nunzia & Giuseppe O. Longo (2012): *Homo immortalis: Una vita quasi infinita*. Milan: Springer-Verlag Italia.

Boothby, Thomas C. et al. (2015): 'Evidence for Extensive Horizontal Gene Transfer from the Draft Genome of a Tardigrade'. *Pnas*, 112 (52):15976–15981.

Borges, Jorge Luis (2004): *The Aleph and Other Stories* (edited by Andrew Hurley). New York: Penguin Classics.

Bostrom, Nick & Julian Savulescu (eds) (2009): *Human Enhancement*. Oxford: Oxford University Press.

Coenen, Christopher, Mirjam Schuijff, Martijntje Smits, Pim Klaassen, Leonhard Hennen, Michael Rader & Gregor Wolbring (Commissioned by the Science and Technology Options Assessment) (2009): *Human Enhancement Study*. Brussels: European Parliament.

Conrad, Peter & Antonio Maturo (eds) (2009): *The Medicalization of Life: Salute & Società, Volume 2*. Milan: Franco Angeli.

Cosmacini, Giorgio (2003): *La vita nelle mani, Storia della chirurgia*. Bari: Laterza.

D'Agostino, Alfonso (2004): 'Il patto col diavolo nelle letterature medievali: Elementi per un'analisi narrativa'. *Studi medievali*, 45 (2):699–770.

DeGrazia, David (2013): 'Moral Enhancement, Freedom and What We (Should) Value in Moral Behaviour'. *Journal of Medical Ethics*. Available online at: http://jme.bmj.com/content/early/2013/01/24/medethics-2012–101157.full.pdf+html.

Douglas, Thomas (2008): 'Moral Enhancement'. *Journal of Applied Philosophy*, 25 (3):228–245.

EGE (The European Group on Ethics in Science and New Technologies to the European Commission) (2005): *Opinion no. 20: Ethical Aspects of ICT Implants in the Human Body*. Luxemburg: European Communities.

Fried, Itzhak (2015): 'Brain Stimulation and Memory'. *Brain*, 138 (7):1766–1767.

Friedmann, Theodore (2016): 'An ASGCT Perspective on the National Academies Genome Editing Summit'. *Molecular Therapy*, 24 (1):1–2.

Fukuyama, Francis (2002): *Our Posthuman Future: Consequences of the Biotechnology Revolution*. New York: Picador.

Fukuyama, Francis (2009): 'Transhumanism'. *Foreign Policy, Special Report*, October 23. Available online at: http://foreignpolicy.com/2009/10/23/transhumanism.

Graf, Arturo (1892/2002): *Miti leggende e superstizioni nel Medio Evo*. Milan: Bruno Mondadori.

Haiken, Elizabeth (1997): *Venus Envy: A History of Cosmetic Surgery*. Baltimore: Johns Hopkins University Press.

Heber-Katz, Hellen et al. (2010): 'Lack of p21 Expression Links Cell Cycle Control and Appendage Regeneration in Mice'. *Pnas*, 107 (13):5845–5850.

Hughes, James (2004): *Citizen Cyborg: Why Democratic Societies Must Respond to the Redesigned Human of the Future*. Cambridge, MA: Westview Press.

Hughes, James (2012): 'The Politics of Transhumanism and the Techno-Millennial Imagination, 1626–2030'. *Zygon*, 47 (4):757–776.

Illich, Ivan (1975): 'The Medicalization of Life'. *Journal of Medical Ethics*, 1:73–77.

Jensen, Eric (2008): 'The Dao of Human Cloning: Utopian/Dystopian Hype in the British Press and Popular Films'. *Public Understanding of Science*, 17 (2):123–143.

Jensen, Eric (2014): *The Therapeutic Cloning Debate: Global Science and Journalism in Public Sphere*. Farnham: Ashgate Publishing.

Khunger, Niti (2014): 'Regenerative Medicine in Aesthetic Surgery: Hope or Hype?'. *Journal of Cutaneous and Aesthetic Surgery*, 7 (4):187–188.

Kurzweil, Ray (2005): *The Singularity Is Near: When Humans Transcend Biology*. New York: Viking Press.

Lanphier, Edward et al. (2015): 'Don't Edit the Human Germ Line'. *Nature*, 519 (7544): 410–411.

Longo, Giuseppe O. (2001): *Homo Technologicus*. Rome: Meltemi.

Longo, Giuseppe O. (2003): *Il simbionte: prove di umanità futura*. Rome: Meltemi.

Lucretius (2003): *De Rerum Natura: The Poem on Nature* (translated by Charles Hubert Sisson). New York: Routledge.

Lytal, Cristy (2015): 'USC Scientist Ponders the Possibility of Immortality'. *USC News*, University of Southern California. Available online at: https://news.usc.edu/83760/usc-scientist-ponders-the-possibility-of-immortality.

Masoro, Edward J. & Steven N. Austad (eds) (2006): *Handbook of the Biology of Aging* (6th edn). San Diego: Academic Press.

More, Max (1990, revised 1996): 'Transhumanism: Towards a Futurist Philosophy'. *Extropy*, 6 (1).

Muneoka, Ken, Manjong Han & David M. Gardiner (2008): 'Regrowing Limbs: Can People Regenerate Body Parts?'. *Scientific American*, 298 (4):56–63.

Niiniluoto, Ilkka, Matti Sintonen & Jan Wolenski (eds) (2004): *Handbook of Epistemology*. Dordrecht: Kluwer Academic Publishers.

Persson, Ingmar & Julian Savulescu (2012a): 'Moral Enhancement, Freedom and the God Machine'. *The Monist*, 95 (3):399–421.

Persson, Ingmar & Julian Savulescu (2012b): *Unfit for the Future: The Need for Moral Enhancement*. Oxford: Oxford University Press.

Pettazzoni, Raffaele (1957): *L'essere supremo nelle religioni primitive*. Turin: Einaudi.

Pindar (2015): *Isthmian 5*, in *The Odes of Pindar* (translated by Cecil M. Bowra). London: Penguin Classics

Prattichizzo, Domenico et al. (2010): 'RemoTouch: A System for Remote Touch Experience'. *RO-MAN, 2010 IEEE, Conference Publication*, pp. 676–679.

Rama, Paolo et al. (2010): 'Limbal Stem-Cell Therapy and Long-Term Corneal Regeneration'. *New England Journal of Medicine*, 363:147–155.

Ravussin, Eric et al. (2015): 'A 2-Year Randomized Controlled Trial of Human Caloric Restriction: Feasibility and Effects on Predictors of Health Span and Longevity'. *Journal of Gerontology, Biological Sciences & Medical Sciences*, 70 (9):1097–1104.

Rossi, Paolo (1988): *Storia della scienza moderna e contemporanea*. Turin: UTET.

Rovatti, Pier Aldo (2008): 'Note sulla medicalizzazione della vita'. *Aut-Aut*, 340:3–13.

Rudwin, Maximilian (1931): *The Devil in Legend and Literature*. Chicago: Open Court Publishing Company.

Sandel, Michael J. (2009): *The Case against Perfection: Ethics in the Age of Genetic Engineering*. Cambridge, MA: Harvard University Press.

Sebastiani, Paola et al. (2012): 'Genetic Signatures of Exceptional Longevity in Humans'. *Plos One*, 7 (1). Available online at: http://journals.plos.org/plosone/article?id=10.1371/journal.pone.0029848.

Severino, Emanuele (1988): *La tendenza fondamentale del nostro tempo*. Milan: Adelphi.

Severino, Emanuele (2008): *Immortalità e destino*. Milan: Rizzoli.

Sinclair, David A. (2005): 'Toward a Unified Theory of Caloric Restriction and Longevity Regulation'. *Mechanisms of Ageing and Development*, 126 (9):987–1002.

Taylor, Jordyn (2015): 'Can We Microchip Our Kids to Prevent Kidnapping?'. *Observer*, March 18. Available online at: http://observer.com/2015/03/can-we-microchip-our-kids-to-prevent-kidnapping.

van der Kolk, Bessel (2014): *The Body Keeps the Score: Brain, Mind, and Body in the Healing of Trauma*. New York: Viking Press.

Vigarello, Georges (2004): *Histoire de la Beauté: Le Corps et l'Art d'Embellir de la Renaissance à nos Jours*. Paris: Éditions du Seuil.

WHO (2014): *World Health Statistics 2014*. Geneva: World Health Organization Press.

Wiener, Norbert (1950): *The Human Use of Human Beings*. Boston: Houghton Mifflin.

Wiener, Norbert (1964): *God & Golem Inc.* Cambridge, MA: MIT Press.

9   Digital immortality or digital death?

Contemplating digital end-of-life planning

*Carla J. Sofka, Allison Gibson and
Danielle R. Silberman*

Introduction

According to American philosopher Roy W. Perrett, 'concern with death and immortality is, of course, universal and hence the literature is enormous' (Perrett 1987:1). This interdisciplinary literature discusses the question: 'Is there survival after death?' Psychiatrist Robert J. Lifton (1979) utilized the term 'symbolic immortality' to describe efforts to transcend or circumvent death through the following means: biological immortality, achieved through the transmission of genetic material to our descendants; social immortality, achieved through our creations that survive us or in the lives of others we have influenced (e.g., friends, students, clients/patients); natural immortality as one's body returns to the ground and re-enters the cycle of life; and theological immortality (immortality of the soul) or spiritual immortality, a topic of discussion throughout recorded history. Psychologist Robert J. Kastenbaum introduced the term 'assisted immortality' to capture new possibilities for technologically assisted survival and asked readers to consider the following question: 'What would be a meaningful or essential form of survival, and would I make use of a technological assist, if available?' (Kastenbaum 2004:460). This question forms the basis of this chapter about 'digital immortality', which is being written at a time when it has become clear that the increased use of technology, particularly digital and social media, has transformed how we will be remembered and how we grieve.

In their roadmap to the key issues surrounding one's digital afterlife, Evan Carroll and John Romano (2011) acknowledged that technology is evolving at a breakneck pace and noted that when we die, the digital content that we have created becomes our digital legacy: 'passing this legacy on will become more important as the shift to digital continues and as your digital content becomes a richer reflection of you' (Carroll & Romano 2011:3). The notion of digital death, described by Stacey Pitsillides 'as either the death of a living being and the way it affects the digital world, or the death of a digital object and the way it affects a living being' (Pitsillides 2009:131), will be experienced by everyone who interacts in the digital world from one or both of these perspectives. In 2016, achieving digital immortality is feasible in a variety of ways due to advances in computer science, artificial intelligence, and the unprecedented role of digital and social media in everyday life. This chapter will identify the types of digital immortality and strategies for achieving it, summarize data and opinions about digital immortality and its impact on the bereaved, describe related policies and legal issues, and identify resources to assist with planning for one's digital afterlife.

Types of digital immortality

Searching the scholarly literature and the popular press for information on digital immortality revealed a wide range of terms and examples that vary based on the mechanism or medium used to achieve immortality, the intentionality of creating a virtual existence on the part of the deceased, and the degree of interactivity with a survivor that may or may not involve a human surrogate to initiate the interactions. Microsoft researchers Gordon Bell and Jim Gray's definition of digital immortality includes elements of intentionality as well as interactivity:

> [a] continuum from *enduring fame* at one end (*one-way immortality* by preserving and transmitting your ideas) to *endless experience and learning* at the other (two-way immortality which allows 'you', or at least part of you, to communicate with the future), stopping just short of endless life.
> (Bell & Gray 2000:2)

They noted that both types of immortality require part of a person to be cyberized and stored in a more durable media and believed that two-way immortality would be possible within this century.

In its most simplistic form, digital immortality is achieved by virtue of using any type of electronic or digital technology that creates digitally preserved materials. This potentially complex 'digital fingerprint/footprint' consists of public, organizational, pseudonymous, and private types of digital data (Garfinkel & Cox 2009) that are almost impossible to eliminate completely. Elizabeth Dow (2009) used the term 'archival immortality' in a discussion about the traditional preservation of a writer's papers and correspondence; this term implies a somewhat 'passive' type of digital immortality that is achieved by allowing one's digital output (e.g., emails, text messages, social media postings, etc.) and other links to digital artefacts of a person's life (for example, just Google yourself) to be saved in totality.

However, Dow also noted that many people 'construct their donation by consciously saving or destroying certain documents to put a particular spin on their place in history' (Dow 2009:117). The term 'digital curation', first used at a 2001 seminar in London discussing leading edge developments in the field of data curation and digital preservation (Beagrie 2006), captures a person's ability not only to influence the materials that are included in or excluded from one's digital legacy but to alter the way that one might be perceived or remembered. A person's 'digital heritage' has been defined as 'the accumulation and curation of digital data online, which could form the basis of an inexhaustible resource containing the exact documentation of our digital past' (Pitsillides *et al.* 2013:90). Following a person's death, survivors would be able to peruse what Cristiano Maciel and Vinicius Pereira (2015) referred to as one's 'post-mortem digital legacy'.

While advocating for the use of common terminology, a literature review by Debra Bassett (2015) described two distinct categories of data that have been used: (1) digital data (e.g., passwords, account information, digital assets, and digital property) that she suggests be referred to as 'digital legacy', and (2) digital selves (e.g., personal videos, messages, photographs, blogs) that she suggests be referred to as 'digital memories'. Elaine Kasket (2012) used the term 'persisting digital self' to refer to what could be considered the digital equivalent of one's 'durable biography' (Walter 1996). While this chapter will not resolve the challenge of standardizing terminology, options for curating one's digital data will be discussed in a subsequent section.

Bassett (2015) also discussed another important element of digital immortality – the intentionality on the part of the deceased regarding the purposeful planning for a socially active digital afterlife or if their virtual presence after death was accidental. Accidental residents of the digital afterlife have been described in several ways. Candi Cann (2014) defined Internet ghosts as 'program-generated prompts that function as part of a social network application, such as the suggestion to "like" something or to "friend" somebody because one's friend is a friend of someone else' (Cann 2014:13). Another example involves a birthday reminder if a deceased friend's Facebook page has not been memorialized, which may prompt a posting on the deceased's page such as this: 'You live on in our hearts and, apparently, on Facebook as well. Rest in Peace my friend' (R. Stevenson, personal communication, August 17, 2016). Authors have also used terms such as restless dead (Nansen *et al.* 2015), digital ghosts (Briggs & Thomas 2014), and digital zombies (Bassett 2015) to describe being 'posthumously present' (Kasket 2012) on social networking sites, social media, or in other virtual realms. A recent example involves the memorialization of Tamir Rice within *Pokémon Go* by virtue of the Cudell Gazebo (the site where the 12-year-old was shot and killed by police officers in 2014) becoming a Pokestop (Morris 2016).

Accidental immortality can transition into the intentional realm. Several examples from gaming serve as the first illustration. Trevor Owens (2014) shared the story of a son who finds his deceased father's 'ghost driver' in an Xbox game called *Rally Sports Challenge* and 'holds back' from beating the ghost to preserve his father's high score and hence his ongoing 'presence' in the game. William S. Bainbridge (2013) created ancestor veneration avatars (AVAs) 'as a medium for both memorializing deceased persons and exploiting the personalities and wisdom those people had possessed' (Bainbridge 2013:196), an alternative way of 'transcending mortality by symbolically returning the dearly departed to our world via role-playing avatars' (Bainbridge 2013:201).

Based on research as part of the Bereavement in Online Communities Project, Lisa Hensley (2012) noted that virtual world participants experience a complex relationship with online representations of individuals (avatars) and that virtual rituals occur to mourn the real-life deaths of online participants. It behoves us to be mindful that the impact of death in a virtual world has a significant impact on gamers in the 'real world' that is worthy of validation and further study.

Alexandra Sherlock (2013) discussed 'digital resurrection', a term used within the entertainment industry to describe the use of technology to provide symbolic immortality to popular media figures after death (e.g., the commercial that brought Bob Monkhouse, a popular British comedian, 'back to life' in order to raise awareness of the disease – prostate cancer – that had killed him four years earlier; deceased rapper Tupac Shakur performing 'live' on stage with Snoop Dogg). She noted that the duration of this type of symbolic immortality is dependent on those left behind to prolong one's presence through 'digital necromancy' or the reanimation of their digital remains.

Gordon Bell and Jim Gemmell (2009) described four steps in the progression of digital immortality that could potentially be achieved, all of which would be considered intentional. The first two involved: (1) transferring one's non-digital legacy media into digital form, and (2) supplementing one's e-memories with new digital sources. The third involved the ability to interact with an avatar that responds just like the deceased would (two-way immortality as previously noted). The fourth would involve an avatar that learns and changes over time, just as the deceased would have. Bell wrote the following:

> Jim Gray and I used to speculate about the possibility of something worth calling digital immortality, where a digital version of yourself lives on and interacts with posterity. What if, a hundred years from now, your heirs could ask you questions and you could answer?
>
> (Bell & Gemmell 2009:151)

In other words, the use of information generated from steps one and two by an avatar would result in steps three and four, provided that artificial intelligence has advanced sufficiently to allow the avatar to impersonate the deceased and continue to evolve. Robert Kuhn (2016) described virtual immortality as the 'theory that the fullness of our mental selves can be uploaded with first-person perfection to non-biological media so that when our mortal bodies die our mental selves will live on' (Kuhn 2016:26), and noted that techno-futurists do not question whether their vision can be actualized, only when it will occur (with estimates between 10 and 100 years).

Additional terms have been used to convey the idea of virtual immortality: 'posthumous interaction' (Maciel & Pereira 2015) and 'posthumous personhood' (Meese *et al.* 2015). The meaning of these terms and strategies to achieve digital immortality vary based on the processes used to preserve one's digital dust and, if ongoing interaction with the living is the desired goal, the mechanism used to facilitate it (e.g., a human surrogate, autonomous and semi-autonomous software enabling interaction in current events via social media, or artificial intelligence to create a re-enlivened form of the deceased), the degree of interactivity with a survivor that is possible, and whether the 'digitally reanimated' or 'digitally revived' entity is capable of further evolution on a cognitive or emotional level.

Options for achieving digital immortality

A range of options exists for achieving one- or two-way immortality. Bell's MyLifeBits project that began in 1998 is a well-documented example.[1] His concept of 'lifelogging' involves recording your life digitally, providing you with 'the opportunity to bequeath your own ideas, deeds, and personality to posterity in a way never before possible. With such a body of information it will be possible to generate a virtual you even after you are dead' (Bell & Gemmell 2009:6). When describing which pieces of paper from his life would be recorded, Bell stated that his 'goal is to record everything I actually read, not what others send me. It's my choice, not theirs, that counts' (Bell & Gemmell 2009:32). Bell and Gemmell's book, *Total Recall*, outlines a plan of action for starting this process. Lifelogging apps abound (see Fankhauser 2013 or www.postscapes.com/lifelogging-device for reviews), making the task of recording daily life quite simple.[2]

A relatively 'passive' type of immortality can be achieved by using a service that sends emails and/or video communications that were prepared prior to death to the recipient(s) of your choice (e.g., AfterWords; Dead Man's Switch; DeadSocial). Other services facilitate the recording of one's life story (e.g., Afternote) or the sharing of a range of digital assets (e.g., Eterniam). In many cases, digital immortality is accomplished through the efforts of family and/or friends who create memorial websites on their own (e.g., Moore 2014) or with the assistance of a service provider.[3] However, several companies have drawn upon advances in artificial intelligence to create options for a livelier digital afterlife.

Liveson.org, a company that brandishes the catchy slogan: 'When your heart stops beating, you'll keep tweeting', provides an opportunity to create a 'social afterlife' (with the help of an executor who activates the service following your death). After you die, this service analyses your original Twitter feed to learn about your likes, tastes, and syntax, and tweets appear via your LIVESON hashtag as if you were still sending them. An executor to your Liveson 'will' decides whether to continue to keep your account 'live'.

While having an active post-mortem presence in the Tweetosphere may be sufficient for some, others have set their sights on a higher level of interaction. The company Eterni.me allows users to collect and preserve their information and create a computer-based avatar that will allow others to access your memories. Eter9 is a social network that allows users to create a 'Virtual Self' called a Counterpart that learns more about each user as (s)he interacts in the social network. Their current advertisement describes cyber eternity/eternizing as a 'way of keeping your thoughts and posts for all time. Are you curious? Come meet your Counterpart and become eternal' (www.eter9.com).

Several scholars are working to achieve Bell and Gemmell's vision of two-way immortality, adding a higher level of 'humanness' to their efforts. Hossein Rahnama, a visiting scholar at the MIT Media Lab, described 'augmented eternity' as a goal

> to bridge the gap between life and death by eternalizing our digital identity ... Your physical being may die, but your digital being will continue to evolve with the purpose of helping people and maintaining your legacy as an evolving being.
>
> (as quoted in Tynan 2016, paras 3–4)

Algorithms would use recorded data to answer questions posed from beyond the grave, creating a 'new form of inter-generational collective intelligence' (Tynan 2016, para. 6). Rahnama notes that 'technology is the easy part. But achieving digital immortality will require overcoming some rather daunting challenges around data privacy' (Tynan 2016, para. 9). AI researcher and medical ethicist Martine Rothblatt described her vision of 'digital consciousness' as follows:

> We cannot ignore the fact that thanks to strides in software and digital technology and the development of ever more sophisticated forms of artificial intelligence, you and I will be able to have an ongoing relationship with our families: exchange memories with them, talk about their hopes and dreams, and share in the delights of holidays, vacations, changing seasons, and everything else that goes with family life – both the good and the bad – long after our flesh and bones have turned to dust.
>
> (Rothblatt 2014:9–10)

She further noted that emotional and intellectual immortality would be made possible through digital clones or 'mindclones' that would use mindfiles updated by mindware, creating a functionally equivalent replica of one's mind based on the thoughts, memories, feelings, beliefs, attitudes, preferences, and values that have been put into it. Working with LifeNaut.com, Rothblatt and her wife, Bina, have participated in a project with the Terasem Movement Foundation (mission: to promote the geoethical use of nanotechnology for human life extension) to create Bina48, a social robot whose interactions are based on information, memories, values, beliefs, and mannerisms that are a composite of several actual persons.[4]

Interviews with AI experts about the feasibility of 'augmented eternity' revealed a range of opinions that varied from deep skepticism to cautious optimism (Tynan 2016). While feasibility is a crucial element to consider, what is known about the opinions of the average person regarding digital immortality? Data from empirical studies supplemented by anecdotal information from various sources will now be presented.

Empirical data and anecdotal opinions about digital immortality and its impact on the bereaved

While discussing his decision to create a memorial website to honor his terminally ill wife's wishes to 'make sure people remember me', Sumit Paul-Choudhury (2011) noted that the fate of a person's digital soul may depend on whether someone is a 'preservationist', who believes that we owe it to our descendants to preserve everything we've done online, or a 'deletionist' who thinks it's vital that the Internet learns to forget. Empirical and anecdotal data, although limited in quantity, provides evidence that opinions: (1) fall in both camps as well as in between; (2) vary based on age; and (3) may be subject to change based on one's personal experience with loss.

Cristiano Maciel and Vinicius Pereira (2015) surveyed teenagers enrolled in integrated secondary and technical education at a public school in Brazil. When asked if they would opt for removal of their user profile, 57.7 percent of the teens said yes, 39.7 percent would opt for non-removal, and 2.6 percent did not know. Qualitative data noted that the wishes of the deceased's relatives should be considered as well as the need to balance whether its availability served as a source of solace to friends and family with concern about the possibility that disrespectful or profane comments could be posted. Carsten Grimm and Sonia Chiasson (2014) reported data from 400 participants between the ages of 18 and 69 who were recruited through crowdsourcing marketplaces from the United States, India, Great Britain, and Asia. Respondents were asked questions regarding their level of concern about preparing their digital footprint for the eventuality of their death and preferences about how their digital footprint should be handled and by whom. Data regarding personal experiences with handling the digital footprint of a deceased relative or friend, receiving automated message from someone who is deceased, or mourning online were not included in their write-up since less than 10 percent of the respondents commented on these experiences.

Although the majority of respondents were unfamiliar with online services related to death, when asked about their preference for the handling of their digital footprint, they had a strong preference for deleting accounts, handing accounts to their next of kin, and deciding individually for each of their accounts. When asked who they would entrust with serving as a digital executor, slightly over half indicated next of kin or friends. The researchers concluded that while death is a topic infrequently considered by mostly younger populations, they are most likely to have accumulated decades of digital data at their time of death: 'for many, this was the first time that the problem of digital death was brought to their attention; this is likely also the case for the general population' (Grimm & Chiasson 2014:9). This research confirmed the need to educate consumers of digital and social media about this topic.

The most recent Digital Death Survey, conducted between November and December 2015 and completed by 250 individuals (Digital Legacy Association 2016), explored attitudes and behaviors toward death and bereavement in today's increasingly digital world. Respondents rated the importance of being able to view a deceased significant other's social media profile as follows: Very important = 29%; Important = 23.5%; A little important = 16.5%; and Not important = 31%. When asked if they would like their own social media profile(s) to remain present online after their own death, 22.8% responded yes; 24% didn't really mind; 19.5% were not sure; and 33.47% responded no. Among those who had viewed the social media profile of a friend or family member after they died, 62.1% reported the experience to be of value, 5.2% found the experience to be upsetting and not of value, and 32.7% reported the experience to be neither of value nor upsetting. An overwhelming majority of the respondents (90+%) have made no plans for their social media accounts (e.g., appointing a Facebook Legacy Contact or a Google Inactive Account Manager) in the event of their death.

In an online survey conducted in the United Kingdom in 2012, only 20% of 2,046 adults aged 18+ had considered what would happen to their online profiles when they died (Perfect Choice Funeral Plans, n.d.). When asked what they would like to have happen, 43% preferred the profiles to be closed down, 20% preferred that they remain available to view but closed to comments, 16% wanted them to remain available to view online forever with commenting enabled, and 20% were not sure. An age difference was discovered regarding the preference for a profile to remain online (45% of 18–24-year-olds vs 25% of those over 55) and knowledge of how to close down an online profile (51% of those aged 18–24 vs 17% over 55).

A qualitative study by Lisa Thomas and Pamela Briggs (2014) provides insight regarding beliefs about digital immortality among a group of older adults (56–76) in a community in the northeast of England. After viewing films about various methods of creating a digital legacy (e.g., lifelogging vs memorialization), participants described their reaction and were asked to consider the value of having a digital social presence after death. Their comments revealed a mixture of potential pros and cons. Participants identified the following benefits: (1) passing on valuable information within the family was important; (2) younger family members could get to know deceased relatives; and (3) people outside the family could access information as a means of evoking memories. Some participants identified the following concerns/ risks: (1) sensitive information should not be seen by everyone and access by non-family members may be inappropriate; (2) technologies that do not directly support face-to-face contact with others during the grieving process may provide less emotional and practical support; (3) technologies could trigger reminders of events someone wishes to forget; (4) accessing information via a QR code on a gravestone may be considered exploitative and in 'bad taste'; (5) someone lacking technological skills may experience digital exclusion; and (6) digital vandalism and trolling (see Phillips 2011) are realities that

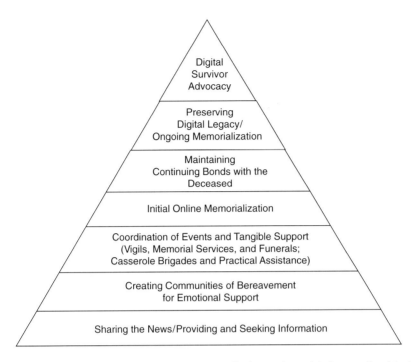

Figure 9.1 Roles of digital and social media in coping with loss and achieving digital immortality

Source: Sofka (2015).

may be even more damaging during times of grief. The authors concluded that these 'technologies were valued by older adults provided they were used in the right context' (Thomas & Briggs 2014:137). Due to concerns about inexperience, providing older adults with opportunities to learn about digital technology will be important.[5]

The scholarly literature and anecdotal evidence supports the fact that thanatechnology (originally defined by Carla J. Sofka in 1997 as 'technological mechanisms that are used to access information or aid in learning about thanatology topics' and subsequently revised in 2012 to include digital technology/social media and the multiple ways that this technology is being used in situations involving impending death, grief, and tragedy) serves a dual role in helping someone to achieve digital immortality and to cope with impending death and grief. While a review of this literature is beyond the scope of this chapter, Figure 9.1 captures these multiple functions.[6]

Does the opportunity to achieve digital immortality have an impact on how we cope with loss? Empirical research documenting the role of thanatechnology in the bereavement process is in its infancy. Although a limited number of studies with small samples have gathered largely qualitative data directly from the bereaved, many publications draw solely upon researcher observations. Generalizable data will only be available following the completion of multiple studies (ideally longitudinal) using standardized instruments with diverse populations. In the absence of empirical data, anecdotal evidence can be used to support the idea that personal experience with grief can impact one's views about preserving one's digital legacy and achieving digital immortality. Bell and Gemmell poignantly describe how the disappearance of their colleague and friend, Jim Gray, has influenced their thinking:

> Ironically, Jim's disappearance is a clear example of something people constantly insist about MyLifeBits: that people must be able to delete anything painful. Based on the decade of personal and professional bits that we've shared with and about Jim, we strongly disagree. While it was painful to be reminded of Jim when he first went missing, those bits are now among the most pleasant we have. Yes, there's still the occasional flash of pain when we run across them, but it [is] usually followed by joy. We just wish there were more of them. Once again, we come back to: Keep everything; you'll wish you had more.
>
> (Bell & Gemmell 2008:14)

In addition to reminding us that reactions to loss change with time, these authors note that rather than erasing painful memories, a person can choose to seal them up since 'what you really want to prevent in these cases is unwanted recall, not retention' (Bell & Gemmell 2009:66).

In 2016, the BBC documentary 'Rest in Pixels' presented various mechanisms for achieving digital immortality, circumstances that influenced people's decision to participate in this quest, and potential consequences of the use of technology for these purposes.[7] One scenario highlighted that the availability of mechanisms to preserve one's digital legacy may be beneficial for people with a limited lifespan. Lucy Watts, who lives with a life-limiting illness, stated that it's 'really therapeutic to share my messages [through social media and blogging] and share my thoughts and memories with the world; I really want to live on in something that's not me'. When describing what influenced his decision to create a pop-up booth where he invited members of the public to record their reflections about what they would like to leave behind when they die and to record messages for their loved ones, James Norris of DeadSocial stated:

> When it comes to being able to say goodbye and pass on our words of wisdom to our friends and family, very few of us gets the chance to do so … I believe that people [should] start to take more ownership over their digital footprint and ensure that it lives on within their digital legacy.

Marius Ursache of Eterni.Me noted that by interacting with an avatar based on one's digital input, people would be able to get advice from someone following their death. Bruce Duncan, connected with the Terasem Movement Foundation and the creation of Bina48, believes that 'if the essence of what it means to be human is based in information and we're able to transfer that information to a new form (technical immortality) ... Everybody's story is worth saving; everybody's story is worth sharing'. While most of the information in this documentary presented digital immortality in a positive light, one anecdote from Dave Bedford of Liveson.org reminds us that digital immortality has the potential to change not only how we react to the death of a loved one, but how we define it:

> I got an e-mail from a guy asking me to bring back his girlfriend that died fairly recently and that he had all of the data from social media and that he had other things – (her) diary and all the stuff of hers and could we use that to bring her back. And that was the first time that I thought we might have got ourselves into a bit of a pickle here because this is serious stuff it's so real.

One fascinating opportunity to conduct research on this topic that does not require gaining human subjects' approval involves reading comments posted online in reaction to news stories, blogs, and videos. Consider the views about augmented eternity that can be gained by comparing the content in Dan Tynan's (2016) article with comments posted by readers. Dr. Alireza Sadeghian, the former chair of computer science at Ryerson, was quoted as follows:

> Imagine the ability to have a conversation with a loved one who is no longer with us, the way people still visit Facebook pages of family members who have passed. In terms of both the technology and the service to humanity this would provide – it would be fantastic.

Now consider the mixed reaction of the reader self-identified as 'Citizenwise': 'If we will be able to do this I cannot decide whether or not it will bring small amounts of joy to some relatives or never ending sadness to many.' In contrast, a reader self-identified as 'gratefullyundead' stated: 'The bastards, I was looking forward to the peace and quiet of death, now that's been Twitterised too.'

In his essay on the feasibility of a digital afterlife, Michael Graziano, a neuroscientist, notes that his interest lies in a practical question: 'Is it even technically possible to duplicate yourself in a computer program? The short answer is: probably, but not for a while' (Graziano 2016, para. 3). He goes on to ask: 'But is it you? Did you cheat death, or merely replace yourself with a creepy copy?' (Graziano 2016, para. 27). Graziano concludes that the answer to this philosophical question is a matter of opinion, suspecting that many people would consider any simulation to be a spooky fake. This ongoing debate promises to be a fascinating one.

Tony Walter, Rachid Hourizi, Wendy Moncur, and Stacey Pitsillides conclude their thought-provoking article on the role of the Internet in death and mourning with the following statement: 'The internet may not, except in unusual circumstances, affect physical death, but it can profoundly and routinely impact the process of social death – both before and after physical death' (Walter *et al.* 2011:296). The same is true regarding the role of thanatechnology in achieving digital immortality.

Digital immortality and digital end-of-life planning: policies and legal/ethical issues

The increased use of technology has transformed how we live and how we will be remembered. Ideally, every person who is active in the digital world should make decisions about the fate of his or her digital footprint in advance of death. In 2009, human–computer interaction (HCI) researchers Michael Massimi and Andrea Charise introduced the term 'thanatosensitive design', encouraging computer scientists and system designers to consider how death impacts the social, technological, and personal dimensions of computing:

> We can easily imagine the proliferation of a person's technologically-mediated identities after death. The shift from material to digital technologies implies a series of attendant issues (privacy, security, archival) which concern individuals who want their unique constellation of personal data – their technological thumbprint – to die with them.
>
> (Massimi & Charise 2009:6)

Wendy Moncur and Annalu Waller (2010) noted the importance of addressing the challenges inherent in the bequest and inheritance of digital artifacts. If preventing access to one's digital dust and the absence of a digital afterlife is truly the goal, it would be wise to communicate that wish to one's next of kin so that 'doing nothing' in terms of digital end-of-life planning has the desired outcome.

Legal and ethical issues have an important role in conversations about digital immortality. One important component of these discussions relates to the deceased user policies developed by digital service providers and social networking sites. These policies provide a protocol for providing a user with the opportunity to take control over what happens to his or her digital legacy in the event of his or her death (Stokes 2015). Available options vary between notifying connected users after you die, appointing someone to have access to all of your online accounts and make decisions on your behalf, or to automatically delete the account of a deceased user. This raises many questions and concerns for a user to consider. For example, do you want your children to see emails from your past after your death? Can you choose if you want your email account to be relinquished to family or deleted? Is the information shared on social media what you want future generations to know about your thoughts and actions in life?

While user policies vary, many tend to offer the 'next of kin' the opportunity to delete the account upon showing proof of death and documenting their relation to the deceased. Researchers Allison Gibson and Danielle R. Silberman (2016) explored deceased user policies for 20 prominent social networking and other online sites (e.g., iTunes, YouTube, Google) and examined the options that were available to an individual who was preparing to end his or her engagement in digitally mediated communication and social media activities at the end of life. They discovered that these sites provide users with very limited opportunities to develop plans in advance for the end of one's online life. Of the sites reviewed, only two – Facebook and Google – provided a mechanism for users to state preferences related to their account before their death. Further, some organizations had no publicly available policy for deceased users on their website. Table 9.1 summarizes Gibson and Silberman's findings for ten prominent services utilized internationally regarding: (1) the availability of a deceased user policy anywhere throughout the website; (2) whether a user can dictate preferences about their account prior to death (similar to that of advanced directives); (3) whether a user's next of kin can dictate a preference for the deceased user's account following the death of the user (which oftentimes does not include the individual user's preference at all); and (4) whether it provided the option to have the deceased user's account memorialized following the death of the user. It is important to note that the remaining ten platforms (for example, iTunes and Snapchat) did not provide any options in cases of deceased users and therefore are not represented in this table.

In April 2013, Google announced the option for users to identify a preference regarding the management of one's account after death. The 'Inactive Account Manager' feature gives users the ability to: (1) tell Google what to do with your Gmail messages and data from several other Google services (i.e., the blogging tool Blogger) if your account becomes inactive for any reason, and (2) to specify to their identified next of kin whether they want them to delete their account and whether they can share certain (or all) data from their Google accounts (Tuerk 2013). While YouTube is a subsidiary of Google, it handles deceased user accounts differently. Although they have a deceased user policy, at this time there are no options to preserve the account by transferring it to one's next of kin or memorializing the account. The account is deleted after a period of inactivity (Eördögh 2012).

Facebook has allowed for the memorialization of accounts of deceased users since 2008; however, this could not be done until the next of kin provided documentation of the individual's death and evidence of his or her relationship to the deceased. In February 2014, Facebook announced the option for users to identify a legacy contact – someone chosen to look after one's account if it is memorialized – in advance of one's death. Once an account is memorialized, the legacy contact would be responsible for your digital immortality and would have the option to write a post that can be pinned to the top of your profile (e.g., information about your death or funeral/

Table 9.1 Policies for end-of-life planning

	Gmail.com/ Google	Hotmaill MSN.com	Yahoo. com	Pinterest. com	Facebook. com	LinkedIn. com	Amazon. com	YouTube. com	Instagram. com	Twitter. com
Policy on deceased user?	√	√	√	√	√	√	√	√	√	√
Can user dictate preference in advance?	√				√					
Can 'next of kin' dictate post-death?	√	√	√	√	√	√	√		√	√
Memorialize account?					√				√	√

Source: Gibson & Silberman (2016).

memorial services), respond to new friend requests, and update your profile picture. Facebook also allowed a user to indicate a preference regarding whether or not the legacy contact has permission to download a copy of everything that the user has shared on Facebook, thus creating a transcript of one's life through status updates (Facebook Help Center 2014).

One important caveat is that many of these social networking sites are relatively new. As digital law develops, technology advances, and even as attitudes toward deceased user policies are further discussed, these policies may continually evolve. One example of a changed policy is that of MSN/Hotmail. In 2010, *Time* magazine reported that upon appropriately notifying the company of the death of a loved one, this popular email provider would send the next of kin a compact disk (CD) of all the emails the user ever sent and received. There are many positive aspects for such an opportunity, such as having access to online account information and the ability to address any outstanding online payments or further inquiries. However, without the ability to dictate preferences in advance, many could argue this practice to be a substantial violation of privacy. The deceased user may not want their email history to be available to surviving family or friends. Currently, sharing a user's email history is no long common practice with this provider. (For a detailed discussion regarding access to a decedent's email in the United States from a legal perspective, consult Cummings 2014.)

If a person is comfortable allowing unlimited access to his or her digital assets, one immediate and simple solution would be to provide your passwords and login information to family and friends for their use following your death. Unfortunately, this violates the terms of agreement of many social media providers and online services that a user 'checks' (in some cases without reading them) when registering for an account.

An estimated 972,000 American Facebook users will die in 2016 (Carroll 2016). A survey of 100 Americans who were asked how they would like to be memorialized revealed that 10 percent would like to be remembered with a Facebook Memorial Page (Une Belle Vie Memorial Urns 2012); this would result in approximately 97,200 memorialized pages in 2016 alone. In the future, Facebook and other social networking sites may adopt the protocol of terminating inactive accounts. If this occurs, expressing one's wishes to memorialize one's account or appointing a Facebook Legacy Contact becomes even more important. Currently, Facebook does not delete inactive accounts; they are only deleted if a violation of the user agreement is documented (Facebook Help Center 2016). However, other providers, such as the blogging website Livejournal, have begun to delete inactive accounts after notifying users via email (Tiku 2012).

What if the deceased did not convey any information or discuss his or her wishes with family or friends? Without an option for users or their next of kin to memorialize the account or transfer the account to a trusted individual, the opportunity to achieve digital immortality or for survivors to preserve a loved one's digital legacy is placed at risk. Blogs such as 'Away for a Bit: Practical Guidance for Managing Digital Estates and Memories' have developed numerous resources to assist individuals and families to begin to think about planning in a digital age.[8] Even with planning, many deceased user policies do not allow families the option to manage someone's account upon notification of their death. To illustrate, following the death of their 16-year-old daughter, Alison Atkin's family wanted to access her online life in order to memorialize and remember her (Fowler 2013). After cracking into her password-protected laptop, her family started logging in to social networking sites as if they were Alison. However, this violated digital privacy law, which stated that the unauthorized use of another user's passwords was considered a breach of user agreement and a violation of the user's privacy. As the family attempted to access Alison's digital remains to facilitate her digital immortality, website and social networking service providers started to block them out. In addition, when passwords require updating, users are often required to select answers to 'secret questions' during this process. Failure to answer correctly may result in being blocked out of an account as well.

These and other legal issues are being discussed in courts in the United States and other countries and by scholars who are interested in the experiences of users dealing with digital death and digital immortality (e.g., Edwards & Harbinja 2013; Locasto *et al.* 2011; Maciel *et al.* 2015). In the United States, the Uniform Fiduciary Access to Digital Assets Act provides a framework through which executors and trustees can access a deceased user's digital life (Reid 2016); to track the ever-changing status of this Act that varies state by state, an enactment status map and legislative tracking tool is available at www.uniformlaws.org. A guide to areas of the law in the United Kingdom that may apply to one's digital legacy is available at www.unlockthelaw.co.uk/digital-legacy-guide-uk.html.

Resources for digital end-of-life planning

As the courts debate these issues and the law catches up with practices in our society to achieve digital mortality, HCI researchers have also presented potential solutions. Locasto *et al.* (2011) proposed an approach to managing a person's digital footprint during life and for dealing with it after a user's death that dealt with issues related to rights of survivorship and transferability as well as identity inheritance. Maciel and Pereira (2013) compared the management of a user's virtual data when alive vs deceased and presented a list of requirements and possibilities to provide users with options for voicing their preferences. In recent years, resources to facilitate the communication of one's wishes regarding digital immortality as well as commercial options to manage digital assets have expanded tremendously due to the increased popularity of this topic and the emergence of the 'digital estate planning' industry, also referred to as digital asset management and digital estate law.[9]

Your Digital Afterlife by Evan Carroll and John Romano (2011) is a practical resource to assist with the identification and management of digital assets. These authors use the term 'lifestream' to describe the 'chronological collection of content that chronicles your digital life' (Carroll & Romano 2011:189) and note numerous elements (digital photos, emails, social media and social networking site postings, etc.) that form a projection of your identity. Carroll and Romano also note that one's personal ideas about the 'value' placed on digital objects are 'both contextual and temporal, changing as situations and time changes' (Carroll & Romano 2011:144).

The following resources are available to help individuals consider their beliefs and values about their digital legacy, to learn about policies and procedures for managing digital assets, and to convey information to family and friends about their wishes. Infographics have been created that compile information about digital assets/digital legacies:

1   www.whoishostingthis.com/blog/2013/12/19/preparing-for-digital-afterlife.
2   www.finder.com.au/infographics/life-insurance/expert-guide-to-protect-yourself-online-before-you-die (guidance for before death).
3   www.finder.com.au/infographics/life-insurance/what-happens-online-when-you-die.

Several blogs/websites specific to the topic of digital death and digital immortality contain free information/tutorials, planning tools, and links to additional resources: Digital Dust (http://digital-era-death-eng.blogspot.com) by Vered (Rose) Shavit; The Digital Beyond (www.thedigitalbeyond.com; includes a resource inventory template) by Evan Carroll and John Romano; DeadSocial (www.deadsocial.org, which includes a Social Media Will template) founded by James Norris; and STEP (www.step.org/digital-assets-public), a worldwide professional association whose members help families plan for and administer digital assets.

For a fee, various companies provide access to: (1) electronic copies of advance directives for health care (e.g., DocuBank) and/or (2) information about digital assets such as online passwords and accounts following verification of one's death by a 'digital executor' appointed by the deceased (e.g., PasswordBox, a 'digital life manager' formerly known as LegacyLocker). The digital estate planning team at Everplans suggest the appointment of a 'cleaner', a confidant that you trust implicitly (without judgment, question, or complaint) to eliminate all of the skeletons in your digital closet that fall into any of the four areas of their DIES chart: dangerous, illegal, embarrassing, and secret (Everplans, n.d.). Regardless of the timing of this type of curation, survivors would merely be able to peruse the contents of your 'post-mortem digital legacy' (a term used by Maciel & Pereira 2015).

Everyone who uses digital technology and has an online presence should carefully consider how and when to get their digital affairs in order. Carla

J. Sofka (2017) proposed that young adults should begin learning about the impact of digital/social media on how we deal with tragedy, death, and grief in partnership with professionals in school systems and parents. There is no doubt that the issue of planning for one's digital legacy is a reality in this digital age.

Conclusion

In his philosophical discussion regarding death, Paul Fairfield posed the following question: 'Is there a life beyond this life, some manner of personal survival that we can believe in or at least hope for without surrendering our reason?' (Fairfield 2015:117). For anyone who has created a digital footprint in life, this chapter has identified one readily attainable type of personal survival after death – digital immortality – and has described opportunities to achieve it that range from one-way immortality, currently attainable by anyone with access to ordinary digital technology and social media, to two-way immortality that is available only to artificial intelligence experts with access to sophisticated social robot prototypes.

Thanatologists have encouraged us for almost 20 years to consider the impact of evolving technology on how our society deals with life-threatening illness, impending death, and coping with tragedy and grief (e.g., Sofka 1997, 2009, 2015, 2016, 2017; Walter *et al.* 2011). In recent years, scholars and researchers in the diverse fields of HCI, communications and communication technology, information science, digital media design, and digital/social media studies (to name only a few) have greatly enriched the discussion of thanatechnology-related issues and the implications that the availability of this technology might have on the lives of anyone considering his or her mortality as well as those who are grieving. In addition, Googling phrases such as 'digital immortality' or 'social media and death' results in an overwhelming number of links to online articles and resources in the mainstream media and popular press too numerous to cite. After perusing these resources, a reader would be wise to consider the following when forming an opinion about the pros and cons of pursuing digital immortality and considering the best strategy to document one's wishes once an informed decision has been made.

As noted in this chapter, empirical data summarizing the wishes of digital and social media users regarding the preservation and availability of their 'digital dust' after death is extremely limited. Opinions range from a strong desire that their digital legacy be preserved and shared to a strong preference that their digital remains be erased. Although a small body of scholarly literature has documented the benefits and potential risks/challenges of digital and social media use among the bereaved, the general public is not likely to have access to this information, limiting their ability make informed decisions about their digital legacy. While the topics discussed in this chapter have gained attention through media stories and a recent documentary on the BBC, rarely do these stories refer readers/viewers to resources designed to facilitate conversations with loved ones about their preferences or to assist with the documentation of their wishes. Creative collaborations between academics/scholars/researchers, clinicians who work with the dying and the bereaved, and the media are strongly encouraged.

Since the user policies of many popular social networking sites and social media apps do not provide a mechanism for account owners to share their wishes with a trusted survivor, this chapter has identified resources that can be used to inform digital and social media users about their options and to facilitate the digital end-of-life planning process. Although useful resources exist to create a basic 'digital/social media will', companies creating digital and social media resources lag behind in the development and implementation of thanatosensitive user policies that provide opportunities for their users to document their wishes directly with each site or app. With the assistance of digital media designers whose work has been previously cited, perhaps this challenge will be eliminated.

Individuals seeking digital immortality currently have a variety of options at their disposal, with the potential for new and exciting (or frightening) opportunities to be developed as technology continues to evolve. Martine Rothblatt reminds us that while our doppelgängers already exist, 'nobody can digitize 100 percent of their life, and hence there will be many differences between what is stored in a brain and what will be stored in a mindfile' (Rothblatt 2014:55). However, she encourages us to use the 1–2 decades before cyberconsciousness is upon us to 'prepare for virtual humanity' (Rothblatt 2014:302). Historically, society's ability to create innovative uses of technology often outpaces our ability to have proactive conversations about the implications of the availability of said technology. The time for conversations about cyberconsciousness has arrived.

It would also be wise to recognize that the value placed on achieving digital immortality and the relative value of one's 'digital dust' is highly subjective. For individuals who conduct research, develop policy, or provide services to individuals who are dealing with decision-making regarding the end of their life or those who are coping with the impact of death and grief in the digital age, the need to form partnerships across academic and professional disciplines to collaborate and effectively navigate what Selena Ellis Gray and Paul Coulton (2013:45) described as the 'sociocultural complexity within this emerging digital ecosystem of loss' has never been higher.

In her review of a book by David Rieff (2016) that contemplates the role of memory in how human beings come to terms with their own mortality, Lauren Murray (2016) stated: 'The need to preserve the memories of the past reflects, in part, a human desire to live beyond our time' (Murray 2016, para. 4). It behoves everyone with a digital fingerprint/footprint to carefully consider your ideal vision of digital immortality, have conversations with important people in your life to determine the compatibility of your preferences, and take the necessary steps to leave digital end-of-life plans that will facilitate this vision becoming your reality.

Notes

1 See: www.microsoft.com/en-us/research/project/mylifebits and http://totalrecallbook. com/links-and-resources.
2 To learn more about the taxonomy that has evolved to describe various degrees of this phenomenon (including 'extreme lifelogging'), see Bell and Gemmell (2012). Information about extreme lifeloggers Steve Mann and Nicholas Felton can be found by Googling their names.
3 See, e.g.: www.everplans.com/articles/the-top-10-online-memorial-websites.
4 To watch a video of Bina48 interacting with Bina Rothblatt, visit: www.youtube. com/watch?v=KYshJRYCArE.
5 The Cyberseniors Connecting Generations campaign provides one model to empower older adults to use technology. Information is available at: http://cyber-seniors.ca/get-involved.
6 This figure, created by Carla J. Sofka (2015), is based on information gathered through original research and reviews of the literature reported in previous publications and presentations (see Sofka 2009, 2015, 2016).
7 See: www.bbc.co.uk/programmes/p03sm61g.
8 See more at https://awayforabit.com/category/digital-afterlife.
9 The resources described in this chapter were identified through Google searches and use of the online services listed on www.thedigitalbeyond.com, a list compiled and updated by Evan Carroll and John Romano. Readers are encouraged to visit this site to learn about the numerous services that are available. Unfortunately, some of the company websites on this list are no longer active, most likely a remnant of the ephemeral nature of companies providing these services.

References

Bainbridge, William S. (2013): 'Perspectives on Virtual Veneration'. *Information Society*, 29 (3):196–202.

Bassett, Debra J. (2015): 'Who Wants to Live Forever? Living, Dying and Grieving in Our Digital Society'. *Social Sciences*, 4 (4):1127–1139.

Beagrie, Neil (2006): 'Digital Curation for Science, Digital Libraries, and Individuals'. *International Journal of Digital Curation*, 1 (1):3–16.

Bell, Gordon & Jim Gemmell (2008): 'Digital Immortality'. Draft of a book chapter that was not used in Bell & Gemmell (2009). The content shared in this chapter with permission.

Bell, Gordon & Jim Gemmell (2009): *Total Recall: How the E-memory Revolution Will Change Everything*. New York: Dutton.

Bell, Gordon & Jim Gemmell (2012): 'Lifelogging Taxonomy: Extreme Lifelogging by 2020'. Available online at: http://totalrecallbook.com/blog/2012/11/1/lifelogging-taxonomy-extreme-lifelogging-by-2020.html.

Bell, Gordon & Jim Gray (2000): 'Digital Immortality'. Technical report for Microsoft Research. Available online at: www.microsoft.com/en-us/research/wp-content/uploads/2016/02/tr-2000-101.pdf.

Briggs, Pamela & Lisa Thomas (2014): 'The Social Value of Digital Ghosts', in Christopher M. Moreman & A. David Lewis (eds): *Digital Death: Mortality and Beyond in the Online Age*. Santa Barbara, CA: Praeger, pp. 125–141.

Cann, Candi K. (2014): *Virtual Afterlives: Grieving the Dead in the Twenty-first Century*. Lexington, KY: University Press of Kentucky.

Carroll, Evan (2016): '972,000 U.S. Facebook Users Will Die in 2016'. Available online at: www.thedigitalbeyond.com/2016/01.

Carroll, Evan & John Romano (2011): *Your Digital Afterlife: When Facebook, Flickr and Twitter Are Your Estate, What's Your Legacy?* Berkeley, CA: New Riders.

Cummings, Rebecca G. (2014): 'The Case Against Access to Decedents' E-mail: Password Protection as an Exercise of the Right to Destroy'. Available online at: https://conservancy.umn.edu/bitstream/handle/11299/163821/Cummings.pdf.

Digital Legacy Association (2016): 'The Digital Legacy and Digital Assets Infographic 2016'. Available online at: http://digitallegacyassociation.org/about/reports.

Dow, Elizabeth H. (2009): *Electronic Records in the Manuscript Repository*. Lanham, MD: Scarecrow Press.

Edwards, Lilian & Edina Harbinja (2013): 'What Happens to My Facebook Profile When I Die?: Legal Issues around Transmission of Digital Assets on Death'. Available online at: http://ssrn.com/abstract=2222163 or http://dx.doi.org/10.2139/ssrn.2222163.

Ellis Gray, Selena & Paul Coulton (2013): 'Living with the Dead: Emergent Post-mortem Digital Curation and Creation Practices', in Cristiano Maciel & Vinicius C. Pereira (eds): *Digital Legacy and Interaction: Post-Mortem Issues*. Cham: Springer International Publishing, pp. 31–47.

Eördögh, Fruzsina (2012): 'What Happens to Your YouTube Videos When You Die?' *The Daily Dot*. Available online at: www.dailydot.com/culture/dead-youtube-videos.

Everplans (n.d.): 'How to Eliminate All the Skeletons in Your Closet'. Available online at: www.everplans.com/articles/how-to-eliminate-all-the-skeletons-in-your-closet-after-you-die.

Facebook Help Center (2014): 'What Is a Legacy Contact?' Available online at: www.facebook.com/help/1568013990080948.

Facebook Help Center (2016): 'Deactivating & Deleting Accounts'. Available online at: www.facebook.com/help/359046244166395.

Fairfield, Paul (2015): *Death: A Philosophical Inquiry*. New York: Routledge.

Fankhauser, Dani (2013): '9 Lifelogging Apps to Log Personal Data'. Available online at: http://mashable.com/2013/09/24/lifelogging-apps/#1ilkoX.VEuqd.

Fowler, Geoffrey A. (2013): 'Life and Death Online: Who Controls a Digital Legacy?'. *Wall Street Journal*, January 5. Available online at: www.wsj.com/articles/SB10001424127887324677204578188220364231346.

Garfinkel, Simon & David Cox (2009): 'Finding and Archiving the Internet Footprint'. Available online at: http://simson.net/clips/academic/2009.BL.InternetFootprint.pdf.

Gibson, Allison & Danielle R. Silberman (2016): 'Preparing your Online Life for End-of-Life'. Poster presented at the Association for Death Education and Counseling's 38th Annual Conference, Minneapolis, Minnesota.

Graziano, Michael (2016): 'Why You Should Believe in the Digital Afterlife'. Available online at: www.theatlantic.com/science/archive/2016/07/what-a-digital-afterlife-would-be-like/491105.

Grimm, Carsten & Sonia Chiasson (2014): 'Survey on the Fate of Digital Footprints after Death'. Available online at: www.internetsociety.org/sites/default/files/03_1-paper.pdf.

Hensley, Lisa (2012): 'Bereavement in Online Communities: Sources of and Support for Disenfranchised Grief', in Carla J. Sofka, Illene Noppe Cupit & Kathleen R. Gilbert (eds): *Dying, Death and Grief in an Online Universe: For Counselors and Educators*. New York: Springer, pp. 119–134.

Kasket, Elaine (2012): 'Continuing Bonds in the Age of Social Networking: Facebook as a Modern Day Medium'. *Bereavement Care*, 31 (2):62–69.

Kastenbaum, Robert J. (2004): *Death, Society, and Human Experience* (8th edn). Boston: Allyn & Bacon.

Kuhn, Robert L. (2016): 'Virtual Immortality'. *Skeptic Magazine*, 21 (2):26–34.

Lifton, Robert J. (1979): *The Broken Connection: On Death and the Continuity of Life.* New York: Simon & Schuster.

Locasto, Michael E., Michael Massimi & Peter J. DePasquale (2011): 'Security and Privacy Considerations in Digital Death', in *Proceedings of the 2011 Workshop on New Security Paradigms*, Marin County, CA, September 12–15, 2011, pp. 1–10.

Maciel, Cristiano & Vinicius C. Pereira (2013): 'The Fate of Digital Legacy in Software Engineers' View: Technical and Cultural Aspects', in Cristiano Maciel & Vinicius C. Pereira (eds): *Digital Legacy and Interactions: Post-Mortem Issues.* Cham: Springer International, pp. 1–30.

Maciel, Cristiano & Vinicius C. Pereira (2015): 'Post-Mortem Digital Legacy: Possibilities in HCI', in Masaaki Kurosu (ed.): *Human-Computer Interaction: Users and Contexts.* New York: Springer, pp. 339–349.

Maciel, Cristiano, Vinicius C. Pereira & Monica Sztern (2015): 'Internet Users' Legal and Technical Perspectives on Digital Legacy Management for Post-mortem Interaction', in Sakae Yamamoto (ed.): *HIMI 2015, Part I, LNCS 9172.* Cham: Springer International, pp. 627–639.

Massimi, Michael & Andrea Charise (2009): 'Dying, Death and Mortality: Towards Thanatosensitivity in HCI'. Available online at: www.chi2009.org/altchisystem/submissions/submission_mmassimi_0.pdf.

Meese, James, Bjorn Nansen, Tamara Kohn, Michael Arnold & Martin Gibbs (2015): 'Posthumous Personhood and the Affordances of Digital Media'. *Mortality*, 20:408–420.

Moncur, Wendy & Annalu Waller (2010): 'Digital Inheritance'. Available online at: www.academia.edu/461818/Digital_Inheritance.

Moore, Rebecca (2014): 'Mythopoesis, Digital Democracy and the Legacy of the Jonestown Website', in Christopher M. Moreman & A. David Lewis (eds): *Digital Death: Mortality and Beyond in the Online Age.* Santa Barbara, CA: Praeger, pp. 143–158.

Morris, David Z. (2016): 'Pokemon Go Memorializes Tamir Rice, 12 Year Old Shot by Cleveland Police'. Available online at: http://fortune.com/2016/07/23/pokemon-go-tamir-rice.

Murray, Lauren (2016): 'Book Review: *In Praise of Forgetting* by David Rieff'. Available online at: http://blogs.lse.ac.uk/lsereviewofbooks/2016/07/01/book-review-in-praise-of-forgetting-historical-memory-and-its-ironies-by-david-rieff.

Nansen, Bjorn, Michael Arnold, Martin Gibbs & Tamara Kohn (2015): 'The Restless Dead in the Digital Cemetery', in Christopher M. Moreman & A. David Lewis (eds): *Digital Death: Mortality and Beyond in the Online Age.* Santa Barbara, CA: Praeger, pp. 111–124.

Owens, Trevor (2014): 'Ghosts of Races Past: Son Finds Father's Ghost in Game'. Play the Past (blog). Available online at: www.playthepast.org/?p=4886.

Paul-Choudhury, Sumit (2011): 'Digital Legacy: The Fate of Your Online Soul'. Available online at: www.newscientist.com/article/mg21028091.400-digital-legacy-the-fate-of-your-online-soul.

Perfect Choice Funeral Plans (n.d.): 'Would You Want to Live Online Forever?'. Available online at: www.perfectchoicefunerals.com/about-perfect-choice/funeral-plan-news/what-happens-to-your-online-profiles-when-you-die/index.aspx.

Perrett, Roy W. (1987): *Death and Immortality.* Dordrecht: Martinus Nijhoff Publishers.

Phillips, Whitney (2011): 'LOLing at Tragedy: Facebook Trolls, Memorial Pages and Resistance to Grief Online'. *First Mind*, 16 (12). Available online at: http://firstmonday.org/ojs/index.php/fm/article/view/3168/3115.

Pitsillides, Stacey, Saavas Katsikides & Martin Conreen (2009): 'Digital Death'. Paper presented at the Virtuality and Society International Workshop, Athens, Greece. Available online at: https://issuu.com/stelios_giama/docs/iov09_proceedings.

Pitsillides, Stacey, Mike Waller & Duncan Fairfax (2013): 'Digital Death: What Role Does Digital Information Play in the Way We Are (Re)membered?', in Steven Warburton & Stylianos Hatzipanagos (eds): *Digital Identity and Social Media*. Hershey, PA: Information Science Reference, pp. 75–90.

Reid, Stephanie (2016): 'Estate Planning in the Digital Age'. Available online at: www.thedigitalbeyond.com/2016/06/estate-planning-in-the-digital-age.

Rieff, David (2016): *In Praise of Forgetting: Historical Memory and its Ironies*. New Haven, CT: Yale University Press.

Rothblatt, Martine (2014): *Virtually Human: The Promise – and the Peril – of Digital Immortality*. New York: St. Martin's Press.

Sherlock, Alexandra (2013): 'Larger Than Life: Digital Resurrection and the Re-Enchantment of Society'. *Information Society*, 29 (3):164–176.

Sofka, Carla J. (1997): 'Social Support "Internetworks", Caskets for Sale, and More: Thanatology and the Information Superhighway'. *Death Studies*, 21 (6):553–574.

Sofka, Carla J. (2009): 'Adolescents, Technology, and the Internet: Coping with Loss in the Digital World', in Charles Corr & David Balk (eds): *Adolescents and Death*. New York: Springer, pp. 155–173.

Sofka, Carla J. (2015): 'Using Digital and Social Media in Your Work with the Dying and Bereaved'. Webinar presented for the Association for Death Education and Counseling.

Sofka, Carla J. (2016): 'Digital Survivor Advocacy: Fighting So You May Never Know Tragedy', in Susan E. Elswick (ed.): *Data Collection: Methods, Ethical Issues and Future Directions*. Hauppauge, NY: Nova Science Publishers.

Sofka, Carla J. (2017): 'Role of Digital and Social Media in Supporting Bereaved Students', in Jacqueline Brown & Shane Jimerson (eds): *Supporting Bereaved Students at School*. New York: Oxford University Press.

Sofka, Carla J., Kathleen R. Gilbert & Illene Noppe Cupit (2012): *Dying, Death and Grief in an Online Universe: For Counselors and Educators*. New York: Springer.

Stokes, Patrick (2015): 'Deletion as Second Death: The Moral Status of Digital Remains'. *Ethics of Information Technology*, 17:237–248.

Thomas, Lisa & Pamela Briggs (2014): 'An Older Adult Perspective on Digital Legacy', in *Proceedings of the Nodichi 2014*. The 8th Nordic Conference on Human–Computer Interaction: Fun, Fast, Foundational (Helsinki, Finland), pp. 237–246.

Tiku, Nitasha (2012): 'No Emo! LiveJournal Starts Deleting Some Inactive Accounts before Its American Comeback Tour'. *Observer: Business & Tech*, January 27. Retrieved from: http://observer.com/2012/01/livejournal-delete-accounts-american-comeback-inactiveempty-livejournal-accounts-01272012.

Time (2010): 'Tools for Managing Your Online Life after Death'. Available online at: http://content.time.com/time/specials/packages/article/0,28804,1920156_1920150_192045,00.html.

Tuerk, Andreas (2013): 'Plan Your Digital Afterlife with Inactive Account Manager'. Available online at: https://publicpolicy.googleblog.com/2013/04/plan-your-digital-afterlifewith.html.

Tynan, Dan (2016): 'Augmented Eternity: Scientists Aim to Let Us Speak from Beyond the Grave'. *Guardian*, June 23. Available online at: www.theguardian.com/technology/2016/jun/23/artificial-intelligence-digital-immortality-mit-ryerson.

Une Belle Vie Memorial Urns (2012): 'Death & Memorials'. Available online at: www.pinterest.com/pin/376121006352850156.

Walter, Tony (1996): 'A New Model of Grief: Bereavement and Biography'. *Mortality*, 1 (1):7–25.

Walter, Tony, Rachid Hourizi, Wendy Moncur & Stacey Pitsillides (2011): 'Does the Internet Change How We Die and Mourn? Overview and Analysis'. *Omega: Journal of Death and Dying*, 64 (4):275–302.

10 The virtual conquest of death

William Sims Bainbridge[1]

Introduction

Humanity has imagined many means to escape death, and among them are to leave a lasting legacy and to remain famous even centuries after departing this life. Julius Caesar still lives, as we can gaze into his face as represented by sculptures that agree in the prominence of his cheekbones, and read his own words from books he wrote, for example his analysis that Druidic ideas about reincarnation made the Druids more formidable warriors, because they believed heroic deaths would not be final (Caesar 1919:338–339). Of course, ordinary ancient Roman citizens did not enjoy Caesar's status, and we remember the names of very few of them. However, many of them were loved by children who memorialized them after death, a form of immortality that Caesar himself lacked. Within four centuries after his death, Romans had adopted Christianity with its optimistic belief in heaven, yet today one of the motivations for imagining technological forms of immortality is an increasing skepticism about all ancient supernatural beliefs. Influential sociologist Émile Durkheim (1915/1965) argued that God was really a symbolic representation of society, from which we may deduce that heaven is really the future of society, such that anyone whose influence lives on, also personally lives on.

This chapter will consider the possibility that modern Internet-based technologies may allow at least a slight improvement in the possibility for ordinary people to have increased fame, for example through massively multiplayer online games in which they can be living players, or avatars of persons who have already died. More convincingly, it can be said that this technology helps people explore alternative meanings of death, and could become a venue for remembrance of the deceased. After an introductory section, this chapter will offer three examples in which specific deceased people are symbolically resurrected as avatars inside virtual worlds. In each case the person was an extremely ambitious religious leader who sought power during life, as a form of 'immortality', and who possessed powerful visions that promised transcendence of the limits of material reality.

Science and technology have extended the human lifespan, without as yet conquering death. That task still lies in the province of religion, perhaps, however, eroded by scientific progress. In the debate over whether religion will vanish through secularization, or survive because it performs essential functions, the third possibility that religion may be transformed by science and technology is often ignored (Bainbridge 2007a, 2015). As manifested through the Internet, industrial robots, and the growing saturation of the world with sensors and computer chips, information technology is transforming human life (Bainbridge 2004a). Yet some of the most revolutionary social media were developed in the almost complete absence of social science, for example Facebook, YouTube, and that virtual nation with millions of citizens, the online game *World of Warcraft* (Bainbridge 2010c). The original inventors of sociology imagined redesigning society on the basis of its principles, even replacing religion with sociology (Comte 1883), yet social engineering did not become a respected profession.

Admittedly modest in scope, this chapter takes that path. We shall explore three massively multiplayer online games (MMOs), not to study the behavior of their human inhabitants, but to explore how the technology might be used for new quasi-religious purposes related to immortality (Bainbridge 2007b, 2010b).

The potential of electronic avatars

Online virtual worlds offer three different but compatible ways through which human beings may seek to transcend death, the first two of which are already technically feasible, and the third is still in early development. First, by role-playing a character in an environment where simulated death is quite common, we deal psychologically with our own tortured emotions about mortality. Second, by entering a virtual world through an avatar based on a selected deceased person, we memorialize that individual as if through a religious ritual (Fortes 1961; Gibbs *et al.* 2012). Third, most virtual worlds include simulated people called 'non-player characters' (NPCs), which through artificial intelligence may evolve in future into realistic simulations of people (Merrick & Maher 2009), thus potentially being used as reincarnations based on specific deceased persons.

This chapter explores these cultural and technological developments by running avatars based on three deceased religious innovators in three historically grounded virtual worlds: (1) *Dark Age of Camelot*, based on sixth-century northwestern Europe; (2) *The Secret World*, based on contemporary but historically oriented New England, Egypt, and Transylvania; and (3) *A Tale in the Desert*, which simulates ancient Egypt. These three are marketed as games, but they vary greatly in character as well as popularity. The three were selected from about four dozen that have been studied by the author because they connect more directly to traditional human cultures, and thus are more realistic environments than many of the fantasy or science fiction gameworlds. Each combination of a religious innovator with a virtual world is designed to explore fundamental issues.

The first example employs an avatar based on Mary Ann MacLean (1931–2005), the Oracle in the Process Church of the Final Judgement, a polytheistic religious movement that was derived from psychoanalysis and Scientology, and which sought to withdraw from modern society (Bainbridge 1978; Wyllie 2009). Her avatar will seek transcendence in the ancient legends about fabled Camelot, thus placing her in a familiar narrative. Basic mechanics of virtual worlds will be described, so that readers unfamiliar with them can begin to see both their potential and the areas where innovation would be required to give them new social functions. *Dark Age of Camelot* illustrates a common feature of online gameworlds, a war between factions of players who are relatively safe in their home realms, but face virtual death when they venture more widely. The realms are Albion (Britain), Midgard (Scandinavia), and Hibernia (Ireland).

The second example illustrates that avatars may be used to memorialize deceased family members, in this case the author's great-grandfather, William Folwell Bainbridge (1843–1915). He was a Baptist clergyman and social scientist who wrote three books based on 1879–1880 field research on American missions in Asia, one of which was a novel that metaphorically resurrected his deceased daughter as the heroine, thus already developing the concept of veneration of the deceased through avatars long ago (Bainbridge 1883). The virtual world he explores represents areas of the real world in which he actually lived and where he sought personal immortality through his writings. Like *Dark Age of Camelot*, *The Secret World* contains three factions, each avatar belonging to one of them: Illuminati (Brooklyn, New York), Templar (London, England), or Dragon (Seoul, Korea). They are not opponents, however, having formed an alliance against evil supernatural forces that are invading their supposedly real world.

The third example of a religious innovator is H. Spencer Lewis (1883–1939), the founder of the AMORC Rosicrucians, who is currently buried beneath a small pyramid in the Egyptian-themed Rosicrucian Park in California, memorialized through monuments he built himself. He will be reborn in a virtual ancient Egypt, where he possesses the equivalent of Rosicrucian Park plus a virtual slave, yet with the irony that the entire virtual world was scheduled for almost immediate destruction. *A Tale in the Desert* contains neither factions nor combat, but involves the cooperative construction of ancient Egypt, in a series of *tellings*, each well over a year long and ending with annihilation, preparing the way for the next telling. The research reported here was done over the final three months of the Sixth Telling.

The subfield of sociology and social psychology most immediately relevant for exploring a virtual world through an avatar is naturally *role theories* and related methodologies like *psychodrama* and *ethnomethodology*. In role-playing research methods, a fundamental tension exists between the self and the role. In so-called *method acting*, a theater actor merges with the character, becoming one both consciously and subconsciously (Stanislavski 1988). The role has already been scripted by the playwright, and the actor must subordinate personal feelings that belong in the real world to those the character would have in the particular fictional scene. In contrast, psychodrama subordinates the role to the needs of the actor, allowing free expression of genuine feelings as a step toward personal improvement (Borgatta *et al.* 1975; Moreno 1944; Moreno & Toeman 1942).

A standard concept in sociological analysis is what Erving Goffman (1961) called *role distance*, the extent to which a person perceives or acts in a way somewhat separate from the role being played at the moment. This becomes problematic in *reflexive methods* (Gouldner 1970; Lemert & Piccone 1982), often called *phenomenology* (Husserl 1965; Schütz 1967) or *ethnomethodology* (Garfinkel 1967). An ethnomethodologist may be subjectively distant from the other people in the situation under study, even often deceiving them or at the very least concealing the fact that a research project is in progress. That implies great role distance. However, ethnomethodological research also holds traditional social science theories at a distance, beginning each field excursion without preconceptions but prepared to distil observations into new concepts using some form of *grounded theory* (Glaser & Strauss 1967). The related phenomenological perspective treats nothing as real unless it is directly experienced by the researcher, thus paradoxically operating at zero role distance.

Perhaps because so many competing schools of thought have analyzed role-playing, most of them have little if any influence in the creation of virtual worlds or other forms of social media. All too often, computer scientists writing about self-presentation in virtual environments will cite only one work, by Goffman (1956), but nothing else. A notable exception is the work of Shanyang Zhao (2005), who fully understands the vast *symbolic interaction* tradition Goffman worked in and applies it to telepresence. That goes all the way back to a classic work by Charles Horton Cooley (1902), which even used electronic metaphors to understand how personal identity is constructed through social interaction. Many of today's leading researchers of avatars and online games do, however, draw upon role theories they have selected from this diverse collection (Bainbridge 2013; Nardi 2010). A prominent example is the concept of the *protean self*, proposed decades ago by Robert Jay Lifton (1968), who argued that our world has become so complex and chaotic that it is impossible to remain constant from situation to situation, requiring one to hop from one role-self to another as the context changes. This idea has morphed into the *proteus effect*, in which people are psychologically influenced by experiences their avatars undergo in computer simulations (Blascovich & Bailenson 2011; Yee 2014; Yee *et al.* 2009).

Reliving the Dark Ages

Each of the three deceased religious leaders who are revived as avatars for this chapter is not merely a person but a representation of a cosmic principle, at least as the author understands them. Mary Ann MacLean sought power and meaning in her life by exerting psychological power over the people closest to her, through building powerful intimate relations that she herself controlled, while remaining anonymous with respect to the larger world that surrounded her and her associates. She thus represents *power through intimacy*. Each of the cosmic principles is challenged, to some extent, by the demands made by the particular virtual world. In her case, the greatest contradiction was the game's need to kill simulated animals, when in real life she was an ardent antivivisectionist and once smashed a television set when it was displaying a bullfight. In a sense, this chapter seeks to explore the emotional meaning of death, with technologies that may be able to blur the line between life and death, without actually providing immortality.

The Process Church of the Final Judgement originated in London through what some leaders consciously called *religious engineering*, then transferred to the United States and Canada, where members wore flamboyant costumes on the streets and scripted elaborate rituals inside their communes. The theology explicitly stated that the universe was a game created when God split himself into four competing supernatural players: Lucifer, Jehovah, Christ, and Satan. What Processeans called the Game of the Gods had given rise to the far inferior Human Game. Now, Processeans were becoming avatars of specific gods in order to escape the Human Game and prepare for a millenarian End and a New Beginning. It had been founded by Mary Ann MacLean in partnership with Robert de Grimston, she a combined avatar of Jehovah and Satan, and he an avatar of Lucifer and Christ. In 1974 the couple split in conjunction with a schism of the group. His faction sought to maintain the old polytheistic culture, but quickly failed. Her faction became monotheistically Jehovian, rejecting even Christ, and in greatly altered form exists today. I imagine that she was frustrated by these developments, and in death would seek a renewal of her early hopes.

This section of the chapter will consider in some detail the process of entering a virtual world through an avatar, which means finding a way to create a story focused on the deceased individual, in a way that harmonizes with the larger narrative of the computerized environment. Emulating Mary Ann through an avatar presented a significant challenge, because I actually had relatively little direct information about her. While I had come to know Robert de Grimston well over the period of a year in Boston and Toronto, I never met Mary Ann. Both from my interviews with members and from recent publications, I knew that she was both reclusive and exercised great psychological power over her subordinates, more like a mysterious cosmic force than a person. Thus, I would need to craft a narrative that would make the particular virtual world meaningful for her, conceptualized in this way. I had extensive prior experience with *Dark Age of Camelot* (DAoC) and believed it was ideal for the purpose.

At her death, Mary Ann had seen her movement go through many amazing challenges, but I naturally thought back to the early years and imagined her seeking to revive something like the original Process in the virtual world where she herself would be revived. Of course, the real woman might have had a very different set of late-life goals, and those who knew her well would make very different choices were they to undertake this kind of virtual memorialization. If she had to launch the Process all over again, from scratch, logically she would need to find a man to take the place of Robert de Grimston, over whom she could exercise power through intimacy.

In the context of popular mythology for a virtual Camelot, one character stands much taller than all the others: King Arthur (Alcock 1971; Ashe 1968; Ashton 1974). She would not select Merlin, because he would be a rival for leadership of a magical cult, and all the others were simply not sufficiently legendary. The Mary Ann avatar could not immediately rush to Camelot and propose to Arthur, however, because she needed to become familiar with the Dark Age culture and prove at least some degree of competence in handling the virtual environment. Thus, I planned to have her thoroughly complete all the early stages of advancement and go to Camelot only after she had reached experience level 20 of the maximum 50 programmed into DAoC.

After creating a new player account for *Dark Age of Camelot*, the next step is to select which of the three realms Mary Ann will belong to, which of many ethnic groups and class specializations, and some other details of the avatar. Clearly, she needed to be a citizen of Albion, because Camelot was its capital. Since the real woman was from Scotland, her ethnic group would be Highland, which entitled her to wear a plaid tartan. Only two very low-resolution pictures of her are available online, and anyway DAoC offers limited capacity to craft realistic avatar forms. An autobiography by a Processean describes Mary Ann as she appeared in 1966, having eyes that were 'bright green and penetrating' and 'wavy, wiry, copper-brown hair' (Verney 2011:17, 39), which indeed the interface allowed the avatar to have. Each avatar must have a class, defined by a set of abilities, and the obvious choice for Mary Ann was Heretic:

> Heretics are a cleric class that has renounced the Church and become an adherent of Arawn, the lord of the underworld. As evil Clerics, they fit into the hybrid category, with both the use of combat styles and high-damage focus spells.[2]

New avatars generally enter a gameworld in a tutorial area, a low-danger region where a series of simple missions gives the player experience handling the virtual environment and some sense of the mythology that provides meaning. Mary Ann found herself standing near Sir Remson, Mayor of Holtham in Constantine's Sound, an area near the sea. He explains, 'We are locked in a bloody war against the loathsome forces of Hibernia and the barbaric hordes of Midgard.' The mayor is an NPC, of the sort who stands in one place but moves a bit to seem realistic, appearing very much like the avatar of another player, but serving a very specific purpose and operated by rather simple computer programming. He is a *quest-giver*, who assigns missions to a player who interacts with him, while other friendly NPCs are trainers who periodically help the player's avatar gain skills, or vendors who sell virtual armor and other goods for virtual money. These NPCs are access points to the game's database, while appearing to be people.

Briefly, Sir Remson increases role distance by going *out of character* (OOC) to explain how some parts of the user interface for the game software work, then goes back into character to assign a simple mission to kill three bears in a field to the northeast, then goes OOC again to explain how the game's map system works. Much of the NPC communication takes place through special windows that open temporarily on the computer screen, but both friendly and enemy NPCs can also communicate through the text chat that players use to communicate with each other. The OOC concept applies to players whenever they are communicating about their real lives, in contrast to in-character role-playing in which they pretend to be the person represented by their avatar.

After completing the tutorial zone at level 15 of experience through a dozen hours of exploration and combat, May Ann performed several missions deep underground in the Tomb of Mithra nearer to Camelot, a maze of tunnels and crypts filled not only with living Mithra cultists, but also reincarnated zombies. Several times she herself was killed. She would be restored to life back in town, taking damage and losing experience that could be regained only by returning to the place she had died and praying before a temporary tombstone bearing her own name. She achieved level 20 by completing her most heroic quest, killing three ancient Roman generals who had returned to half-life as NPCs: Favonius Facilis, Virilis, and Anilius. These names seem to have been based on real Roman military officers who participated in the occupation of Britain prior to the days of Arthur, although Favonius Facilis was only a centurion, not a general.[3]

After this glorious accomplishment, Mary Ann rode to Camelot, over a fortified drawbridge across a stream and through one of the main gates of the city. Only after she had entered the majestic castle that held the fabled Round Table, did she learn the horrible truth: Arthur was nowhere to be found, because *Dark Age of Camelot* depicts the terrible times following his death:

> Aye, the sun has lost some of its fire with the loss of Arthur Pendragon. Aye, our enemies bark at the gates of our fair realm. Merlin is seen no more and the Knights of the Round Table are scattered. And yet, the dream of Camelot remains, and there are those among us who still follow Arthur's code of chivalry. Our knights are the finest in the world, and our mages carry on the traditions of the master wizard, Merlin. But our enemies swarm around us, and Morgana's evil sorcery raises the dead. These are dark times, indeed, yet not hopeless. We but need new blood – dauntless men and women to defend our lands and to rid the countryside of the plague of bandits and monsters belligerent to humankind. See here the many wonders of Albion and choose your path to glory.[4]

Thus, Mary Ann's quest to resurrect the Process Church in partnership with King Arthur ended in a cruel joke. His avatar had already died, so her death in the real world had not allowed her to join him in Camelot. We may well doubt whether King Arthur ever actually lived, or perhaps may have been a late Roman warrior named Artorius who never wore a crown. Had Mary Ann entered this virtual world as a member of Midgard, she could have met the resurrection of a real person outside the city of Jordheim, named Snorri Sturluson. He was an actual Icelandic historian who wrote the *Prose Edda* around the year 1200 and believed that pagan gods are mythologized versions of real historical figures, the theory of legends technically called *euhemerism* (Sturluson 1916). Not only is this a variant of role theory, but the Snorri Sturluson in *Dark Age of Camelot* is an automatic NPC quest-giver, thus a crude example of how in the far future humans might be resurrected in virtual worlds by means of artificial intelligence (Bainbridge 2004b).

Lands of horror

If the previous incarnation ended with a cruel joke, this one is more completely tragic. William Folwell Bainbridge, the person emulated here, sought to become the world's most prominent interpreter of the Bible and the human history contained within its pages. Yet in so doing he lost connections with his own family, thus forsaking the most normal way in which people seek immortality, through their children. As a cosmic principle, he represented *transcendence through prophecy*. If he could explain the fundamental mysteries of the Judeo-Christian tradition, he could appropriate all its glory for himself. In this case the contradiction is especially extreme, placing him inside a virtual world that explicitly denies Christian faith concerning immortality.

The highly acclaimed Norwegian MMO, *The Secret World*, depicts three areas of the real world that are associated with powerful cultural traditions that emphasize horror and conflict with conventional religion. The region designed for very experienced players is vampiric Transylvania, which contains the virtual tomb of Dracula. Players of middle experience explore the tombs of Egypt, battling Aten cultists as well as reanimated mummies. Arguably the most horrible of the regions is the first, the Maine sea coast in New England, which draws heavily upon the long tradition of American horror literature. There are specific references to Nathaniel Hawthorne, H. P. Lovecraft, Edgar Allan Poe, Washington Irving, and an indirect reference to the living writer Stephen King, represented by a reclusive NPC quest-giver, Sam Krieg, who lives in a lighthouse. When the real Stephen King dies, the game designers can rename this NPC to allow him to live again.

To be sure, Poe and Irving were not New Englanders, although Irving is buried just across the border. Yet it is reasonable to consider the most powerful form of horror literature depicted in *The Secret World* to be New England Horror, not only because the MMO uses Maine as the locale, but because the genre is much closer to the world inhabited by the original audience for the literature, while Egypt and Transylvania were distant realms and thus less directly meaningful. For a decade William Folwell Bainbridge was the minister of a New England church, First Baptist in Providence, Rhode Island, a city with an ironic religious name. For simplicity's sake, we can call his avatar Folwell, perhaps meaning 'follow well', and thus requiring the person operating the avatar to follow Stanislavski's dictum in becoming the character. The original William Folwell Bainbridge died in Cambridge, Massachusetts, and then had the unusual if unfelt real-world experience of having his brain dissected by his surgeon son, who was looking for a medical cause of religious obsessions. He had explored Egypt, as well, back in 1867, and had actually fired his revolver inside the pharaoh's burial chamber in the great pyramid, but simply to hear the echo rather than to restore a mummy to death.

The fundamental principle of New England horror can be described as Protestantism after God has been removed, defining Protestantism in terms of asceticism and self-control as suggested by sociologist Max Weber (1930), but with an emphasis on the fears that motivate these qualities. Consider the secret motto of *Moby-Dick*, which author Herman Melville dedicated to Nathaniel Hawthorne: 'I do not baptize you in the name of the Father, Son, and Holy Ghost – but in the name of the Devil' (Melville 1892; Parker 2002:16). The primary assumptions of *The Secret World* are that benevolent gods do not exist, but many horrifying supernatural beings described in folklore do exist. Periodically, they burst through protective barriers into our world, and are doing so now, but without the awareness of the world's leaders. To combat them, the secret societies have formed an alliance, including the Illuminati to which the Folwell avatar belonged.

The Illuminati was the correct faction, not only because it was headquartered in the United States, specifically in Brooklyn, where William Folwell Bainbridge had been the chief clergyman in the Brooklyn City Mission Society in the 1880s, but because the Illuminati supposedly had early called New England their home. The Templars would have been the second choice, because William Folwell Bainbridge had lived for a while in London. The Dragons headquartered in Korea might have been a distant third, because he had never visited there. However, in China in 1879 he had visited his cousin, John Nevius, who was the Protestant missionary who developed the famous Nevius Plan that was partly responsible for the success of Christianity in Korea (Bainbridge 1882b). Nevius himself could be a good subject for a Dragon avatar in *The Secret World*, because among his works was a research study of spirit possession in Asia (Nevius 1896).

I ran Folwell for 153 hours in *The Secret World*, exploring all the major territories available in the early history of this MMO, and experiencing one quest after another that concerned death and connected in symbolic ways with the real person on whom the avatar was based. For example, many intellectually interesting missions take place at Innsmouth Academy, a fictional boarding school described thus on the game's website: 'With a skeleton in every closet and deals with various devils inked into the very blueprints of the buildings, the Academy is an occult powder keg primed to explode – as it very nearly has during attacks in its past'.[5]

There are several Academy connections to the real William Folwell Bainbridge, including missions related to a Yazidi death-curse, because he had actually lived with the Yazidi for a while in Kurdistan in 1880. Many of his descendants attended New England boarding schools, and he had sent his son to Mohegan Lake Military Academy, just outside New England, where his son sent his grandson a generation later, but this boarding school died in 1934. His book, *Along the Lines at the Front*, is the most scientific of his works, and it conceptualizes missionary work through analogies with military strategy (Bainbridge 1882a). Mohegan used military discipline to reinforce Protestant values, which the school's 1886 catalogue said 'inculcates and enforces habits of self-control, accuracy, close attention and prompt obedience'.[6]

The most fundamental way to gain status in *The Secret World*, or indeed in almost any MMO, is to kill NPCs defined as enemies. This reminds us of the fact that Julius Caesar was a battlefield murderer, who also was himself murdered, even as he analyzed the propensity of Druidism to encourage warriors to risk their lives. As pathological as it may sound, killing can be an emotional release for fear about one's own death, even as the Gauls were forced to kill in self-defense when Caesar invaded their lands. Every popular violent MMO allows the player's avatar to resurrect, but requires extensive metaphoric killing, thus emotionally connecting in powerful ways with human feelings about mortality.

Indeed, Folwell killed fully 5,650 virtual enemies, distributed across 20 general categories, itemized in Table 10.1, with some descriptions quoted from the game. The first two categories, 2,657 zombies and 555 familiars, were especially common in New England, zombies lurking everywhere and familiars clustered around the boarding school. The third most common enemy killed, 522 cursed Egyptian cultists, is the closest to normal people, worshipping death but themselves still living. Looking down the list in Table 10.1, the only other living human enemies are the 70 filthy humans, who have been driven mad and are rotting, but still seem to be alive and not fully transformed into inhuman monsters, as for example in the case of the 104 wendigos. One can debate whether the 319 ghouls are still human, but like the 136 mummies they seem to be reanimated corpses. The monsters attacking Innsmouth Academy are a metaphor for the principle that immortality is a bad thing, polluting the natural cycle of generations in which children replace their parents, and all of *The Secret World* endorses death at a proper time in life.

Rosicrucian resurrection

H. Spencer Lewis, the avatar of this section, was the leader of a Rosicrucian hierarchical organization that had a very public face as the continuation of ancient Egyptian religious principles, while internally functioning as an esoteric secret society. Thus, status within the organization, and within the wider

Table 10.1 The 5,650 enemies killed by Folwell in *The Secret World*

Enemy	Description	Killed
Zombies	Animated corpses lacking self-awareness	2,657
Familiars	Wayward former companions of students of magic	555
Cursed Cultists	Death-worshipping followers of Aten, the Egyptian Sun God	522
Ghouls	Undead inhabitants of burial grounds or deserts	319
Draug	'The cause of a hundred ghost ship tales'	282
A'kab	'They were the cold, pale things of native myths'	248
Locusts	'A monstrous reborn Plague swarms across the desert'	199
Mummies	Embalmed ancient Egyptians, revived by a curse	136
Rakshasa	Man-eating demons from the Hindu-Buddhist tradition	116
Spectres	'Creatures with terrible mass and terrifying physicality'	109
Wendigo	'The vestiges of humans who turned to cannibalism'	104
Spirits	'The flickering lights of the foolish fire'	74
Filthy Humans	Infected with an epidemic disease that drove them mad	70
Scorpions	Dinosaur-sized, gushing vile, green poison	69
Hellspawn	Soldiers of Satan's army in Transylvania	41
Golems	Monstrous humanoids created from inanimate matter	39
Deep Ones	'Natives of the cold black depths of the Atlantic'	33
Shades	Evil ghosts that have escaped the underworld	33
Scarecrows	'A manifestation of fear and hatred'	30
Revanants	'All they crave is misery, pestilence and death'	14

Rosicrucian subculture, was crucial to him, almost as if he sought to gain pharaonic status in a resurrected ancient Egypt. Thus he represents the principle of *organizational status ambition*. The virtual world he inhabits allows no killing, but could permit slavery, and we can imagine a resurrected Lewis seeking to lord over others as a pharaoh might. As a strategy for immortality, the pharaonic method had some success, but within limits. One is reminded of the oft-cited poem by Percy Bysshe Shelley, titled 'Ozymandias', which portrays a ruined heroic statue, probably of Pharaoh Rameses II, which was intended to achieve immortality:

> And on the pedestal these words appear:
> 'My name is Ozymandias, king of kings:
> Look on my works, ye Mighty, and despair!'
> Nothing beside remains. Round the decay
> Of that colossal wreck, boundless and bare
> The lone and level sands stretch far away.

In 1972, aware that the Process was influenced by the Ritual Magick and Rosicrucian traditions, I visited Rosicrucian Park in San Jose, California, photographed the many outdoor displays, subscribed to an AMORC correspondence course, and did about the same for the competing Rosicrucian Fellowship further south in the same state. Visiting the rosicrucianpark.org website over four decades later I see that a labyrinth has been added, learn that an alchemy museum is planned, and read this appealing description of the place: 'The Park offers a mysterious and beautiful combination of Egyptian and Moorish architecture set among broad lawns, rose gardens, statuary, and sparkling fountains'.[7]

Visitors to Rosicrucian Park in California in 1972 were offered a deeply mystical experience when they entered a simulated Egyptian tomb underground: A recording provided narration in the voice of long-dead H. Spencer Lewis. Today's museum website mentions AMORC but says almost nothing about it, or indeed about Rosicrucianism more generally. For some insight, one must separately locate amorc.org. There one learns that this particular brand of self-avowed mysticism supposedly originated in the Eighteenth Dynasty in about 1500 BC in Egypt, locked in the cultural background ever since, until Harvey Spencer Lewis visited a group of French Rosicrucians:

> They initiated him and entrusted him with the mission to reactivate the Order in the United-States, so it could be reintroduced later in Europe when circumstances would be more favorable (the First World War was already looming on the horizon).[8]

AMORC stands for 'Ancient and Mystical Order Rosae Crucis', thus beginning with a claim of antiquity, while incorporating Latin symbols of rose and cross, and both formal names carry modern trademark protection.

The many Rosicrucian groups tend to be highly eclectic culturally, while claiming to possess secret doctrines and even magical powers (McIntosh 2011), but AMORC most visibly exploited public fascination with ancient Egypt by boldly claiming to revive its esoteric practices. Given his ancient Egyptian affectations, H. Spencer Lewis would have approved of an avatar based on him in that re-creation of ancient Egypt, *A Tale in the Desert*. I had studied this virtual world periodically, starting with an avatar named Renhotep, July 2009 to March 2010 during the Fourth Telling, using a different avatar in September and October 2013 in the Sixth Telling, then re-creating Renhotep late in the Sixth Telling in January 2015. The Hspencer avatar representing H. Spencer Lewis joined him in June 2015 until both were destroyed in the conclusion of their telling on September 8, 2015.

The plan was to use Renhotep as the slave of Hspencer. Superficially, this unequal social relationship supported Lewis's own desire to lord over other people, rising above them in spiritual status. For our purposes, it let Renhotep simulate an NPC, despite the fact he was operated by a human being – the standard technology development method called the 'Wizard of Oz' technique in computer science. Essentially, everything Renhotep did for Hspencer could have been done by a robot, because his work was entirely the collection and preparation of manufacturing materials and objects that allowed Hspencer to have a modest virtual equivalent of Rosicrucian Park. Thus current technology might really be sufficient to render a slave immortal within a virtual world, still lacking the ability to emulate freedom.

Much of Renhotep's work consisted of gathering materials, processing them (such as cutting tree limbs to make boards), and constructing products that Hspencer wanted. On the few occasions when the software system and game rules required Hspencer to do any work himself, Renhotep would prepare all the materials then place them in a huge-capacity warehouse he built, for Hspencer to pick up when he felt the urge.

When Hspencer decided to be reincarnated in ancient Egypt, Renhotep had already built a 'compound', a sand-colored building containing many basic pieces of virtual construction equipment, including a flax comb, distaff, and loom for making fabrics such as linen and canvas. He also had not only an industrial wood plane for cutting tree logs into boards, but also a more advanced carpentry shop, not to mention two different kinds of kiln, a glazier's bench, and a terrarium for breeding sacred scarab beetles. His land was right beside the Nile river, just north of a crossing point, and there was room in the area for several other structures. The first order Hspencer gave to Renhotep was to construct a guild hall, between the compound and the north–south road. Renhotep started by setting up a small building site, which required four pieces of rope plus a sheet of canvas, then added 300 boards and 500 bricks to make a starter hall suitable for as many as ten members. To make bricks, he had first to make brick racks, essentially a mold for casting six sun-dried bricks at a time and requiring four boards. Each set of six bricks required him to gather three units of mud, one unit of sand, and two units of straw, which were produced by gathering two units of grass and drying them in the sun. The brick racks wore out after a few uses, so this was hard work for Renhotep, if not for Hspencer.

The guild hall was beautiful, in ancient Egyptian style, decorated with lotus columns and winged sun symbols. Hspencer was not yet ready to recruit followers, but one passing Egyptian with the classical name Cheops did join and was given initiate rank. Both Hspencer and Renhotep held elder rank, which served a very useful practical purpose. Renhotep was able to change the ownership rule on all his equipment, transferring everything to the guild, so that both he and Hspencer could use it. To start gaining status in the Egyptian social system, Hspencer had to do some grubby manual labor, such as building his own compound between the guild hall and Renhotep's compound. As much as the rules permitted, Renhotep prepared the materials for Hspencer. A hard-working construction players' guild named zFree, to which Renhotep belonged, had constructed huge Pyramids of Heaven across the wide Egyptian sands, and Hspencer was gratified to learn that when he meditated for the first time at each one he gained one level of game experience, without the need for any manual labor.

Renhotep was already level 17, without the benefit of pyramid meditations, and by various lazy means Hspencer reached level 13, but these were plebeian ranks in a social system that required many months of hard work to ascend.

As is typically the case, members of radical religious movements gain subjective social status from their involvement, and leaders may feel superior to all the rest of humanity, even if the outside world does not accord them great honor (Bainbridge 1997; Stark & Bainbridge 1985). In his studies, mainly using the *Tale*'s wiki at www.atitd.org, Hspencer discovered that this ancient Egypt had many modernistic fantasy elements, for example Raeli mosaics and a device looking for all the world like a flying saucer called a Raeli Gliderport that fires robot aircraft that soar around in artistic trajectories. He imagined, I suspect accurately, that this was inspired by the Raëlian Movement oriented toward supernatural extraterrestrials (Palmer 2004).

The wiki explained what materials Renhotep would need to give him, few of which they already had in storage, to make the saucer and two gliders, including 200 units of concrete and 250 Raeli tiles. Producing all these materials himself would be hopeless for Renhotep, because he had not yet learned metalworking nor had any of the necessary equipment, not to mention everything required to manufacture Raeli tiles. However, he had begged the leaders of the exclusive Palm Valley guild to allow him to join, and it freely gave him most of what was needed. This illustrates the great value of social cooperation in *Tale*, and the fact that by combining their labor and resources individuals could create much more complex technology than any of them could alone.

Once Renhotep had given him the necessary materials, Hspencer was able to build the gliderport very quickly. He could use it in either of two ways to gain a level of experience: refine it so that the gliders flew complex paths and shot out glorious colors so that other ancient Egyptians would rate it one of the best, thereby passing it as a Test, or simply demolish it without entering any competition, earning only an experience point. For weeks he could not decide, but eventually Hspencer grew tired of it and demolished it, reaching level 14 and avoiding the risk of receiving insults rather than praise from the common people.

Somehow, Hspencer did not seem to be enhancing Renhotep's spiritual life. Then history intervened. August 2015 would be the last full month for the Sixth Telling, during which seven special guilds built monuments for the seven disciplines that constituted the main line of experience advancement for avatars. Each monument would memorialize the names of those who contributed to its construction, thus offering a traditional form of nominal immortality. Renhotep abandoned Hspencer, rushing off to join the guilds devoted to the seven disciplines listed in Table 10.2.

The seven disciplines in *Tale* represent a cultural division of labor; each requires completing seven increasingly difficult missions, and only really dedicated players attempt to excel in them all. For example, the *Tale* wiki summarizes Worship thus: 'demonstrating reverence and fidelity to the gods. In Egypt religion is a communal activity, and the Tests of Worship emphasize and reward group teamwork. Worship is also associated with agriculture'.[9] The most common Worship mission requires two players to cooperate, ideally under the supervision of a third, more advanced player, in doing a ritual

Table 10.2   The seven disciplines, with population statistics for August 30, 2015

Discipline	Description from the game's Wiki	Guild members	Students	Pharaoh's Oracles
Architecture	The construction of magnificent buildings	55	379	13
Art and Music	Enriching Egypt with works of creativity	40	113	16
Harmony	Understanding and coordinating with one's fellow Egyptians	37	341	45
Human Body	Achieving physical excellence	56	435	31
Leadership	Securing the trust and cooperation of others	40	285	17
Thought	The achievement of mental fitness	49	133	13
Worship	Demonstrating reverence and fidelity to the gods	37	565	11

honoring gods in this order: Horus, Isis, Osiris, Thoth, Ra, Bastet, and Amun. Renhotep was already an Initiate of six of the seven disciplines, lacking only Worship because Hspencer was supposed to take care of his religious needs. Humble peasant that he was, he did not initially realize that in fact he was not eligible to be memorialized by a monument, because despite all his hard work and progress up the experience ladder, he had never actually passed a Test in any of the disciplines.

Passing one Test in a discipline gives one the status of Student; passing two Tests in the same discipline makes one a Prentice; and additional passing takes one up through Journeyman, Scribe, Master, Sage, and with seven passes to Pharaoh's Oracle.[10] Table 10.2 shows how many virtual Egyptians had reached the lowly Student and exalted Oracle ranks, although only a few earned monumental status in the last days of this Egypt. Thus the slave Renhotep was not eligible for veneration, nor was his socially isolated master Hspencer, and neither achieved the symbolic immortality gained by the 113 elite avatars whose names were actually inscribed across the seven Egyptian monuments.

Conclusion

In this chapter it has been shown how avatars in online gameworlds may be used to memorialize, assess, and gain inspiration from deceased persons. Case studies placed three unconventional religious leaders who lived in the nineteenth and twentieth centuries in three twenty-first-century virtual worlds that were selected to be appropriate environments for appreciation of the chosen individuals. This trio of personalities illustrates symbolic attempts to gain immortality that might be called *cosmic principles*: power through intimacy, transcendence through prophecy, and organizational status ambition. The worlds themselves are also revivals of dead societies: Dark Age northwestern Europe, nineteenth- and twentieth-century American literature, and ancient Egypt. All three games contain much virtual death, even nonviolent *A Tale in the Desert* because all inhabitants die at the end of each telling, so they can encourage thoughtful players to contemplate the meaning of mortality and explore a variety of philosophies about death. The immortality achieved through the three avatars of deceased religious innovators is obviously of a rather limited kind, but for that very reason can offer insights about the path forward: (1) Progress in the areas of science and technology that can mitigate the finality of death is likely to be incremental or episodic, thus requiring definitions, expectations, and investments to evolve over a period of many years. (2) At the present time, given the many possibilities and uncertainties, it is worth exploring life extension and symbolic revival in a variety of different technological modalities. (3) Some forms of technological immortality will require effort on the part of other people, for example the surviving family members who operate ancestor veneration avatars. (4) Technology-based immortality is likely to have complex relationships with religion, which traditionally had the responsibility to offer symbolic transcendence of mortality.

We cannot know how science and religion will evolve over the future centuries, whether as partners or opponents. However, the information technologies that have emerged in recent years, and became spectacularly influential in popular culture, allow us to explore possibilities and may inspire innovators to develop a revolutionary synthesis. Many questions can be the subjects of near-term social-psychological research, even as the supporting technology advances. When online game players kill virtual enemies, or watch their own avatars die, what are the consequences for their orientations toward their own eventual real deaths? How does operating an avatar based on a deceased person compare with prayer or traditional forms of memorialization in venerating that departed individual? As the artificial intelligence improves that operates non-player characters in online games, or robots in the physical world, will people come to treat them as real, especially if they represent deceased humans?

In principle, online virtual worlds could be used as laboratories for rather more systematic experimentation with technological means of immortality than the conceptually based but admittedly superficial explorations described here. But in the context of sociological role theory, the avatar technology can suggest new perspectives on the meaning of human existence, in a civilization that may move beyond religion. Atheism implies not only the non-existence of God, but of the human soul as well, unless the soul is given a new, non-supernatural definition (Bainbridge 2010a). In role theory, a person is a collection of roles, so immortality would mean merely the perpetuation of those roles in a social system that survives the individual person. Information theory subsumes role theory, but considers a person to be a complex, dynamic pattern of information, with each role serving the same function as a subroutine in a computer program that incorporated many other kinds of coding as well.

In principle, then, data about a personality could be captured through all the methods of social and psychological science, then emulated by artificial intelligence through a robot in the material world or an avatar in a virtual world (Bainbridge 2014a, 2014b, 2016a, 2016b). To the extent that the computer program behaves as a specific deceased human would have behaved, then it offers a realistic form of immortality (Turing 1950). Such theories and speculations about the future of technology are difficult to assess, but anyone who wishes to can create an avatar like those described here, and immediately experience virtual veneration of the dead, providing at least a limited degree of immortality to the deceased.

Notes

1 The views expressed in this chapter do not necessarily represent the views of the National Science Foundation or the United States.
2 camelotherald.wikia.com/wiki/Class, accessed June 7, 2015.
3 romaninscriptionsofbritain.org/inscriptions/200, accessed June 28, 2015.
4 camelotherald.wikia.com/wiki/Albion, accessed June 28, 2015.
5 www.thesecretworld.com/world/locations/academy.
6 *Annual Catalogue of Mohegan Lake School* (Albany, NY: Reynolds and Wilcox, 1886), p. 9.
7 www.rosicrucianpark.org/about, accessed August 5, 2015.
8 www.amorc.org/amorc-presentation-english, accessed August 5, 2015.
9 www.atitd.org/wiki/tale6/Discipline, accessed August 11, 2015.
10 www.atitd.org/wiki/tale6/New_Player_Guide, www.atitd.org/wiki/tale6/The_Monument_Guide, accessed August 18.

References

Alcock, Leslie (1971): *Arthur's Britain*. Harmondsworth: Penguin Books.

Ashe, Geoffrey (ed.) (1968): *The Quest for Arthur's Britain*. London: Paladin.

Ashton, Graham (1974): *The Realm of King Arthur*. Newport, Isle of Wight: Dixon.

Bainbridge, William Folwell (1882a): *Along the Lines at the Front: A General Survey of Baptist Home and Foreign Missions*. Philadelphia: American Baptist Publication Society.

Bainbridge, William Folwell (1882b): *Around the World Tour of Christian Missions*. New York: Blackall.

Bainbridge, William Folwell (1883): *Self-Giving: A Story of Christian Missions*. Boston: D. Lothrup.

Bainbridge, William Sims (1978): *Satan's Power: A Deviant Psychotherapy Cult*. Berkeley, CA: University of California Press.

Bainbridge, William Sims (1997): *The Sociology of Religious Movements*. New York: Routledge.

Bainbridge, William Sims (ed.) (2004a): *Encyclopedia of Human–Computer Interaction*. Great Barrington, MA: Berkshire.

Bainbridge, William Sims (2004b): 'Progress toward Cyberimmortality', in Immortality Institute (ed.): *The Scientific Conquest of Death: Essays on Infinite Lifespans*. Allen, TX: Libros En Red, pp. 107–122.

Bainbridge, William Sims (2007a): *Across the Secular Abyss*. Lanham, MD: Lexington.

Bainbridge, William Sims (2007b): 'The Scientific Research Potential of Virtual Worlds'. *Science* 317:472–476.

Bainbridge, William Sims (2010a): 'Cognitive Science and the New Atheism', in Amarnath Amarasingam (ed.): *Religion and the New Atheism*. Leiden: Brill, pp. 79–96.

Bainbridge, William Sims (ed.) (2010b): *Online Multiplayer Games*. San Rafael, CA: Morgan & Claypool.

Bainbridge, William Sims (2010c): *The Warcraft Civilization*. Cambridge, MA: MIT Press.

Bainbridge, William Sims (2013): *eGods: Faith Versus Fantasy in Computer Gaming*. New York: Oxford University Press.

Bainbridge, William Sims (2014a): *An Information Technology Surrogate for Religion: The Veneration of Deceased Family Members in Online Games*. New York: Palgrave/Macmillan.

Bainbridge, William Sims (2014b): *Personality Capture and Emulation*. London: Springer.

Bainbridge, William Sims (2015): 'The Paganization Process'. *Interdisciplinary Journal of Research on Religion*, 11:14.

Bainbridge, William Sims (2016a): *Star Worlds*. Ann Arbor, MI: University of Michigan Press.

Bainbridge, William Sims (2016b): *Virtual Sociocultural Convergence*. London: Springer.

Blascovich, Jim & Jeremy Bailenson (2011): *Infinite Reality: The Hidden Blueprint of Our Virtual Lives*. New York: William Morrow.

Borgatta, Edgar F., Robert Boguslaw & Martin R. Haskell (1975): 'On the Work of Jacob L. Moreno'. *Sociometry*, 38 (1):148–161.

Caesar, Gaius Julius (1919): *The Gallic War*. New York: G. P. Putnam's Sons.

Comte, Auguste (1883): *The Catechism of Positive Religion*. London: Trübner.

Cooley, Charles Horton (1902): *Human Nature and the Social Order*. New York: C. Scribner's Sons.

Durkheim, Émile (1915/1965): *The Elementary Forms of the Religious Life*. New York: Free Press.

Fortes, Meyer (1961): 'Pietas in Ancestor Worship'. *Journal of the Royal Anthropological Institute of Great Britain and Ireland*, 91 (2):166–191.

Garfinkel, Harold (1967): *Studies in Ethnomethodology*. Englewood Cliffs, NJ: Prentice-Hall.

Gibbs, Martin, Jopji Mori, Michael Arnold & Tamara Kohn (2012): 'Tombstones, Uncanny Monuments and Epic Quests: Memorials in World of Warcraft'. *Game Studies*, 12 (1).

Glaser, Barney G. & Anselm L. Strauss (1967): *The Discovery of Grounded Theory*. Chicago: Aldine.

Goffman, Erving (1956): *The Presentation of Self in Everyday Life*. Edinburgh: University of Edinburgh Social Sciences Research Centre.

Goffman, Erving (1961): *Encounters: Two Studies in the Sociology of Interaction*. Indianapolis: Bobbs-Merrill.

Gouldner, Alvin W. (1970): *The Coming Crisis of Western Sociology*. New York: Basic Books.

Husserl, Edmund (1965): *Cartesian Meditations*. The Hague: Martinus Nijhoff.

Lemert, Charles & Paul Piccone (1982): 'Gouldner's Theoretical Method and Reflexive Sociology'. *Theory and Society*, 11 (6):733–757.

Lifton, Robert Jay (1968): 'Protean Man'. *Partisan Review*, Winter:13–27.

McIntosh, Christopher (2011): *The Rose Cross and the Age of Reason: Eighteenth-Century Rosicrucianism in Central Europe and Its Relationship to the Enlightenment*. Albany, NY: State University of New York Press.

Melville, Herman (1892): *Moby-Dick, or The White Whale*. Boston: St. Botolph Society.

Merrick, Kathryn E. & Mary Lou Maher (2009): *Motivated Reinforcement Learning: Curious Characters for Multiuser Games*. New York: Springer.

Moreno, Jacob L. (1944): 'Psychodrama and Therapeutic Motion Pictures'. *Sociometry*, 7 (2):230–244.

Moreno, Jacob L. & Zerka Toeman (1942): 'The Group Approach in Psychodrama'. *Sociometry*, 5 (2):191–195.

Nardi, Bonnie (2010): *My Life as a Night Elf Priest: An Anthropological Account of World of Warcraft*. Ann Arbor, MI: University of Michigan Press.

Nevius, John Livingston (1896): *Demon Possession and Allied Themes: Being an Inductive Study of Phenomena of Our Own Times*. New York: Fleming H. Revell.

Palmer, Susan J. (2004): *Aliens Adored: Rael's UFO Religion*. New Brunswick, NJ: Rutgers University Press.

Parker, Hershel (2002): *Herman Melville, Volume 2*. Baltimore: Johns Hopkins University Press.

Schütz, Alfred (1967): *The Phenomenology of the Social World*. Evanston, IL: Northwestern University Press.

Stanislavski, Constantin (1988): *An Actor Prepares*. New York: Routledge.

Stark, Rodney & William Sims Bainbridge (1985): *The Future of Religion*. Berkeley, CA: University of California Press.

Sturluson, Snorri (1916): *The Prose Edda*. New York: Oxford University Press.

Turing, Alan (1950): 'Computing Machinery and Intelligence'. *Mind*, 59:433–460.

Verney, Sabrina (2011): *Xtul: An Experience of the Process*. Baltimore: PublishAmerica.

Weber, Max (1930): *The Protestant Ethic and the Spirit of Capitalism*. London: G. Allen & Unwin.

Wyllie, Timothy (2009): *Love Sex Fear Death: The Inside Story of the Process Church of the Final Judgment*. Port Townsend, WA: Feral House.

Yee, Nick (2014): *The Proteus Paradox*. New Haven, CT: Yale University Press.

Yee, Nick, Jeremy N. Bailenson & Nicolas Ducheneaut (2009): 'The Proteus Effect: Implications of Transformed Digital Self-Representation on Online and Offline Behavior'. *Communication Research*, 36 (2):285–312.

Zhao, Shanyang (2005): 'The Digital Self: Through the Looking Glass of Telecopresent Others'. *Symbolic Interaction*, 28(3):387–405.

11   The proliferation of postselves in American civic and popular cultures[1]

Michael C. Kearl

Introduction

The Gershwin Centennial Celebration of the San Antonio Symphony was a remarkable event as it featured George Gershwin himself. Though dead since 1937, he 'performed' on a 1912 concert grand player piano, flown in from Denver, with rolls that precisely preserved his keystrokes. As the music was about to begin, a spotlight moved across stage as if following Gershwin as he was taking his seat. An attendant even brought a glass of wine, placing it above the keyboard for him to drink.

Gershwin was neither the first nor last deceased person in recent years to engage with the living. Prime-time television is full of programmes and commercials featuring spirits, channelling mediums, angels, and dissected corpses. Annually rank-ordered is the earnings of deceased celebrities by Forbes and their recognisability and likeability 'Dead Q' scores by Marketing Evaluations Inc. Halls of fame proliferate. James Dean and Marilyn Monroe achieve the philatelic immortality previously reserved for founding fathers, victorious military figures, and presidents. And concurrent with the screening of Tim Burton's *Corpse Bride* was the national tour of Gunther von Hagen's 'Body Worlds', featuring skinned and variously dissected plastinated cadavers.

The intent here is to speculate on the interrelationships between these and other apparently unrelated phenomena. From the only country to put men on the moon and park a spacecraft on an asteroid 196 million miles away, whose scientists have mapped the human genome and who investigate the most elemental components of matter, we find a population with renewed interests in immortality and novel connections with its deceased members.

The presumed disappearance of the dead in late modern life

There is an irreversible evolution from savage societies to our own: little by little, the dead cease to exist. They are thrown out of the group's symbolic circulation. They are no longer beings with a full role to play, worthy partners in exchange, and we make this obvious by exiling them further and further away from the group of the living.

(Baudrillard 1993:126)

Reflected in the Jean Baudrillard passage above is the thesis that late modernity has banished the dead from everyday life. One inference is that the dead do not exist because humanity eventually outgrows its needs to believe in the illusions of an afterlife and to attribute unintended or inexplicable events to ancestral meddling. In addition, there is a sense of disconnect with a perceived irrelevant past, accounting for the profound degree of historical ignorance (Kearl 2001). Memories of the deceased evaporate within a generation or two along with their traditional statuses as role models and reference groups.

Further, the modern adult mind, programmed with the scientific insights of inevitable extinction not only of all life forms but of the post-Big Bang universe itself, has reached psychologists' final developmental stage of death understandings, when one maturely grasps the inevitability, irreversibility, and finality of finitude – particularly with increasing education, decreasing religion, and the here-and-now orientation fostered by materialism.

Finally, the supposed disappearance of the dead also owes something to the changing nature and visibility of death itself. With the longevity revolution, death increasingly arrives with advance warning only to the oldest segments of society, to those who have lived full and complete lives and who now live largely segregated from other, younger age groups. With lives no longer ending 'prematurely' to the unprepared, the ghostly embodiments of social frustrations occasioned by incompletely lived lives have largely disappeared. The dead, like the contemporary old, supposedly occupy a 'roleless role'.

The transcendence motive and its cultural shapings

> Man cannot live without a continuous confidence in something indestructible within himself.
>
> (Franz Kafka cited in Choron 1964:15)

On the other hand, there are various psychological, sociological, and cultural forces at work that continue to keep the dead very much alive. The human primate has always been infested with lice and ghosts – the former the consequence of our biological nature, the latter because of our symbolic essence. For the only creature aware of its inevitable demise, its death-transcending drive is seen to underlie not only its psychic health but also the creation and maintenance of entire cultural orders (Bauman 1992; Becker 1973; Lifton 1979).

The quest for immortality runs deeply throughout the earliest known Western stories (Hentsch 2004), whose themes involve not speculation of the existence of an afterlife but rather how to keep the dead in their place (Walter 1996:13). Underlying Western civilisation is Christianity's synthesis of these stories, featuring its grand assumption of immortal existence. The cultural consequences of challenging and possibly voiding this basic assumption are profound. St Paul observed 'if the dead are not raised ... our Gospel is null and void ... and your faith has nothing in it' (1 Corinthians 15:13). What have changed are the array of death-transcending strategies and the proliferation of postselves. Here Edwin S. Shneidman's (1973) concept of the 'postself' is expanded to include all engagements between deceased individuals and the living, whether based on their intended legacies or the designs of others. Since the time of the concept's coinage, technological innovations, legal expansion of posthumous rights, and capitalism's commodification of symbolic immortality have expanded considerably the roles of the dead in everyday life.

American exceptionalism

If we follow our reading of Jean Baudrillard's line of reasoning, it would seem logical to conclude that the death ethos of the United States – one of the most economically advanced, scientifically inclined, and materialistic of nations – should resemble those of other highly developed Western cultures. However, as is evident in Figure 11.1, such is not the case. Various surveys show that more than seven out of ten Americans fully expect an afterlife. This proportion has been on the increase at least over the past three decades, particularly among Catholics, Jews, and those with no religious affiliation (Greeley & Hout 1999) – a proportion unexplained by demographic changes (e.g. the ageing of the population).

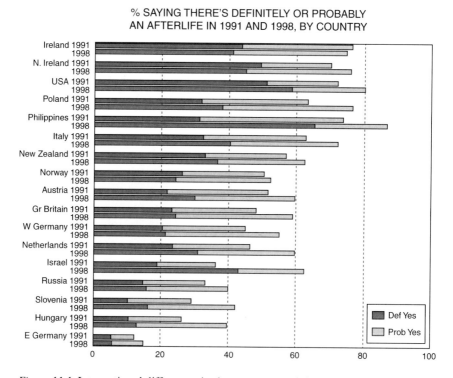

Figure 11.1 International differences in the percentage of the adult public believing in life after death

Source: ISSP (1991, 1998).

Table 11.1 'How often have you felt as though you were really in touch with someone who had died'? Percentage saying at least once – with DKs omitted

	Men	*Women*	*Total once+*
USA	37	42	40
New Zealand	30	37	34
Slovenia	26	36	32
Israel	27	34	31
Ireland	26	33	29
Austria	35	32	28
Poland	24	32	28
Great Britain	23	33	28
Philippines	28	27	27
Netherlands	23	25	24
West Germany	21	26	23
Italy	15	27	21
Hungary	16	23	20
East Germany	12	21	17
Northern Ireland	15	17	16
Russia	11	16	14
Norway	9	17	13

Source: ISSP (1991).

Not only do Americans lead the developed world in confidence in an afterlife but, according to this cross-national study of religious beliefs (ISSP
1998), they led all surveyed countries in the percentage believing in the
existence of heaven (86%) and are basically tied with Cypriots for the greatest percentage believing in hell (74%, compared to 14% of Swedes, 22% of
French, 33% of British, and 59% of Italians). Further, when asked if one
has felt personally in touch with someone who had died, Americans again
top the chart of international respondents with four in ten having experienced such connection (see Table 11.1). Such findings prompted George
Gallup Jr to observe how 'one of the most dramatic – yet perhaps least
noticed – developments of the late 20th and early 21st century has been
the explosion of interest among the U.S. populace in spiritual matters'
(Gallup 2001).

The American story is unique in its cultural challenges to death's finality. For Europeans, the New World was the place for second chances, for
personal rebirths, and quests for immortality. It was where Ponce de León
searched for the fountain of youth and is the current home of the anti-
ageing Methuselah Foundation. It was from where sprouted the Church of
Latter-day Saints with its certitude in the continuation of familial relations
through eternity, Scientology with its belief in an immortal soul that under-
goes countless reincarnations, and from where emerged the Spiritualism
movement with its conviction that the dead could communicate with the
living (Braude 2001).

The immortalist zeitgeist was to nurture and be nurtured by American ingenuity. Thomas Edison, the epitome of American inventiveness, wrote of dying bodies being deserted by a swarm of highly charged energies that enter into space and another cycle of existence, detectable by 'an instrument so delicate as to be affected by our personality as it survives in the next life' (Lescarboura 1920). Eighty-five years later, Raymond Kuzweil, recipient of the Lemelson-MIT prize and the 1999 National Medal of Technology Award, predicted immortality to be but a few decades away for a software-based humanity. He envisions cybernetically enhanced humans genetically improved through Internet downloads and through whose bodies course billions of 'nanobots', molecular-level robots, that reverse the ageing process by continuously modifying brain cells, muscles, arteries, and bone (Kurzweil 2005).

In recent years, quantum physicists have demonstrated a phenomenon called 'entanglement', where particles can be in two places at once and change in one simultaneously alters the other. Researchers have not only slowed light to the speed of a train but have brought it to a dead stop, stored it and then released it as if it were an ordinary material particle. Certainly, such activities are no more mystical than a person's essence surviving in some form after death. The present era holds considerable parallels to the mid nineteenth century and the 1920s (periods Swatos & Gissurarson 1997 argue are one and the same epoch, the golden age of Western spiritualism), when pseudo-science flourished as prestige in science grew, together producing then and now an anything-is-possible mindset. If dead pets can be cloned and perhaps woolly mammoths be resurrected, why cannot deceased loved ones continue to live?

We should note the relative non-exclusivity of most Americans' criteria for eternal life. In this religious country without a state-sanctioned faith, according to a 2008 Pew national survey, two-thirds of the religiously affiliated believe many religions can lead to eternal life, with a majority of Christians understanding that this includes non-Christian faiths (Pew Forum on Religion and Public Life 2008). The individualist creed underlying this unrestrictive mindset has engendered a do-it-yourself approach to both material and spiritual matters, at times viewing the two as interrelated. During the nineteenth century, for instance, subscribers to spiritualism included many leaders of the abolitionist, feminist, Temperance, and labour reform movements (Buescher 2003). For both Spiritualists and Mormons, the dead were to be liberated by the living (leading to the latter's difficulties with various Jewish groups in 1995 over its postmortem baptisms of Holocaust victims).

Finally, Americans' belief in an afterlife plays an underlying role in the so-called 'culture wars'. In 2006, the difference in afterlife expectations between Democrats and Republicans was greater than any year since 1973, with Republicans 13 percentage points more likely to believe. To control for the fact that 10 per cent of Republicans were more likely also to be strongly religious. Table 11.2 shows the party differences among those not strongly religious in the correlation between afterlife beliefs and attitudes towards abortion (agreeing that women should have the right to a legal abortion

Table 11.2 The effects of party identification and beliefs in afterlife on culture war battleline issues among those strongly and not strongly religious

Believe in afterlife?	Democrats[a]		Independents		Republicans[a]	
	Yes	No/undecided	Yes	No/undecided	Yes	No/undecided
Strongly religious						
% Favouring abortion[b]	54.2	58.6	36.3	39.3	34.5	54.9
% Favouring euthanasia[c]	56.9	66.7	46.0	66.7	46.8	81.3
% Saying homosexuality not wrong at all[d]	28.1	25.0	14.8	5.0 (n.s.)	12.3	29.4
Not strongly religious						
% Favouring abortion[b]	54.2	58.6	36.3	39.3	34.5	54.9
% Favouring euthanasia[c]	79.8	78.6	70.7	76.0	72.0	83.5
% Saying homosexuality not wrong at all[d]	47.2	47.4	34.9	33.0	30.8	42.9

Source: Davis & Smith (2007).

Notes:
a Responses to 'Generally speaking, do you usually think of yourself as a Republican, Democrat, Independent, or what?' Category 'independent lean Democrat' combined with 'strong Democrat' and 'Democrat'. Category 'independent lean Republican' similarly combined with 'strong Republican' and 'Republican'.
b 'Do you think that a woman should have the right to a legal abortion if she wants it for any reason?'
c 'When a person has a disease that cannot be cured, do you think doctors should be allowed by law to end the patient's life by some painless means if the patient and his family request it?'
d 'What about sexual relations between two adults of the same sex – do you think it is always wrong, almost always wrong, wrong only sometimes, or not wrong at all?'

if she 'wants it for any reason'), euthanasia, homosexuality, and belief in evolution. With the exception of evolution, afterlife beliefs have little or no effect on the attitudes of Democrats and Independents. Among Republicans, however, the effects are considerable, with the afterlife non-believers closely resembling the Democrats. And while beliefs in an afterlife have little correlation with agreement about Darwinian tenets among Independents, sizeable differences are produced in the minds of Republicans and Democrats. In the Discussion, I will return to the significance of these correlations.

In sum, in contradiction to the claim that late modern secular cultures have extinguished the role of the dead in everyday life, I argue that extreme individualism, capitalism, and technological innovations together have increased their number, visibility, and influence. My proposal is that American culture can best be understood in terms of its core salvific goal of death control and its embracement of the hereafter: its immortalist ethos.

The proliferation of postselves

With these points in mind, I turn to current death-transcending trends in American popular and civic cultures as well as their commodification in the service economy.

Postselves in popular culture

Popular culture is often where deep cultural trends are crystallised and given clear expression. The 'success' of an artistic motif owes as much to public receptivity towards its message as to the work's artistic merits. Consider the socio-cultural context producing the audience receptivity to the immortalist ethos in mass media. In cinema, the spiritual genre of popular movies has grossed hundreds of millions of dollars, with such blockbusters as the *Star Wars* trilogy capturing and restoring to American culture the archetypal sacred sense. Over the past two decades not only are there more roles for the dead in mainstream productions but their task in the plotline has largely shifted from instilling terror to becoming guardians of the living: *Field of Dreams* (1989), *Ghost* (1990), *Ghost Dad* (1990), *Casper* (1995), *City of Angels* (1998), *What Dreams May Come* (1998), *Meet Joe Black* (1998), *Jack Frost* (1999), *City of Angels* (1998), *Sixth Sense* (1999), *The Gift* (2000), *What Lies Beneath* (2000), and *Dragonfly* (2002). In addition, the deceased now perform with the living, perhaps beginning with Woody Allen's *Zelig* (1983) and perfected in *Forrest Gump* (1994), wherein John Kennedy, George Wallace, Lyndon Johnson, John Lennon, and Elvis Presley are put to work from the grave.

Cinematic success leads to television imitations, and no longer in the latter medium are attempts made by the living to connect with the dead limited to Shirley MacLaine New Age cable specials, but rather, these attempts have become prime-time fare. Almost nightly, one can watch John Edward reunite 'people in the physical world with their loved ones who have crossed over'. Facing plummeting ratings in spring 2002, ABC television aired *Contact: Talking to the Dead*, featuring psychic George Anderson's interviews with the deceased loved ones of Vanna White and Mackenzie Phillips as well as the murdered wife of Robert Blake. In the fall of that year appeared spiritual medium James Van Praagh's *Beyond*, following his CBS miniseries *Living With the Dead*. The central message from the great beyond: one never dies. In 2005, NBC premiered its *Medium* series, 'inspired by the non-fictional story of research medium Allison Dubois ... who begins to suspect that she can talk to dead people, see the future in her dreams and read people's thoughts' (nbc.com).

Table 11.3 *Forbes*'s richest deceased celebrities

2000 rank	Name	Forbes's richest deceased celebrities	
		2000 earnings	*2007 earnings*
1	Elvis Presley	$35 million	$49 million
2	Charles Schulz	$20 million plus	$35 million
3	John Lennon	$20 million	$44 million
4	Theodor 'Dr. Seuss' Geisel	$17 million	$13 million
5	Jimi Hendrix	$10 million plus	(did not make top 13)
6	Bob Marley	$10 million	$ 4 million
7	Andy Warhol	$ 8 million	$15 million
8	J. R. R. Tolkien	$ 7 million	(did not make top 13)
9	Frank Sinatra	$ 6 million	(did not make top 13)
10	Jerry Garcia	$ 5 million	(did not make top 13)

Source: Fong & Lau (2001); Goldman & Paine (2007).

Deceased celebrities have proven to be great pitchmen as they are highly regarded and never embarrass the sponsors. The trend in television began in 1991 when Elton John performed for Louis Armstrong, James Cagney, and Humphrey Bogart in a Diet Coke commercial. By the mid-1990s, Babe Ruth was receiving 100 endorsement deals a year and was, followed by James Dean, the most popular client of the Curtis Management Group.

This Indianapolis firm markets 'late greats' on behalf of the descendants (who, in some states, own the rights to the deceased's image for 70 years). Its website opens with an image of James Dean with the quotation, 'If a man can bridge the gap between life and death … if he can live on after he's dead, then maybe he was a great man'. Clients of 2009 include such disparate individuals as Gen. George Patton, Mark Twain, Jean Harlow, Ed Sullivan, Malcolm X, Oscar Wilde, Amelia Earhart, Will Rogers, and Tiny Tim. In 1997, 25 years after his death and 50 years after his debut with the Brooklyn Dodgers, Jackie Robinson became the first deceased athlete to adorn Wheaties cereal boxes. So great had the earnings of the dead become that in 2000 *Forbes* began its annual rankings of the 'top-earning dead celebrities' (see Table 11.3).

Though the dead have released albums since at least the 1970s, there is a new twist: their songs are no longer simply remastered archival retrievals but rather are postmortem performances made with the living. Natalie Cole sings with her long-deceased father Nat; the surviving Beatles reunite with John Lennon to perform 'Free as a Bird' and 'Real Love'.

Postselves in civic culture

To fortify the illusion of our own immortality, the deathlessness of others must be acknowledged – and of the groups responsible for maintaining their memories and those of one's self. For most, the chief hope for being remembered after death was by one's descendants. With changes in modern family systems, however, that assumption has often been invalidated. Modern repressions of death terror are now made possible through identifications with the death-defying powers of other social groups.

Increasingly, organisations are rescuing from oblivion the memories of their deceased members. Halls of fame multiply as social groups attempt to affirm their sovereign status (hence the national, state, city, organisational, and professional levels of halls) by conferring immortality to their elect. Of the 213 halls of fame identified from Victor J. Danilov's (1997) detailed inventory, the web, and contacts from a local newspaper, all but four were founded after the Second World War and roughly one-half since 1980. Through time-transcending rituals for their special (and often deceased) members, groups establish special claims to legitimacy and respect in part by their ability to protect their members' identities and deeds from time's oblivion. Cities and towns are always willing to host these halls of fame, hoping for increased revenues from tourist dollars – especially during the annual ceremonies for new inductees.

Such affirmations of sovereign status through death-transcending capacities are most evident with the nation-state, the broadest of social integrators. Consider the Social Security Administration's creation of an online deceased Americans database, the Social Security Death Index, which totalled over 83 million individuals in 2009. In addition, beyond its monuments and other memorialisations for the political saints, there is the federal funding of various genealogical resources such as the Statue of Liberty-Ellis Island Foundation's online passenger arrival records, whose database contains information on over 25 million immigrants.

Consider also how political immortality is conferred philatelically. Between 1847 and 2000, the United States issued nearly 3,500 distinct stamps. Generally, such symbolic immortality was reserved for a select group of the political elite, typically featuring the busts or heads of the founding fathers, presidents, and generals. In the last quarter of the twentieth century, I have observed a veritable explosion in the number and backgrounds of Americans so honoured – even those from such historically disenfranchised groups as women (with only 19 so commemorated through 1970) and African Americans (the first appearing in 1940).

Since 1980, the number and diversity of individuals so honoured reflects an affirmative action programme for a political afterlife, featuring the likes of Elvis Presley, Marilyn Monroe, James Dean, and Malcolm X (one of the Black Heritage series). Through the 1990s nine sets of the 'Legends of American Music' series were issued, along with 'Legends of the West', 'Legendary Football Coaches', 'Comedians', 'Legends of Hollywood', and 'Stars of the Silent Screen'.

In addition to halls of fame, electronic databases, and postage stamps, other death-transcending activities of civic groups have included political rituals of resurrection and immortalisation. As evidenced by attempts to recover identifying DNA from long-fallen unknown warriors from the Second World War and Vietnam, the Justice Department's reopening of Emmitt Till's case one half-century after his infamous murder, and the political debates of the 1970s over the restoration of citizenship to Robert E. Lee and Eugene V. Debs as well as the current attempts to grant a presidential pardon for Jack Johnson (the country's first black heavyweight boxing champion who was convicted in 1913 for violating the Mann Act by having consensual relations with a white woman), the American government has long been in the business of preserving the identities, rights, and citizenship status of its deceased members (Kearl & Rinaldi 1983). Three days following the 9/11 terrorist attacks on America, Representative Serrano introduced HR 2897 to

> provide for the granting of posthumous citizenship to certain aliens lawfully admitted for permanent residence who died as a result of the hijackings of four commercial aircraft, the attacks on the World Trade Center, or the attack on the Pentagon, on September 11, 2001, and for other purposes.

The nation-state has no monopoly over such bestowals of symbolic immortality. A historically recent trend of professional groups, particularly in the arts, is the 'Lifetime Achievement Awards' ritual. Here simultaneously acknowledged and fused are the ways individuals' biographies contribute to the illusion of immortality of the group. Unlike funerals, recipients are often alive for the celebrations of their lives – albeit proximate to death. Examples (year founded: first recipient) include the Grammy Awards (1962: Bing Crosby), American Film Institute (1973: John Ford), and the Horror Writers Association (1987: Fritz Leiber; Frank Belknap Long; Clifford D. Simak).

From Columbine High School to the sprouting of roadside memorials across the nation, attempts to personalise death and to preserve the identities of the deceased can be observed. The Oklahoma City National Memorial Center features a field of 168 empty chairs, placed in nine rows according to the floor on which one died, each seat etched with the name of a victim. The AIDS Memorial Quilt comprises over 44,000 individualised 3×6-foot panels to individualise each and every victim of the epidemic.

The growing reaffirmations of the rights of the dead were dramatised by the Native American Graves Protection and Repatriation Act. In August 1989, the World Archaeological Congress, in association with the International Indian Treaty Council, the World Council of Indigenous Peoples, and American Indians Against Desecration, held at the University of South Dakota the first inter-congress on 'Archaeological Ethics and the Treatment of the Dead', all framing the issue in terms of human rights. The same year, the Smithsonian Institution agreed to return the skeletal remains of thousands of American Indians to their tribes for reburial in their homelands.

Finally, in addition to simply being remembered, the dead are also being accorded greater social powers in the worlds of the living. Consider the political lengthening of the rights accorded to postselves. The Constitution authorised Congress to give authors and inventors the exclusive right to their works for a 'limited' time. In 1790, copyrights lasted 14 years. Two centuries later in 1998 the Sonny Bono Copyright Term Extension Act lengthened protection by 20 years, to 70 years after the death of the inventor or author if known. (Works owned by corporations are protected for 95 years.)

Commodifications of the afterlife

Given the increasing visibility of postselves in the public realm, especially those who continue to make money posthumously, it should come as little surprise that this demand would be recognised by the private sector. Capitalism has not been oblivious to ways in which to profit from this metaphysical zeal. Indeed, full-blown transcendence markets have come into existence to enhance individuals' prospects for being remembered – and for the living to profit from their existence. To protect the persona of the deceased, the first postmortem celebrity rights law was passed in California (Civil Code s. 3344.1) in 1984. Presently, 28 states extend the right of publicity past death, allowing the deceased's image and likeness to be inherited (the descendible right of publicity) like property for up to one century. In Indiana, the inheritable extends to name, voice, gestures, distinctive appearances, signature, and mannerisms.

In addition to the preservation of personas, new industries have arisen to preserve individuals' physical essence. Companies like Geneternity (whose mission is 'to serve humanity's interest in immortality') preserve DNA samples of the departed. Kentucky bookbinder and printer, Timothy Hawley Books, offers a line of what it calls 'bibliocadavers' – bound volumes whose blank or printed pages are created from a pulp containing the ashes of a loved one. The cremains of loved ones are also transformed into living coral reefs by Eternal Reefs, Inc., high-quality diamonds by LifeGem, and into customised granite-like slabs by Relict Memorials.

Some desire not only the preservation of their personas but the actual resurrection of their selves after crossing over. Since 1967, over 90 Americans have been cryonically suspended at the moment of death, for possible renascence in the distant future when a cure has been found for their demise. For those who cannot afford full body freezing, discount cryonics centres like Alcor Life Extension Foundation have come into existence that just preserve heads, which await eventual body transplants.

Such commodifications of the dead are not limited to one's self or family members, illustrated by the international publicity in 1987 given to Michael Jackson's attempts to buy the remains of Joseph Merrick, the so-called 'Elephant Man'. One can now purchase a biological connection with those already immortalised. For instance, consider one of the collector pen lines of the Krone Company, the Lincoln pen, which contains a molecule of the president's DNA from an authenticated snippet of his hair. When Ed Headrick, the inventor of the modern Frisbee, died during the summer of 2002, his son reported that his father's wish was for his ashes to be moulded into commemorative Frisbees. The family observed his request and now markets the 'Steady Ed Memorial Discs'.

Symbolic immortality is less macabre and more easily marketable. Americans are a charitable people, but not all can afford having a building or major charity named after them. Fundraisers for schools, municipal facilities, and myriad causes have discovered that such illusions of immortality can be broken down into numerous parts. For the new $165.5 million Seattle Central Library, for instance, donors contributed $45 million to have their monikers affixed to 24 named spaces. Two decades ago at the Ann Arbor Michigan Theater, one could have one's name on a concession stand for $12,000, a light fixture for $250, or an aisle sign for $100 (Fuchsberg 1987).

There are growing desires to design postselves that remain active players in the world of the living. In the early 1990s, Cards From Beyond, a Fairport, NY company, offered deceased individuals the ability to send cards to loved ones for holidays and anniversaries. A decade later, Loving Pup Productions provided 'Timeless Mail', a posthumous email service: 'You care about your family, friends, and loved ones, show you care by leaving them each an e-mail to be delivered after you pass on.' How about receiving a phone call from a deceased relative? With AT&T Labs' Natural Voices speech software, voice cloning is now a reality.

For those wishing not only to connect with but to exercise control over the living along the lines of their values, the legal institution provides opportunities. Estate lawyers report growing numbers of clientele desiring to control posthumously the life plans of the living, motivating *Time* magazine to publish 'Ruling from the Grave: Through incentive trusts, you can lead wayward young heirs to fruitful lives' (Kadlec 2002).

The post-9/11 politics of the afterlife

> The faithful shall enter paradise, and the unbelievers shall be condemned to eternal hellfire.
>
> – Koranic verse

The above quotation portrays the cultural context of 9/11/01. With the terrorists' attacks on the American symbols of financial and military might – on the day matching the nation's emergency telephone number followed by the first year of the West's new millennium – Americans were shaken to the core. Within moments, thousands of living beings simultaneously entered the spirit world, leaving little corporeal evidence of their existence seconds earlier. Never had so many Americans simultaneously perished in such compressed space, let alone in their homeland.

Evidence of American immortalism can be seen in the speed with which the press gravitated to the afterlife component of the zealot's motivations, how these individuals were motivated by the promise of a glorious afterlife in exchange for giving up their lives to exterminate infidels. There were many interpretative frames available, such as capitalism's injustices in the Third World (i.e. Bhopal) or the ways in which Western powers carved up their colonial holdings into self-defeating states. Instead, the American press focused on stories like that of West Bank suicide bomber Raed Barghouti, who reportedly told his family how he would spend eternity with great Islamic leaders and be tended to by 72 virgins (Caldwell 2001), and how other shahids-to-be anticipated their actions would allow them to bring 70 relatives with them to heaven.

A Republican was at the helm of power. Much has been made about the rise of the Religious Right and its influence over the Republican Party and the national agenda during the administration of George W. Bush. According to a national survey conducted the year following the attacks (Pew Research Center for the People and the Press 2002), belief in one's faith's exclusivity in providing eternal life ranged from 32 per cent among conservative Republicans (53 per cent among Republican Evangelicals) to 11 per cent of liberal Democrats. In Table 11.2 one can see the potency of belief in an afterlife in shaping Republicans' positions towards the major battlelines in America's 'culture wars'. Looking at those strongly religious, observe how afterlife beliefs have little effect on Democrats' support for abortion while Republican disbelievers are two-thirds more likely to support women's rights to an abortion for any reason than Republicans believing in an afterlife. Similarly, only among Republicans does belief in an afterlife produce significant differences in support for homosexual relations. Finally, the more conservative the party identification, the larger the effect of afterlife beliefs on support for euthanasia.

Such effects of afterlife beliefs on these core moral issues are even more interesting among those who are not strongly religious (which is the case for 65 per cent of Democrats and 53 per cent of Republicans). Among these individuals, the belief in life after death has virtually no effect either on Democrats' or Independents' support of abortion, euthanasia, or homosexual relations. For Republicans, on the other hand, afterlife beliefs suppress support for these issues by 11 to 20 percentage points.

Given the increased presence of the dead in American civic and popular cultures prior to 9/11, the publicity given to the terrorists' immortal motivations strengthened the Republican Party's hand in the country's culture wars. Afterlife beliefs assumed a dramatic increase in political saliency; Christian notions of desirable eternal lives being reserved for those having lived morally worthy lives had to be reaffirmed. And given the cognitive connections between this fundamental outlook with the moral issues of the time, we have better insight into why Terri Schiavo, gay marriage, and the administration's restrictions on stem cell research and attempts to redefine 'abortion' to include birth control received the considerable cultural attention that they did.

Discussion

Contrary to the thesis that late modern selves have outgrown the need for immortality beliefs and that there is no place for the dead in late modern societies, it is argued that an immortalist zeitgeist now permeates American civic and popular cultures, underlying a number of curious and seemingly disparate phenomena. It is not unique but rather an extreme case of trends occurring throughout much of the West (Figure 11.1 revealed how afterlife beliefs increased during the 1990s in all but one of the countries surveyed), prompting Glennys Howarth's (2000) observation of the blurring of boundaries between the living and the dead.

There are a number of factors accounting for American exceptionalism to the culture's pursuits towards death transcendence. These include the religious foundations underlying the nation's founding and the New World symbolising the possibilities for personal rebirth and spatialising mythic associations with the West's hyperborean and fountain themes of superlongevity (Gruman 2003:30, 32–33). Additionally, the ethos of individualism, self-sufficiency, and personal responsibility for salvation was unleashed upon a rare frontier. Analysts of the American character often cite the implications of not being bogged down by history; here fates were no longer pre-programmed by the legacies of feudalism, aristocracy, or by ancestral deeds and rivalries. In this land bereft of reminders of the accomplishments of scores of generations past, the proverbial slate was clean for leaving one's own mark on time.

American militarism adds to this cultural chemistry. Wars produce an abundance of spirits and postlife beliefs. High-water marks in the American spiritualism movement, for instance, followed the Civil War, the First World War, and the Vietnam War. A spiritual realm is required to overcome the natural death fears of the combatants. As Bertrand Russell observed one half-century ago:

> as the Mohammedans first proved, belief in Paradise has considerable military value as reinforcing natural pugnacity. We should therefore admit that militarists are wise in encouraging the belief in immortality, always supposing that this belief does not become so profound as to produce indifference to the affairs of the world.
>
> (Russell 1957:91)

Attempting to counter the finality of death, from this perspective, the Bush administration censored photographs of military coffins being returned to the United States from the conflicts in Iraq and Afghanistan (Milbank 2003).

Much of the evidence of the recent growth in American zeal for death transcendence began in the late 1970s and early 1980s. At the time, connections were already being made linking Americans' extreme individualism with their rejuvenated defiant stance against death. Christopher Lasch observed how the 'irrational terror of old age and death is closely associated with the emergence of the narcissistic personality ... giving rise to attempts to abolish old age and to extend life indefinitely' (Lasch 1979:211). In 'The Me Decade and the Third Great Awakening', Tom Wolfe noted the dissolution of 'man's age-old belief in serial immortality', where most generations 'have lived as if they are living their ancestors' lives and their offspring's lives and perhaps their neighbors' lives as well' (Wolfe 1976:39). Such framing of existence no longer sufficed for the new predominant personality type. Science's insights that cells and creatures are not programmed to die nor that extinction is the fate of all species provided compensation for primates who think about time-lessness and eternity. In sum, the death consolation of the genetic form of symbolic immortality was waning, being replaced by mimetic immortality to shore up the transcendent reaffirmations of religion.

It was also during this era that the human environment was increasingly becoming a McLuhanian electronic envelope, whose lineaments became understood as various information systems and whose essence was increasingly one of Jean Baudrillard's simulacra. Given the interwoven nature of self and society, the understood essence of selfhood was to be profoundly changed as well. Instead of being corporeal mechanisms, modern selves are becoming seen as attention- and identity-seeking social algorithms whose distinctive 'programs' influence the programming of others' lives and the logics of institutional systems. And, just as individuals cannot erase their residues in cyberspace, neither does their existence conclude with physical extinction. One's images, behaviours, words, beliefs, and accomplishments exist indefinitely in this new electronic world, available to be paused, reversed, and fast-forwarded.

These cultural solutions to the problem of transcendence fit well with American capitalism's need to counter the scientific materialism of its chief twentieth-century ideological rival, communism. One highly publicised battleline during the Cold War was drawn when the Soviet Union officially proclaimed the finality of death (Kluckhohn 1962), even banning Sir Arthur Conan Doyle's 1892 *The Adventures of Sherlock Holmes* because of its references to occultism and spiritualism. Nevertheless, communist regimes were to embalm and place on public display the physical remains of founding fathers (e.g. Vladimir Lenin, who used to have the companionship of Josef Stalin in the Red Square Mausoleum; Mao Tse-tung (who had wished cremation) in Beijing; Ho Chi Minh in Hanoi; Georgi Dimitrov, founder of communist Bulgaria (until cremated in 1990 after regime overthrow); Kim Il Sung in Pyongyang, North Korea). It turned out to be an interesting balancing act of the United States, supposedly a secular nation, walking the tightrope when immortalising its elite and to do so without the non-putrefying saints of the Catholic Church and the Communist Party.

Conclusion

Four decades after Arnold Toynbee (1969:131) observed how 'death is un-American', ethicist Arthur Caplan proclaimed: 'It's not immoral to want to be immortal' (Caplan 2008). Crystallised between the pronouncements, two fronts in the culture's war against death were drawn: one in the here-and-now and the other in the hereafter. With regard to the former, the United States has witnessed growing public demands for the nation-state to kill (or at least give forewarning to) whatever kills us, whether Taliban fighters, lethal microbes, stray asteroids, dangerous chemicals or foods, death genes, or unexpected earthquakes and tsunamis. This has led to further expansion of the medical-military-industrial complex, the proliferation of warning labels, demands for risk-free environments, and dramatic improvements in life expectancy. Well over three-quarters of the American federal budget is currently devoted to military and medical endeavours and to assisting those most likely to die (e.g. the old; in 2003, the portion of the federal budget going just to Social Security, Medicare, and Medicaid was 42 per cent). Like the classical Egyptians, this high civilisation has become increasingly oriented towards conquering the finality of death through new death-transcending technologies.

This contrasts with Americans' deep faith in being able to transcend death. Like Abraham Maslow's needs-based hierarchy of motivations of the living, there exists a hierarchy of post-mortem objectives that range across simply being a part of others' DNA (or genetic immortality), being remembered (mnemetic immortality), being able to influence others' behaviours and beliefs (mimetic immortality), and finally, being able to continue as a fully conscious social actor (sentient immortality). Though traditional religious beliefs offer hope for the latter, a growing multitude of secular symbolic forms have demonstrably delivered all the others. For this reason, Edwin S. Shneidman's (1973) concept of the 'postself' is broadened to include these other forms, not just individuals' anticipations of and actions towards how they will be posthumously remembered. Since its coinage, so many laws and industries have emerged around the social status and commodification of deceased individuals that the concept requires broadening. The extreme individualism of the American character rejects death's finality and its consignment to oblivion. In the new market-driven and media-saturated culture, even revisionist biographical memories and infamy can be preferable to being forgotten.

Note

1 Chapter previously published as Michael C. Kearl (2010): 'The proliferation of postselves in American civic and popular cultures'. *Mortality*, 15 (1): 47–63, DOI: 10.1080/13576270903537591.

References

Baudrillard, Jean (1993): *Symbolic Exchange and Death*. London: Sage Publications.
Bauman, Zygmunt (1992): *Mortality, Immortality and Other Life Strategies*. Stanford, CA: Stanford University Press.
Becker, Ernest (1973): *The Denial of Death*. New York: Free Press.

Braude, Ann (2001): *Radical Spirits: Spiritualism and Women's Rights in Nineteenth-Century America*. Indianapolis: Indiana University Press.

Buescher, John B. (2003): *The Other Side of Salvation: Spiritualism and the Nineteenth-Century Religious Experience*. Boston, MA: Skinner House Books.

Caldwell, J. (2001): 'Suicide Bombings Tear at the Heart of Islam'. *Irish Examiner*, 18 September. Available online at: http://archives.tcm.ie/irishexaminer/2001/09/18/story12963.asp.

Caplan, Arthur (2008): 'It's Not Immoral to Want to Be Immortal'. Msnbc.com, 25 April. Available online at: www.msnbc.msn.com/id/23562623.

Choron, Jacques (1964): *Death and Modern Man*. New York: Collier Books.

Danilov, Victor J. (1997): *Hall of Fame Museums: A Reference Guide*. Westport, CT: Greenwood Press.

Davis, James A. & Tom W. Smith (2007): 'General Social Surveys, 1972–2006' (machine-readable file). Principal Investigator: James A. Davis; Director and Co-Principal Investigator, Tom W. Smith; Co-principal Investigator, Peter V. Marsden. Sponsored by the National Science Foundation. Chicago, IL: National Opinion Research Center (producer); Storrs, CT: The Roper Center for Public Opinion Research Center, University of Connecticut (distributor).

Fong, Mei & Debra Lau (2001): 'Earnings from the Crypt'. *Forbes*, 28 February. Available online at: www.forbes.com/2001/02/28/crypt.html.

Fuchsberg, Gil (1987): 'For the Right Price, Just about Anything Can Bear Your Name'. *Wall Street Journal*, 21 September, pp. 1, 14.

Gallup, George, Jr (2001): 'Tuesday Briefing: Religion Update'. Forbes.com, 31 July.

Goldman, Lea & Jake Paine (2007): 'Top Earning Dead Celebrities'. *Forbes*, 29 October. Available online at: www.forbes.com/media/2007/10/26/top-dead-celebrity-biz-media-deadcelebs07-cz_lg_1029celeb.html.

Greeley, Andrew M. & Michael Hout (1999): 'Americans' Increasing Belief in Life after Death: Religious Competition and Acculturation'. *American Sociological Review*, 64 (6):813–835.

Gruman, Gerald (2003): *A History of Ideas about the Prolongation of Life: Classics in Longevity and Aging*. New York: Springer.

Hentsch, Thierry (2004): *Truth or Death: The Quest for Immortality in the Western Narrative Tradition*. Vancouver, BC: Talonbooks.

Howarth, Glennys (2000): 'Dismantling the Boundaries between Life and Death'. *Mortality*, 5 (2):127–138.

International Social Survey Program (ISSP) (1991): *International Social Survey Program: Religion, 1991*. Cologne: Zentralarchiv für Empirische Sozialforschung.

International Social Survey Program (ISSP) (1994): *International Social Survey Program: Religion, 1994*. Cologne: Zentralarchiv für Empirische Sozialforschung.

International Social Survey Program (ISSP) (1998): *International Social Survey Program: Religion, 1998*. Cologne: Zentralarchiv für Empirische Sozialforschung.

Kadlec, Daniel (2002): 'Ruling from the Grave'. *Time*, 22 April.

Kearl, Michael C. (2001): 'An Investigation into Collective Historical Knowledge and Implications of Its Ignorance'. *Texas Journal of Ideas, History and Culture*, 23:4–13.

Kearl, Michael C. & Anoel Rinaldi (1983): 'The Political Uses of the Dead as Symbols in Contemporary Civil Religions'. *Social Forces*, 61:693–708.

Kluckhohn, Richard (ed.) (1962): *Culture and Behavior: Collected Essays of Clyde Kluckhohn*. New York: Free Press.

Kurzweil, Raymond (2005): *The Singularity Is Near: When Humans Transcend Biology*. New York: Viking.

Lasch, Christopher (1979): *The Culture of Narcissism: American Life in an Age of Diminishing Expectations*. New York: W. W. Norton & Co.

Lescarboura, Austin C. (1920): 'Edison's Views on Life and Death: An Interview with the Famous Inventor Regarding His Attempt to Communicate with the Next World'. *Scientific American*, 123 (18):446.

Lifton, Robert J. (1979): *The Broken Connection: On Death and the Continuity of Life*. New York: Simon & Schuster.

Milbank, Dana (2003): 'Curtains Ordered for Media Coverage of Returning Coffins'. *Washington Post*, 21 October, p. A23.

Pew Forum on Religion and Public Life (2008): 'Many Americans Say Other Faiths Can Lead to Eternal Life', 18 December. Available online at: www.pewforum.org/2008/12/18/many-americans-say-other-faiths-can-lead-to-eternal-life.

Pew Research Center for the People and the Press (2002): 'Americans Struggle with Religion's Role at Home and Abroad', 20 March. Available online at: http://people-press.org.

Russell, Bertrand (1957): *Why I Am Not a Christian*. London: Allen & Unwin.

Safire, William (2001): 'For a Muslim Legion'. *New York Times*, 1 October, p. A23.

Shneidman, Edwin S. (1995): 'The Postself', in John.B. Williamson & Edwin S. Shnediman (eds): *Death: Current Perspectives* (4th edn). Menlo Park, CA: Mayfield (adapted from: Edwin S. Shneidman (1973): *Death of Man*. New York: Quadrangle).

Swatos, William H. & Loftur R. Gissurarson (1997): *Icelandic Spiritualism: Mediumship and Modernity in Iceland*. New Brunswick, NJ: Transaction.

Thiessen, Mark (2004): 'Jewish Group: Mormons Still Baptize Dead'. *AP Online*, Available online at: http://story.news.yahoo.com/news?tmpl=story&cid=519&ncid=519&e=6&u=/ap/20040410/ap_on_re_ us/baptizing_the_dead.

Toynbee, Arnold (1969): *Man's Concern with Death*. St. Louis, MO: McGraw-Hill.

Walter, Tony (1996): *The Eclipse of Eternity: A Sociology of the Afterlife*. New York: St. Martin's Press.

Wolfe, Tom (1976): 'The Me Decade and the Third Great Awakening'. *New York Magazine*, 23 August, pp. 26–40.

Word, Ron (2003): 'Abortion Doctor's Killer Expects Reward'. *AP Online*, 2 September. Available online at: www.encyclopedia.com/doc/1P1-79097390.html.

Index

Note: Book titles are in italics.

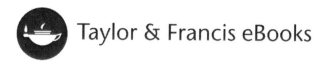

Taylor & Francis eBooks

Helping you to choose the right eBooks for your Library

Add Routledge titles to your library's digital collection today. Taylor and Francis ebooks contains over 50,000 titles in the Humanities, Social Sciences, Behavioural Sciences, Built Environment and Law.

Choose from a range of subject packages or create your own!

Benefits for you

» Free MARC records
» COUNTER-compliant usage statistics
» Flexible purchase and pricing options
» All titles DRM-free.

REQUEST YOUR FREE INSTITUTIONAL TRIAL TODAY

Free Trials Available
We offer free trials to qualifying academic, corporate and government customers.

Benefits for your user

» Off-site, anytime access via Athens or referring URL
» Print or copy pages or chapters
» Full content search
» Bookmark, highlight and annotate text
» Access to thousands of pages of quality research at the click of a button.

eCollections – Choose from over 30 subject eCollections, including:

Archaeology	Language Learning
Architecture	Law
Asian Studies	Literature
Business & Management	Media & Communication
Classical Studies	Middle East Studies
Construction	Music
Creative & Media Arts	Philosophy
Criminology & Criminal Justice	Planning
Economics	Politics
Education	Psychology & Mental Health
Energy	Religion
Engineering	Security
English Language & Linguistics	Social Work
Environment & Sustainability	Sociology
Geography	Sport
Health Studies	Theatre & Performance
History	Tourism, Hospitality & Events

For more information, pricing enquiries or to order a free trial, please contact your local sales team: www.tandfebooks.com/page/sales

The home of Routledge books

www.tandfebooks.com